Hysterectomy for
Benign Disease

FEMALE PELVIC SURGERY VIDEO ATLAS SERIES

Series Editor:

Mickey Karram, MD

Director of Urogynecology

The Christ Hospital

Clinical Professor of Obstetrics and Gynecology

University of Cincinnati

Cincinnati, Ohio

Other Volumes in the Female Pelvic Surgery Video Atlas Series

Basic, Advanced, and Robotic Laparoscopic Surgery

Tommaso Falcone & Jeffrey M. Goldberg, Editors

Maternal Emergencies in Obstetrics

Baha Sibai, Editor

Pelvic Organ Prolapse

Mickey Karram & Christopher Maher, Editors

Posterior Pelvic Floor Abnormalities

Tracy L. Hull, Editor

Urinary Incontinence

Roger Dmochowski & Mickey Karram, Editors

Urologic Surgery for the Gynecologist and Urogynecologist

John B. Gebhart, Editor

Vaginal Surgery for the Urologist

Victor Nitti, Editor

FEMALE PELVIC SURGERY VIDEO ATLAS SERIES
Mickey Karram, Series Editor

Hysterectomy for Benign Disease

Mark D. Walters, MD
Professor and Vice Chair of Gynecology
Department of Obstetrics and Gynecology
Obstetrics, Gynecology, and Women's Health Institute
Cleveland Clinic
Cleveland, Ohio

Matthew D. Barber, MD, MHS
Vice Chair of Clinical Research
Associate Professor of Surgery
Department of Obstetrics and Gynecology
Obstetrics, Gynecology, and Women's Health Institute
Cleveland Clinic
Cleveland, Ohio

Illustrated by **Joe Chovan, Milford, Ohio**

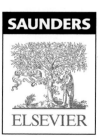

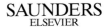

SAUNDERS
ELSEVIER

1600 John F. Kennedy Blvd.
Ste 1800
Philadelphia, PA 19103-2899

HYSTERECTOMY FOR BENIGN DISEASE (A Volume in the Female   ISBN: 978-1-4160-6271-4
Pelvic Surgery Video Atlas Series edited by Mickey Karram, MD)

Library of Congress Cataloging-in-Publication Data

Walters, Mark D.
  Hysterectomy for benign disease / Mark D. Walters, Matthew D. Barber; illustrated by Joe Chovan.
      p. ; cm.—(Female pelvic surgery)
  Includes bibliographical references and index.
  ISBN 978-1-4160-6271-4 (hardcover : alk. paper) 1. Hysterectomy. 2. Uterus—Surgery.
I. Barber, Matthew D. II. Title. III. Series: Female pelvic surgery.
  [DNLM: 1. Hysterectomy. 2. Uterine Diseases—surgery. WP 468 W233h 2010]
  RG391.W38 2010
  618.1′453—dc22
                                                                            2010011653

Senior Acquisitions Editor: Rebecca S. Gaertner
Senior Developmental Editor: Arlene Chappelle
Publishing Services Manager: Patricia Tannian
Senior Project Manager: Sharon Corell
Design Direction: Lou Forgione
Marketing Manager: Radha Mawrie
Multimedia Producer: Dan Martinez

Printed in the United States of America

Last digit is the print number: 9 8 7 6 5 4 3 2 1

To ginny, with my everlasting love

–Mark D. Walters

To my wife, Heather, for all her love and support, and to my children, Samantha, Sydney, and Adam, who fill me with pride and joy

–Matthew D. Barber

Contributors

Matthew D. Barber, MD, MHS
Vice Chair of Clinical Research, Associate Professor of Surgery, Department of Obstetrics and Gynecology, Obstetrics, Gynecology, and Women's Health Institute, Cleveland Clinic, Cleveland, Ohio
Anatomy of the Uterus and Its Surgical Removal; Epidemiology and Indications of Hysterectomy: Changing Trends; Outcomes of Hysterectomy; Difficult Vaginal Hysterectomy; Complications of Hysterectomy

Linda D. Bradley, MD
Vice Chair of Obstetrics, Gynecology and Women's Health Institute, Director, Center for Menstrual Disorders,, Fibroids & Hysteroscopic Services, Department of Obstetrics and Gynecology, Obstetrics, Gynecology, and Women's Health Institute, Cleveland Clinic, Cleveland, Ohio
Alternative Treatments to Hysterectomy

Gouri B. Diwadkar, MD
Fellow, Female Pelvic Medicine and Reconstructive Surgery, Department of Obstetrics and Gynecology, Obstetrics, Gynecology, and Women's Health Institute, Cleveland Clinic, Cleveland, Ohio
Teaching and Learning Gynecologic Surgery

Pedro F. Escobar, MD
Assistant Professor of Surgery, Section of Gynecologic Oncology, Department of Obstetrics and Gynecology, Obstetrics, Gynecology, and Women's Health Institute, Cleveland Clinic, Cleveland, Ohio
Laparoscopic and Robotic-Assisted Total and Supracervical Hysterectomy

Tommaso Falcone, MD
Vice Chairman, Office of Professional Staff Affairs, Professor and Chairman, Obstetrics and Gynecology, Obstetrics, Gynecology and Women's Health Institute, Cleveland Clinic, Cleveland, Ohio
Preoperative and Perioperative Considerations and Choosing the Route of Hysterectomy

J. Eric Jelovsek, MD
Assistant Professor of Surgery, Associate Staff, Center of Urogynecology and Reconstructive Pelvic Surgery, Co-Site Director OB/GYN Residency, Department of Obstetrics and Gynecology, Obstetrics, Gynecology, and Women's Health Institute, Cleveland Clinic, Cleveland, Ohio
Teaching and Learning Gynecologic Surgery

Marie Fidela R. Paraiso, MD
Section Head, Center of Urogynecology and Reconstructive Pelvic Surgery, Co-Director, Female Pelvic Medicine and Reconstructive Surgery, Director of the Pelvic Floor Disorders Center, Lakewood Hospital; Assistant Professor of Surgery, Department of Obstetrics and Gynecology, Obstetrics, Gynecology, and Women's Health Institute, Cleveland Clinic, Cleveland, Ohio
Laparoscopic and Robotic-Assisted Total and Supracervical Hysterectomy

Amy J. Park, MD
Director of Benign Gynecology, Section of Female Pelvic Medicine and Reconstructive Surgery, Washington Hospital Center; Assistant Professor, Departments of Obstetrics/Gynecology and Urology, Georgetown University School of Medicine, Washington, DC
Anatomy of the Uterus and Its Surgical Removal

Beri M. Ridgeway, MD
Staff, Center of Urogynecology and Reconstructive Surgery, Department of Obstetrics and Gynecology, Obstetrics, Gynecology, and Women's Health Institute, Cleveland Clinic, Cleveland, Ohio
Abdominal Hysterectomy

Anthony P. Tizzano, MD
Wooster Clinic, Wooster, Ohio
The Evolution of Uterine Surgery and Hysterectomy

Rebecca S. Uranga, MD
Resident, Department of Obstetrics and Gynecology, Dartmouth-Hitchcock Medical Center, Lebanon, New Hampshire
Prophylactic Oophorectomy at Hysterectomy

Mark D. Walters, MD
Professor and Vice Chair of Gynecology, Department of Obstetrics and Gynecology, Obstetrics, Gynecology, and Women's Health Institute, Cleveland Clinic, Cleveland, Ohio
The Evolution of Uterine Surgery and Hysterectomy; Preoperative and Perioperative Considerations and Choosing the Route of Hysterectomy; Outcomes of Hysterectomy; Vaginal Hysterectomy and Trachelectomy: Basic Surgical Techniques; Complications of Hysterectomy

James L. Whiteside, MD
Assistant Professor, Dartmouth-Hitchcock Medical Center, Dartmouth Medical School, Lebanon, New Hampshire
Prophylactic Oophorectomy at Hysterectomy

Devorah R. Wieder, MD, MPH
Associate Staff, Center for Specialized Women's Health, Obstetrics, Gynecology, and Women's Health Institute, Cleveland Clinic, Cleveland, Ohio
Alternative Treatments to Hysterectomy

Video Contributors

Chi Chiung Grace Chen, MD
Assistant Professor, Department of Gynecology and Obstetrics, Johns Hopkins Bayview Medical Center, Baltimore, Maryland
Video: *Uterine Morcellation Techniques*

Anna C. Frick, MD
Obstetrics, Gynecology and Women's Health Institute, Cleveland Clinic, Cleveland, Ohio
Video: *Vaginal Hysterectomy; Anterior Cul-de-sac Entry; Electrosurgical Device-Assisted Vaginal Hysterectomy; Difficult Anterior Entry; Difficult Posterior Entry; Uterovaginal Prolapse*

John B. Gebhart, MD, MS
Department of Obstetrics and Gynecology, Mayo Clinic, Rochester, Minnesota
Video: *Techniques in Vaginal Oophorectomy; Transvaginal Cystotomy Repair*

Mickey Karram, MD
Director of Urogynecology, The Christ Hospital; Clinical Professor of Obstetrics and Gynecology, University of Cincinnati, Cincinnati, Ohio
Video: *TAH, Endometriosis; Vaginal Trachelectomy; Intentional Cystotomy with Passage of Ureteral Catheters*

Rosanne M. Kho, MD
Department of Obstetrics and Gynecology, Mayo Clinic, Scottsdale, Arizona
Video: *Techniques in Vaginal Oophorectomy*

Javier F. Magrina, MD
Department of Obstetrics and Gynecology, Mayo Clinic, Scottsdale, Arizona
Video: *Techniques in Vaginal Oophorectomy*

Tristi W. Muir, MD
Director, Division of Female Pelvic Medicine and Reconstructive Surgery, University of Texas Medical Branch, Galveston, Texas
Video: *Vaginal Bilateral Salpingo-oophorectomy*

Preface

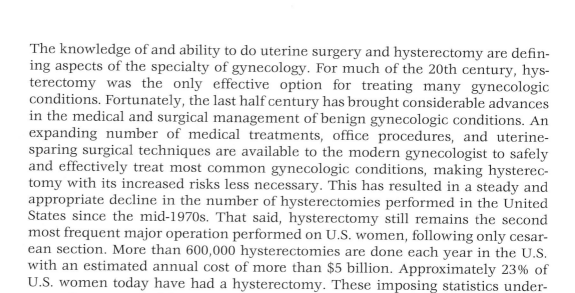

The knowledge of and ability to do uterine surgery and hysterectomy are defining aspects of the specialty of gynecology. For much of the 20th century, hysterectomy was the only effective option for treating many gynecologic conditions. Fortunately, the last half century has brought considerable advances in the medical and surgical management of benign gynecologic conditions. An expanding number of medical treatments, office procedures, and uterine-sparing surgical techniques are available to the modern gynecologist to safely and effectively treat most common gynecologic conditions, making hysterectomy with its increased risks less necessary. This has resulted in a steady and appropriate decline in the number of hysterectomies performed in the United States since the mid-1970s. That said, hysterectomy still remains the second most frequent major operation performed on U.S. women, following only cesarean section. More than 600,000 hysterectomies are done each year in the U.S. with an estimated annual cost of more than $5 billion. Approximately 23% of U.S. women today have had a hysterectomy. These imposing statistics underscore the great need for continued and up-to-date education on this important subject.

Hysterectomy remains a popular and important option in spite of the growing number of alternative therapies because it is a highly effective and permanent treatment for many of the most common benign gynecologic conditions including abnormal uterine bleeding, uterine fibroids, dysmenorrhea, and endometriosis. It is the procedure of choice for these conditions when other less invasive options have failed. Additionally, technologic advances and surgical innovation have increased the availability of minimally invasive options to hysterectomy, including vaginal, laparoscopic, and robotic approaches, resulting in decreasing risk and an improved patient experience. For these reasons, hysterectomy will remain an essential gynecologic treatment for the foreseeable future.

A number of excellent and distinguished texts and atlases of gynecologic surgery currently are available. What makes this book unique is its specific and comprehensive focus on hysterectomy. Our goal for this video atlas is to provide a comprehensive clinical resource for the gynecologic surgeon and obstetrician-gynecologist trainee, addressing this most fundamental of gynecologic procedures. With this goal in mind, we have included a broad array of clinically relevant hysterectomy-related topics, including a thorough discussion of the surgical techniques of abdominal, vaginal, laparoscopic, and robotic hysterectomy and the many hysterectomy alternatives. We include many concise real-life case presentations and discussions with corresponding narrated videos.

Also included are interesting discussions of the historical evolution of uterine surgery and hysterectomy, pelvic anatomy related specifically to hysterectomy, the changing trends of hysterectomy and its indications, an in depth discussion of the pros and cons of different routes of hysterectomy and oophorectomy, an evidence-based discussion of preoperative and postoperative care, and strategies for preventing and managing hysterectomy complications.

Given the decline over the last several decades in the number of hysterectomies and other surgical cases available to residents, coupled with the increase in the number of surgical alternatives for managing gynecologic disease, there is a clear need for more effective and efficient methods for teaching gynecologic surgery. The final chapter of this text is dedicated to teaching and learning gynecologic surgery, a topic rarely found in surgical texts in spite of its importance. The chapter includes discussions of modern learning theory as it applies to teaching surgical techniques and the use of surgical simulation and mental imagery to improve outcomes. A description and video on giving effective feedback to trainees about their performance will be of value to both OB/GYN faculty who train residents and practicing surgeons learning a new technique.

The format of the *Female Pelvic Surgery Video Atlas Series* with its combination of case-based presentations, detailed topic discussions, numerous illustrations, and hours of complementary video footage is an ideal way to present all of these topics and make them readily accessible. We hope that this book will meet the training needs for residents in obstetrics and gynecology and prove to be a valuable resource for physicians who teach medical students, residents, and fellows. We also hope that practicing OB/GYNs will find it interesting and useful as they strive to take better care of their patients.

Mark D. Walters, MD
Matthew D. Barber, MD, MHS

Contents

1 The Evolution of Uterine Surgery and Hysterectomy   **1**

Anthony Tizzano, MD, and Mark D. Walters, MD

2 Anatomy of the Uterus and Its Surgical Removal   **31**

Amy J. Park, MD, and Matthew D. Barber, MD, MHS

Video Demonstrations:
- 2-1   Anterior Abdominal Wall   *34*
  - Amy J. Park, MD, Matthew D. Barber, MD, MHS, and Tommaso Falcone, MD
- 2-2   Anatomy of the Uterus and Adnexa   *42*
  - Amy J. Park, MD, Matthew D. Barber, MD, MHS, and Tommaso Falcone, MD
- 2-3   Vasculature   *46*
  - Amy J. Park, MD, Matthew D. Barber, MD, MHS, and Tommaso Falcone, MD
- 2-4   Lower Urinary Tract   *53*
  - Amy J. Park, MD, Matthew D. Barber, MD, MHS, and Tommaso Falcone, MD
- 2-5   Avascular Planes of the Pelvis   *55*
  - Amy J. Park, MD, Matthew D. Barber, MD, MHS, and Tommaso Falcone, MD

3 Epidemiology and Indications of Hysterectomy: Changing Trends   **65**

Matthew D. Barber, MD, MHS

4 Preoperative and Perioperative Considerations and Choosing the Route of Hysterectomy   **77**

Mark D. Walters, MD, and Tommaso Falcone, MD

5 Outcomes of Hysterectomy   **89**

Matthew D. Barber, MD, MHS, and Mark D. Walters, MD

6 Abdominal Hysterectomy   **103**

Beri Ridgeway, MD

Video Demonstrations:
- 6-1   Total Abdominal Hysterectomy, Basic Techniques   *104*
  - Beri M. Ridgeway, MD

6-2   TAH, Endometriosis   *115*
Mickey Karram, MD

6-3   Total Abdominal Hysterectomy, Fibroid Uterus   *117*
Beri M. Ridgeway, MD

7 Vaginal Hysterectomy and Trachelectomy: Basic Surgical Techniques   **123**

Mark D. Walters, MD

Video Demonstrations:

7-1   Vaginal Hysterectomy   *124*
Anna C. Frick, MD, and Mark D. Walters, MD

7-2   Anterior Cul-de-Sac Entry   *127*
Anna C. Frick, MD, and Mark D. Walters, MD

7-3   Electrosurgical Device-Assisted Vaginal Hysterectomy   *132*
Anna C. Frick, MD, and Mark D. Walters, MD

7-4   Vaginal Trachelectomy   *132*
Mickey Karram, MD

8 Difficult Vaginal Hysterectomy   **135**

Matthew D. Barber, MD, MHS

Video Demonstrations:

8-1   Uterine Morcellation Techniques   *140*
Gouri B. Diwadkar, MD, Chi Chiung Grace Chen, MD, Marie Fidela R. Paraiso, MD, and Mark D Walters, MD

8-2   Difficult Anterior Entry   *150*
Anna C. Frick, MD, Matthew D. Barber, MD, MHS, and Mark D. Walters, MD

8-3   Difficult Posterior Entry   *152*
Anna C. Frick, MD, Matthew D. Barber, MD, MHS, and Mark D. Walters, MD

8-4   Uterovaginal Prolapse   *157*
Anna C. Frick, MD, Matthew D. Barber, MD, MHS, and Mark D. Walters, MD

9 Prophylactic Oophorectomy at Hysterectomy   **161**

James L. Whiteside, MD, and Rebecca S. Uranga, MD

Video Demonstrations:

9-1   Techniques in Vaginal Oophorectomy   *165*
John B. Gebhart, MD, MS, Rosanne M. Kho, MD, and Javier F. Magrina, MD

9-2   Vaginal Bilateral Salpino-oophorectomy   *166*
Tristi W. Muir, MD, and Mark D. Walters, MD

10 Laparoscopic and Robotic-Assisted Total and Supracervical Hysterectomy   **179**

Marie Fidela R. Paraiso, MD, and Pedro F. Escobar, MD

Video Demonstrations:

10-1   Conventional Total Laparoscopic Hysterectomy (4 video clips)   *181*
Marie Fidela R. Paraiso, MD

(a)   Sealing and Transection of Left Infundibulopelvic Ligament
(b)   Development of Bladder Flap
(c)   Uterine Vessel Ligation
(d)   Colpotomy

10-2   Robotic-Assisted Laparoscopic Supracervical Hysterectomy
(4 video clips)   *187*
Marie Fidela R. Paraiso, MD
(a)   Development of Bladder Flap and Sealing of Right Uterine Vessels
(b)   Transection of the Upper Pedicles on the Left Uterine Corpus
(c)   Transection of the Uterine Corpus from the Cervix
(d)   Closure of the Cervical Os

11 Complications of Hysterectomy   195

Mark D. Walters, MD, and Matthew D. Barber, MD, MHS

Video Demonstrations:
11-1   Transvaginal Cystotomy Repair   *204*
John B. Gebhart, MD, MS
11-2   Intentional Cystotomy with Passage of Ureteral Catheters   *207*
Mickey Karram, MD

12 Alternative Treatments to Hysterectomy   213

Linda D. Bradley, MD, and Devorah R. Wieder, MD, MPH

Video Demonstration:
12-1   Operative Hysteroscopic Myomectomy   *221*
Linda D. Bradley, MD

13 Teaching and Learning Gynecologic Surgery   249

Gouri B. Diwadkar, MD, and J. Eric Jelovsek, MD

Video Demonstrations:
13-1   Knot-Tying: A Guide to Tying Surgical Knots and Common Knot-Tying Mistakes   *253*
Gouri B. Diwadkar, MD, and J. Eric Jelovsek, MD
13-2   Feedback in Surgical Training   *258*
Anna C. Frick, MD, and J. Eric Jelovsek, MD

Index   267

The Evolution of Uterine Surgery and Hysterectomy

Anthony P. Tizzano M.D.
Mark D. Walters M.D.

"What cannot be cured with medicines is cured by the knife, what cannot be cured by the knife is cured by fire, and what fire cannot cure is incurable."

Hippocrates

The evolution of uterine surgery is an intriguing story whereby original procedures and theories would fall from favor only to be successfully resurrected and popularized by subsequent generations. Prior to the nineteenth century an inadequate understanding of pelvic anatomy and physiology plagued practitioners. Moreover, despite a surgeon's best efforts, early attempts at uterine surgery were often foiled by an ignorance of asepsis, the absence of anesthesia, faulty suture materials, inadequate instrumentation, and suboptimal exposure. As a result, any consistent success was delayed until the midnineteenth century. Particularly intriguing was the development of an amazing variety of innovative instruments of remarkable craftsmanship and materials that paralleled the many surgical advances.

This chapter is an attempt to touch upon the milestones leading to successful trachelectomy and hysterectomy and to acknowledge the many pioneers who paved the way. The author's selection of important milestones is listed in Table 1-1. Kindly note that this chapter emphasizes American and some European contributions and benchmarks that influenced contemporary thought, patient care and surgical practices. Throughout the chapter an effort is made to identify individuals who were first to perform a particular operation or technique. However, a number of variables confound the process including whether or not the procedure was purposefully planned or the result of intraoperative necessity or misadventure. Also important are whether or not the patient survived the actual operation and had a full recovery and whether there is documentation (clinical or pathologic) that verifies all the surgical details.

Clearly we owe a great debt of gratitude to these and many others who established the foundation for successful pelvic surgery and ultimately for our specialty. Perhaps Kelly, an avid historian and bibliophile, summarized it best by stating, "No group should ever neglect to honor the forebears upon whom their contributions are based. Great is the loss to anyone who neglects to study the lives of those he follows." We are particularly grateful for the works of Dr. Thomas Baskett, Dr. James V. Ricci, and Dr. Harold Speert, whose extensive research on the subject made this chapter possible.

Table 1-1 Timeline of Milestones Related to Uterine Surgery

100 CE	First good description of the human uterus: *De Morbis Mulierum* by Soranus.
1507	Earliest authentic account of vaginal excision of the uterus in a case of prolapse: Giacomo Berengario da Carpi.
1561	First accurate description of the human oviduct: *Observationes Anatomicae* by Gabriele Falloppio.
1663	First work on operative gynecology: *Heel-konstige aanmerkkingen betreffende de gebreeken der vrouwen* by Hendrick van Roonhuyze.
1672	First accurate account of the female reproductive organs and ovarian follicles—"graafian follicles:" *De Mulierum Organis Generationi Inservientibus* by Regnier de Graaf.
1737	Description of the peritoneum and the posterior cul-de-sac: *A Description of the Peritoneum* by James Douglas.
1774	The finest work on uterine anatomy to date: *Anatomy of the Gravid Uterus* by William Hunter.
1801	Friedrich Benjamin Osiander performed the first partial trachelectomy by means of a knife for the treatment of cervical cancer.
1812	Although planning to perform a trachelectomy for cancer, G.B. Paletta inadvertently performed the first vaginal hysterectomy; the patient died 3 days later.
1813	Conrad Langenbeck performed the first intentional complete vaginal extirpation of the uterus for prolapse with cervical ulceration, using an apparent extraperitoneal approach, after which the patient survived.
1822	J.M. Sauter of Baden, Germany, performed the first planned and successfully executed complete vaginal hysterectomy for cervical cancer.
1826	First American textbook on gynecology: *A Treatise on the Diseases of Females* by William Potts Dewees.
1829	Earliest report of a successful trachelectomy in America: *Case of a successful excision of the cervix uteri in a scirrhous state* by John B. Strachan.
1846	First deliberate abdominal supracervical hysterectomy in America for fibroids (with the correct preoperative diagnosis) was performed by John Bellinger of Charleston, South Carolina. The patient died on the fifth postoperative day.
1849	Anders Adolf Retzius described the prevesical space.
1850	First successful vaginal hysterectomy performed in America by Paul F. Eve of Augusta, Georgia.
1852	Hugh Lenox Hodge detailed the use of his pessary for the correction of uterine displacement.
1853	Walter Burnham of Massachusetts performed the world's first successful (albeit unplanned) abdominal supracervical hysterectomy. *Extirpation of the uterus and ovaries for sarcomatous disease* (Nelsons Am Lancet 1853;7:147). It was done with the patient under chloroform anesthesia; the patient survived.
1853	Gilman Kimball performed the first deliberate and successful abdominal supracervical hysterectomy for a fibroid uterus. (Kimball G: Successful case of extirpation of the uterus. Boston Med Surg J 1855;52:249–255.)
1861	Samuel Chopin performed the first successful vaginal hysterectomy for prolapse in America.
1861	James Marion Sims described method for trachelectomy: *Amputation of the cervix uteri*.
1863	Earliest successful excision of the uterus and ovaries for tumor. *Exstirpation de l'uterus et des ovaries* by Eugene Koeberle.
1868	First attempt at cesarean hysterectomy in America by Horatio Robinson Storer of Boston.
1876	First successful cesarean hysterectomy by Edorado Porro of Pavia, Italy.
1878	First carefully planned and successful abdominal hysterectomy for cancer using Lister's antiseptic method. *Eine neue Methode der exstirpation des ganzen uterus* by Wilhelm Alexander Freund. Freund also introduced "compression forceps" (clamps) to vaginal hysterectomy to secure vascular pedicles.
1890	Freidrich Trendelenburg described his manner for positioning patients to enhance exposure.

Table 1-1 Timeline of Milestones Related to Uterine Surgery—cont'd

1893	Karl August Schuchardt described his mediolateral incision to enhance exposure for radical vaginal hysterectomy in cases of cervical cancer. He performed the first radical hysterectomies for cervical cancer. (Garrison FH, Morton LT: *Morton's Medical Bibliography*, 5th ed. Aldershot, England, Scholar Press, 1991.)
1895	The first radical hysterectomy for invasive cervical cancer by John Goodrich Clark at Johns Hopkins Hospital.
1895	Alwin Mackenrodt provided a comprehensive and accurate description of the pelvic connective tissue and its relationship to pelvic prolapse.
1898	Howard Atwood Kelly's text *Operative Gynecology* published. Provided the foundation for the specialty in America.
1900	Hermann Johannes Pfannensteil introduced a transverse incision for laparotomy.
1900	Ernst Wertheim described his radical operation for cervical and uterine cancer.
1901	Alfred Ernest Maylard advocated an oblique transection of the rectus muscles to improve exposure.
1906	Albert Doderlein and S. Kronig described their technique for vaginal hysterectomy beginning with an anterior colpotomy incision.
1908	Friedrich Schauta described his method for radical vaginal hysterectomy in cases of carcinoma of the cervix.
1911	Max Brödel chaired the world's first Department of Medical Illustration at Johns Hopkins University.
1915	William Edward Fothergill modified Archibald Donald's operation for complete uterine prolapse: *Anterior colporrhaphy and its combination with amputation of the cervix*, the so-called Manchester operation.
1915	Arnold Sturmdorf introduced his tracheloplasty technique.
1928	Edward H. Richardson reported his simplified technique for abdominal hysterectomy, using the uterosacral and cardinal ligaments in vaginal cuff closure.
1934	Nobel Sproat Heaney described his technique for vaginal hysterectomy using a clamp, needle holder, and retractor of his own design. His method for suturing the vaginal cuff in a manner that incorporates peritoneum, vessels, and ligaments is eponymously termed the "Heaney stitch."
1941	A.F. Lash described the coring method for reducing the size of the uterus to facilitate vaginal hysterectomy.
1941	Leonid Sergius Cherney proposed a modified low transverse abdominal incision, whereby the rectus muscle is reflected off its insertion into the posterior pubis, to maximize access to the space of Retzius.
1946	Richard Wesley TeLinde published his *Operative Gynecology*, which remains the standard American work on the subject under successive authors.
1972	Allen and associates first reported that perioperative prophylactic antibiotics (cephalothin versus placebo) reduce major infection rate after abdominal hysterectomy.
1989	Reich described the first laparoscopic hysterectomy.

Antiquity

"Never as yet have I gone astray, whether in treatment or in prognosis, as have so many physicians of great reputation. If anyone wishes to gain fame ... all that he needs is to accept what I have been able to establish."

Claudius Galen

The foundation of all surgical specialties is predicated on an accurate and thorough understanding of the pertinent anatomy. Magnificent prehistoric drawings on the walls of caves and carvings of human figures have been dated as far back as 40,000 to 16,000 BCE However, it was not until many millennia later that any real effort was devoted to the study and illustration of human anatomy. The earliest descriptions of the uterus are gleaned from the Ebers Papyrus (1500 BCE), which depicts the uterus as an independent animal, capable of movement within the abdomen and pelvis of its host. Similar accounts in other documents correspondingly describe the uterus as a salamander, crocodile, or tortoise (Fig. 1-1).

Accounts by Hippocrates (460–377 BCE) regarding the uterus portray the organ as going wild when not sufficiently nourished with male semen. During the second century CE the eminent Greek physician Aretaeus reinforced this animalistic concept stating in his *Causes and Indications of Acute and Chronic Diseases*:

> *In the middle of the flanks of women lies the womb, a female viscus closely resembling an animal, for it moves hither and thither in the flanks, also upwards in a direct line to below the cartilage of the thorax, and also obliquely to the right or the left, either to the liver or the spleen; and it is likewise subject to prolapse downwards; and in a word is all together erratic. It delights also in fragrant odors and advances towards them, and it has an aversion to fetid odors and flees from them; and on the whole the womb is like an animal within an animal.*
>
> Aretaeus

This animalistic concept of the uterus was subsequently replaced, during the Common Era, by the notion that the uterine cavity comprised seven separate compartments—three on either side and one elongated compartment in the center. The so-called "seven cell doctrine" proposed that male embryos developed in cells on the right, females developed on the left, and from the center cell hermaphrodites were produced. This and other similar theories remained popular throughout the Middle Ages until cadaver dissections would prove otherwise.

Perhaps the earliest acceptable description of the uterus came from Soranus of Ephesus (98–138 CE), a learned and leading medical figure of the early

Figure 1-1 An eighteenth century umbilical cord clamp mounted on a tortoise representing the uterus.

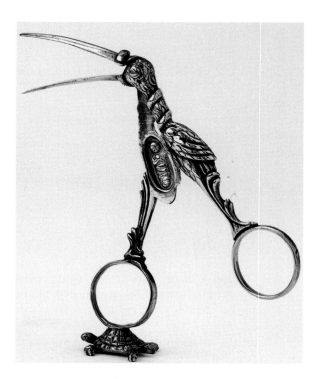

second century CE. Soranus is best known for his text on the diseases of women, *De Morbis Mulierum*, which ultimately provided a basis for gynecologic texts up to the seventeenth century. He suggested that a prolapsed uterus that had become gangrenous could be safely excised without harm to the patient but otherwise a pessary should be employed to restore the prolapse. His description of the uterus is clearly based on cadaver dissections as evidenced in his elaborate description regarding adjacent organs in the pelvis. Soranus related his concept of the uterus and appreciation for its surrounding structures in his narrative, "What Is the Nature of the Uterus and of the Vagina?"

> *The uterus (metra) is also termed hystera and delphys. It is termed metra because it is the mother of all the embryos borne of it or because it makes mothers of those who possess it: or, according to some people, because it possesses a metre of time in regard to menstruation and childbirth. And it is termed hystera because afterwards it yields up its products, at least broadly speaking. And it is termed delphys because it is able to procreate brothers and sisters.*
>
> *The uterus is situated in the large space between the hips, between the bladder and the rectum, lying above the rectum and sometimes completely, sometimes partly, beneath the bladder, because of the variability of the uterus. For in children the uterus is smaller than the bladder (and lies, therefore, wholly beneath it). But in virgins in their prime of puberty, it is equal to the size of the superimposed bladder, whereas in women who are older and have already been deflowered and even more in those who have already been pregnant, it is so much bigger that in most cases it rests upon the end of the colon.*
>
> *By thin membranes the uterus is connected above with the bladder, below with the rectum, laterally and posteriorly with the excrescences of the hips and the os sacrum. When these membranes are contracted by an inflammation, the uterus is drawn up and bent to the side, but when they are weakened and relaxed, the uterus prolapses. Although the uterus is not an animal (as it appeared to some people), it is, nevertheless, similar in certain respects, having a sense of touch, so that it is contracted by cooling agents but relaxed by loosening ones.*
>
> *The shape of the uterus is not curved as in dumb animals, but is similar in shape to a cupping vessel. For beginning with a rounded and broad end at the fundus, it is drawn together proportionally into the isthmus, neck and finally a narrow orifice. The orifice lies in the middle of the vagina, for the neck of the uterus is enclosed tightly by the vagina while the outer part ends in the labia. ... In the natural state the orifice is in most cases as large as the external end of the auditory canal. Yet at certain times it is dilated, as in the desire of intercourse for the reception of semen. ... and to an extreme degree till it even admits the hand of a grown-up person. In its natural state in virgins, the orifice is soft and fleshy, similar to the spongy texture of the lung or the softness of the tongue. But in women who have borne children it becomes more callous and, as Herophilus says, similar to the head of an octopus or to the larynx.*
>
> Soranus (from Temkin, 1956)

The ancients are credited with a great many basic instruments fashioned from tin, iron, steel, lead, copper, bronze, wood, and horn. Ferrous metals were likely the most popular, but few survived the oxidation of more than 2000 years. Nonetheless, a surprising number of instruments including scalpels, forceps, and catheters that date to the first century were recovered from archeological digs at Pompeii. Of the instruments recovered, the most impressive are the massive bivalve, trivalve, and quadrivalve vaginal specula which were fabricated from bronze and thus remain nicely preserved.

Arabian medicine texts, despite their large numbers, contained very little with respect to gynecology and are, for the most part, an accumulation of Greek contributions with numerous translations from the Indian, Persian, and Syrian. Perhaps their greatest value was the preservation of Greek medical literature and culture that likely would have all but vanished during the Dark Ages.

Medieval Medicine

Those unfortunate enough to contract The Black Death "ate lunch with their friends and dinner with their ancestors in paradise."

                                                Giovanni Boccaccio

The Medieval Period or Middle Ages marked the end of Arabic supremacy and is commonly referred to as the Age of Faith or Era of Monastatic Medicine, a period whereby confidence in any one individual was replaced by divine trust. As such, St. Benedict, founder of the Benedictine Order, encouraged his monks to tend to the sick but forbade any formal study of medicine. The struggle against leprosy, plagues, and prostitution were the main challenges of the day, and few meaningful contributions were made to the fund of medical knowledge. Moreover, medicine during the period was essentially nonsurgical and the majority of physicians were typically itinerant practitioners, many of whom were likely quacks and charlatans.

The Renaissance

Regarding Leonardo da Vinci "He was like a man who woke up too early, in the darkness, while everyone else was still sleeping."

                                                Dmitri S. Merezhkovsky, 1901

The Renaissance was marked by the rescission of medieval oppression of liberty of thought and inquiry, the rise of universities, the dawn of the printing press, and the subsequent emergence of self-education, which collectively led to the rebirth of medical thinking in general and investigation of human anatomy in particular. These essential elements served to elevate medicine to the next level and would provide for a more clear understanding of female anatomy.

Early on was the work of Leonardo da Vinci (1452–1519), founder of iconographic and physiologic anatomy that served as a foundation for modern anatomic illustration. Da Vinci, "the greatest artist and scientist of the Italian Renaissance produced over 750 sketches portraying all the principal organs of the body" (Garrison and Morton, 1991) and the earliest accurate depiction of the fetus in utero. Unfortunately, his work was appreciated by only a few of his contemporaries and was not published until the end of the nineteenth century. Da Vinci's contemporary, Giacomo Berengario da Carpi (circa 1460–1530?), introduced iconography and independent observation into the teaching of anatomy. His *Commentaria* was the first work since Galen to present a substantial amount of anatomic illustrations based on his own investigations and observation. Da Carpi's work included the most extensive account of the female reproductive organs up to that time (Garrison and Morton, 1991).

Most remarkable, however, was the contribution of Andreas Vesalius (1514–1564), who at the age of 29 published the *Fabrica* in 1543 containing "the most famous anatomical illustrations of all time. His work more than any other, with its extraordinary blend of scientific exposition, art and typography, revolutionized the science of anatomy and the manner in which it was taught" (Garrison and Morton, 1991). Vesalius was among the first to successfully challenge the anatomic teachings of Galen, but more important, he asserted that the physician must perform cadaver dissection firsthand to master the art. An apparently engaging young man, he made human dissection a respected and viable profession. His illustrations include an accurate description of the entire female urogenital tract and its vasculature depicting the left ovarian vein entering the left renal vein for the first time. Vesalius also produced a number of distinguished pupils including Matteo Realdo Colombo (circa 1510–1559), who is credited with earliest use of the term "labia," which he thought were essential in protecting the uterus from the cold, dust, and air; Gabriele Falloppio (1523–1562), who became professor of anatomy at Ferrara, Pisa, and Padua and who is eponymously remembered for the fallopian tube among his many contributions; and Bartolomeo Eustachi (circa 1510/1520–1574) whose fine copper plates, produced in 1552, provided the first accurate delineation of the uterine cavity and cervical canal. Unfortunately they remained unprinted and forgotten in the Vatican Library until the early eighteenth century, when they were recovered and subsequently presented by Pope Clement XI to his physician, who published them in 1714.

Gynecologic surgeries during the Renaissance, although few and far between, were nonetheless a consideration. Jacopo Berengario da Carpi (1470–1550) a pre-Vesalian anatomist and surgeon provided the earliest account of a vaginal hysterectomy performed with a scalpel, by his father, on a prolapsed gangrenous uterus. Later, Berengario himself would perform a vaginal hysterectomy by circumferentially ligating the prolapsed uterus with some very strong twine and tightening the ligature until the organ was severed. The renowned French military surgeon Ambroise Paré (1510–1590) was the first to employ vascular ligatures in place of cautery or boiling oil for hemostasis. However, the use of ligatures quickly fell from favor due to faulty suture materials with insufficient strength and longevity and a likely increased rate of resulting infections and foreign body reactions. More than two centuries would pass before the suture ligature was resurrected, improved and popularized by Lister in the mid-nineteenth century. Although best known for contributions to military medicine, Paré was equally ingenious with respect to his gynecologic therapy. He was the first to employ a pessary fashioned of hammered brass and waxed cork for uterine prolapse, he suggested trachelectomy for cervical cancer, and he devised an imaginative and elaborate fumigation apparatus employing a special elongated pessary of gold or silver with perforations along its length and an open end to introduce medicated steam into the vagina and to ventilate the uterus (Fig. 1-2). He is credited with the development of a great many instruments including vaginal specula of his own design and is said to have excised an inverted uterus and the patient survived (Johnson, 1678). Among the more comprehensive accounts of Renaissance gynecologic surgery is Caspar Stromayr's *Practica Copiosa* (1559), which contains beautifully executed plates depicting diseases of women. Together with the many illustrations of instruments and surgical techniques are several that depict the replacement of a uterine prolapse by placement of a pessary comprising a sponge bound with twine, sealed with wax, and dipped in butter. He also created one of the earliest illustrations of a standing pelvic examination for a woman with prolapse (Fig. 1-3).

Ultimately, despite the many academic advances in areas outside medicine during the Renaissance, the approach to the majority of gynecologic problems changed very little from that which was popular since the classical period.

Seventeenth Century

"We are now at odds with our barber-surgeons who wish to unite with the surgeons of St. Cosmas, our ancient enemies. Those of St. Cosmas are miserable rascals, nearly all tooth-pullers and very ignorant who have attached the barber-surgeons to their string, by making them share their halls and their pretended privileges."

Guy Patin (1601–1672), Dean of Medicine, Paris

Figure 1-2 Fumigation apparatus. A sixteenth century woodcut illustrating Ambroise Paré's uterovaginal fumigation apparatus for the treatment of uterine prolapse. (From Johnson TH (transl.): The Works of Ambroise Paré. London, 1678.)

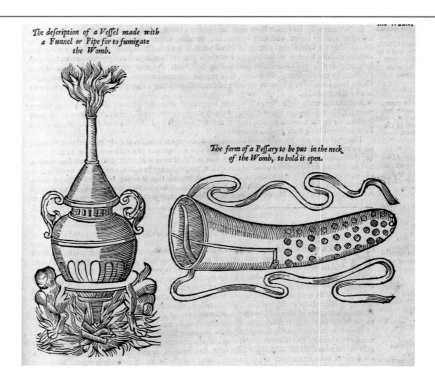

The description of a Vessel made with a Funnel or Pipe for to fumigate the Womb.

The form of a Pessary to be put in the neck of the Womb, to hold it open.

Figure 1-3 Sixteenth century illustration showing examination of women with uterine prolapse. (From Stromayr's Practica Copiosa, 1559, Edited by W. von Brunn, Berlin, 1925.)

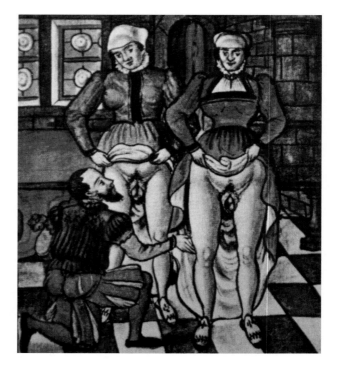

Throughout the seventeenth century, many theories with respect to anatomy, physiology, chemistry, and generation received clarification and a more credible basis for medicine began to emerge. "In medicine, this was the century of 'systems,' speculations and explanations, and surgery consequently remained in the background" (Ricci, 1990, p 99).

The anatomist, Regnier de Graaf (1641–1673), published his work *De Mullierum Organis Generationi* in 1672, which provided the first accurate account of the ovary's gross morphology, anatomic relations, and function (Fig. 1-4).

Figure 1-4 De Graff's illustration of the uterus, vagina, tubes, and ovaries arranged to show clearly the ovarian and hypogastric arteries with their ramifications. (From de Graaf R: De Mulierum Organis Generationi Inservientibus. Leyden, Hackiana, 1672.)

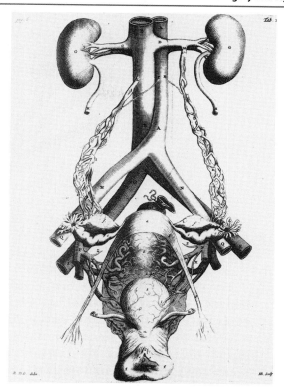

He also provides clear descriptions and illustrations of the uterine vasculature, lymphatic drainage, uterine fibroids, and the ovarian follicle, which was named the "graafian follicle" in his honor.

The first illustrations of gynecologic procedures are nicely portrayed, in a stepwise fashion for the first time, in the engravings by Johannes Scultetus (1595–1645) in his *Armamentarium Chirurgicum* (1655). Included are examples of treatment of imperforate hymen, hematocolpos, and clitoral hypertrophy and the use of a T-binder to control hemorrhage following vaginal surgery. Scultetus advocated and described the use of a vaginal speculum so that afflictions of the rectum, vagina, and uterus could be seen and treated (Fig. 1-5).

Successful surgery during the period was limited and hysterectomy was not a popular method of therapy during the seventeenth century unless the organ had prolapsed and became gangrenous. Instead, classical notions for treating prolapse persisted as evidenced in the writings of Francois Thevenin (?–1656) who favored replacement of the organ followed by placement of a foul-smelling vaginal pack (to drive the organ upward), and application of sweet scents to the mouth and nose to attract the uterus (capable of movement within its host) upward, and thus preventing it from prolapsing. Only if such measures failed or the organ became gangrenous would ligation or extirpation be seriously considered.

Eighteenth Century

"Two inconveniences generally attend the use of the Cautery ... forcing us to neglect it. First, the patient is usually wonderfully terrified of it and second, Mankind in general looks upon it as barbaric to advise it."

Lorenz Heister, 1718

Figure 1-5 Early iron vaginal speculum from the mid-sixteenth century.

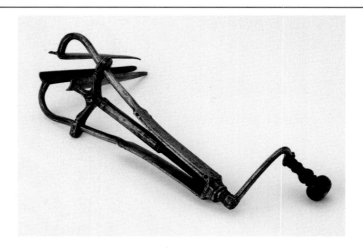

The eighteenth century might best be characterized by the relentless conflict between old and new ideas, the abolition of medievalism, and the beginnings of a new world structure. Although relatively few advances occurred in the realm of medicine, there were many notable contributions made in the fields of natural philosophy, microscopy, physics, and biology. As a result, theories regarding pathologic anatomy and experimental pathology began to surface and eventually provided the foundation for medical thinking from a clinical pathology perspective. Dissection of cadavers to improve one's understanding of anatomy and to facilitate the development of surgical techniques had become commonplace. Accordingly, surgery during the eighteenth century began to rise beyond the skills of individual surgeons with the founding of surgical societies and the publishing of medical journals. Nonetheless, surgeons remained under close public scrutiny at the hands of popular medical caricaturists, such as Thomas Rowlandson (1756–1827), whose flair for satire and caustic pencil found a ready target in the shams, failures, and generally antisocial behavior of the eighteenth century medical practitioner (Fig. 1-6). There were likely some valid reasons for the somewhat less than lofty regard for our profession at that time. "Laws regulating the practice of medicine were poorly defined, often disregarded and never seriously enforced, thus permitting quacks and nostrum-vendors to flourish like locusts." Apparently, Rowlandson considered anatomists of his day to be little more than "an accomplice of the vicious and even murderous body snatchers" (Saffron, 1971). Rowlandson's opinions notwithstanding, a number of significant contributions were made during the century relating to pelvic anatomy. In 1730 James Douglas (1675–1742) provided the first adequate description of the pelvic peritoneum and cul-de-sac as well as describing the vaginal musculature. His work paved the way for early retroperitoneal surgery and the corresponding decrease in peritonitis that commonly plagued pelvic surgery during that time. Justus Gottfried Gunzius (1714–1784) accurately described the uterosacral ligaments and anterior bladder folds and Joannes Fridericus Cassebohm (?–1743) suggested that the fibers derived from the uterus coalesced, giving rise to the round ligaments. In 1774 William Hunter (1718–1783) published his monumental work, *Anatomy of the Gravid Uterus*, providing the best account of uterine anatomy to date and considered by many to be the finest anatomy atlas ever produced (Choulant, 1842).

Among the most popular surgical texts of the seventeenth century was one by Lorenz Heister (1683–1758) a formally educated military surgeon who ultimately became professor of anatomy and surgery at Helmstadt, Germany. The

Figure 1-6 "The Anatomist," an eighteenth century medical caricature by Thomas Rowlandson.

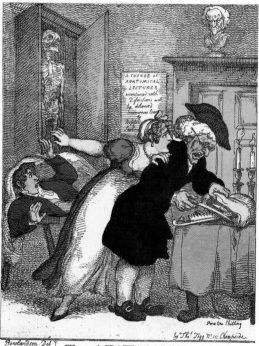

first edition of his work *A General System of Surgery* was published in 1718 and is of particular interest due to its abundant illustrative engravings. He provided the first illustration of a manual examination of the cervix and subsequent removal of an intrauterine mass with specially designed forceps (Fig. 1-7).

During the first half of the century uterine polyps were typically excised, crushed, or cauterized. In 1749 Andre Levret (1703–1780) completed a massive work on polyps of the uterus, throat, and nose that popularized the use of ligatures to snare the polyp. Subsequently, all manner of devices were created to facilitate placement of a ligature about the base of the polyp whereby it could be successfully secured and the polyp removed (Fig. 1-8).

By the latter half of the eighteenth century the surgical instrument trade began to emerge when cutlers began to specialize in the fabrication of steel surgical instruments with handles of wood, ebony, and ivory. Toward the end of the century surgical instrument catalogues had begun to appear containing fundamental instruments from makers such as Perret in 1772, Laundy in 1795, and Savigny in 1798.

Although military surgery enjoyed some advances during the century, gynecology had yet to reach its operative phase. Most of the uterine surgeries up to this time involved emergent removal of protruding or bleeding masses, be they uterine polyps, myomas, cancers, or uterine inversion. Thus, by the close of the eighteenth century there was little verifiable evidence that intentional hysterectomy, be it abdominal or vaginal, had actually been successfully and intentionally done with the patient surviving.

Nineteenth Century

"There are no operations within the domain of surgery more grave, requiring greater courage and skill, or greater fertility of resources."
C.D. Palmer, 1880 (on abdominal hysterectomy for fibroid uterus)

Figure 1-7 Earliest known illustration of an endometrial polypectomy. (From Heister L: Heister's Textbook of Chirurgie. Lurmberg, Germany, J Hoffman Publisher, 1718.)

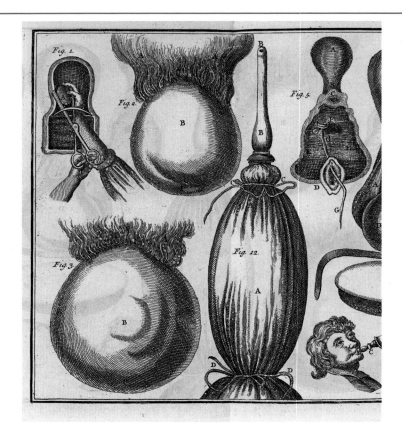

Figure 1-8 An elaborate early nineteenth century uterine polyp snare by the French maker Luer.

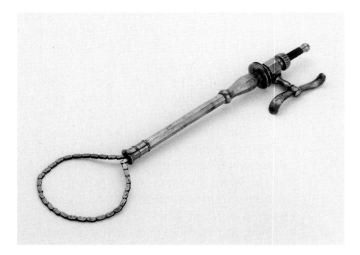

Pelvic Examination

At the beginning of the nineteenth century it seems that it was acceptable to perform a vaginal examination in the upright and supine positions (Fig. 1-9). However, it was frowned upon to expose the genitals unnecessarily and thus patients remained clothed. As a result, most of the recognized pathology was at or beyond the introitus, and diagnosis of pelvic masses, cervical tumors, and determination of the degree of uterovaginal prolapse required careful palpation and was difficult at best.

John C.W. Lever, an accoucheur at Guy's Hospital in London, stated in 1843, that vaginal examination could be done erect or recumbent but the upright

Figure 1-9 An early nineteenth century illustration depicting proper etiquette for pelvic examination. (From Maygrier JP: Nouvelles Demonstrations d'Accouchemens. Paris, 1822.)

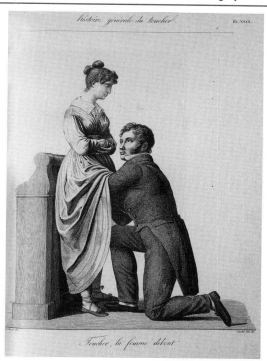

position was more likely to reveal relaxation of the uterine ligaments and prolapse. He provided the following instructions for vaginal examination:

> *The patient lying on her left side with her knees drawn up, and her head slightly inclined, having, as before, evacuated the contents of the bladder and rectum, the examiner kneels at her bedside, and anointing his fore-finger with lard passes it into the vagina: by its assistance he ascertains whether there be any dislocation of the uterus, if it be anteverted, retroverted, or prolapsed; he marks the existence or non-existence of inflammation or irritability, whether the os uteri is prenaturally firm or hard; whether there are any polypoid growths, their consistence, sensibility and place of attachment; he ascertains the weight and size of the uterus by raising the organ with his finger, and he endeavors to discover that the tumor (if one exists), felt by an external examination, is uterine, by placing one hand over the abdominal region, and testing whether the impetus given to the one is communicated to the other."*

J.C.W. Lever (1843, as quoted in Ricci, 1990)

The surgical instrument trade flourished in America during the nineteenth century, initially to satisfy the needs of Civil War surgeons and later to meet the demand of emerging specialties. Accordingly, creativity prospered throughout the remainder of the nineteenth century, resulting in an extensive gynecologic armamentarium. Most remarkable is the evolution of the vaginal speculum over the course of the nineteenth century. Early in the century specula resembled those from the classical era. The device would undergo more than 200 permutations before the introduction of the Graves speculum in 1867. There were many variations of forms seen during the development of vaginal specula and a large variety of materials was employed in their fabrication, with intriguing examples fabricated from lead, iron, copper, silver, brass, tin, pewter, bronze, steel, glass, porcelain, ebony, boxwood, pearwood, horn, bone, and ivory. Following the early trivalve designs an assortment of tubular specula emerged, the first of which was devised in 1816 by Joseph Claude Anselme Récamier (1744–1852), who is credited by some as the founder of the specialty of gynecology. His initial device was made of

Figure 1-10 Cylindrical specula such as this example by Récamier were particularly well suited for the application of leeches and cautery to the cervix.

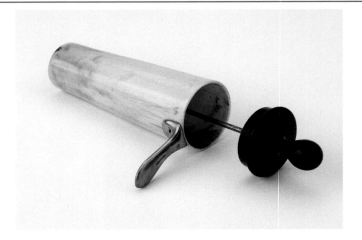

tin that was highly polished to enhance the reflection of light to illuminate the cervix. The tubular design was particularly useful since application of leeches and cautery irons to the cervix required protection for the vaginal mucosa (Fig. 1-10).

Particularly popular was the tubular speculum of William Ferguson (1808–1877) introduced about 1845 and consisting of a glass tube coated with quicksilver and covered with India rubber and then varnish. However, the best known model was the bivalve introduced in 1850 by Edward Gabriel Cusco (1819–1894) and then popularized with a slight modification in 1878 to its present form by T.W. Graves, a general practitioner from Massachusetts. This speculum provided the vaginal surgeon more flexibility and space (compared to tubular specula) to remove cervical masses and operate up in the vagina.

Instruments manufactured prior to 1890 exhibited standards of workmanship, fit, finish, and overall artistry that were later sacrificed in the production of aseptic instruments which required that they be fabricated from steel and then nickel-plated so as to withstand the rigors of sterilization.

Trachelectomy

Prior to the nineteenth century, surgical management of prolapse and cervical malignancy was limited, for the most part, to amputation of the cervix. However, as surgery during the nineteenth century progressed, surgeons attained credibility by requiring, in addition to the usual surgical apprenticeship, a series of formal studies in the areas of internal medicine, anatomy, and pathology. The three requisites for successful surgery—anesthesia, antisepsis, and hemostasis—were yet to emerge. Lacking these essential adjuncts, only the most self-assured surgeons undertook an occasional fistula repair, ovariotomy, vaginal hysterectomy for carcinoma, or abdominal hysterectomy for fibroids.

As new procedures evolved, so did specialized instruments, particularly those intended for fistula repairs and trachelectomy. Given that the treatment of cervical malignancy was an important concern for gynecologists, a number of instruments were introduced including specula, forceps, scissors, and knives specifically designed to facilitate visualization and amputation of the cervix and extirpation of the uterus in the absence of anesthesia and with little hemostasis. At the outset of the nineteenth century excision of the cervix was attempted by surgeons only to be discarded by midcentury in favor of hysterectomy. Trachelectomy for the treatment of cervical malignancy was first given serious

Figure 1-11 A nineteenth century galvanocautery apparatus for trachelectomy.

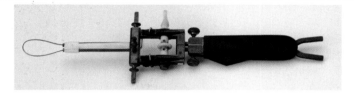

Figure 1-12 An exhibition quality example of Colombat's hysterotome designed for trachelectomy and fashioned from steel, silver, gold, and ivory by the Charriere Company of France (ca. 1860).

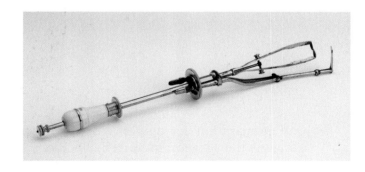

Figure 1-13 Colombat's uterocepts intended for fixation and traction of the cervix in preparation for trachelectomy. (From The American Armamentarium Chirurgicum Catalog of Surgical Instruments. Chicago, George Tiemann & Company, 1889.)

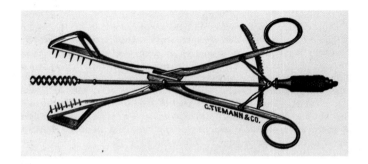

consideration by H.A. Wrisberg in 1787. More than a decade later, on May 5, 1801, Friedrich Benjamin Osiander (1759–1822), while professor of obstetrics at Gottingen, Germany, was the first to perform a partial trachelectomy by removing a large carcinomatous cervix. He delivered the large mass with a pair of Smellie's obstetric forceps, amputated it with Pott's curved fistula knife, and controlled hemostasis with a sponge dusted with styptic powder. Subsequently, in 1829 John B. Strachan of Virginia successfully performed the operation without incident. The trachelectomy operation was typically accomplished by either bistoury, scissors, ecraseur, or galvanocautery (Fig. 1-11). A wide variety of instruments were devised to amputate the cervix—from a simple spoon with a serrated edge developed by Dupuytren to the very elegant and complex trachelectomy instruments devised by Marc Colombat de L'Isere (1797–1851).

Colombat's "uterocepts" was intended for fixation and traction while his "hysterotomist" or "hysterotome" was intended for fixation and excision of the cervix (Figs. 1-12 and 1-13). His hysterotome was a cumbersome vulsellum forceps-knife combination which provided a means for grasping the portio of the cervix securely and then engaging a knife at right angles to the neck of the cervix while rotating the blade about a central axis. With proper traction it is likely that an acceptable conization of the cervix could be produced, hemostasis notwithstanding. His uteroceps provided a means for firmly grasping and crushing the distal portion of the cervix while entering the cervical canal with the central corkscrew-like portion of the instrument to further steady the organ

Figure 1-14 An exhibition quality example of Chassaignac's Screw Ecraseur used for polypectomy and subtotal hysterectomy.

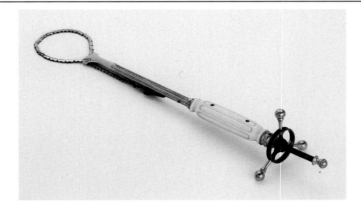

in preparation for surgery. Excision could then be performed by whatever means the surgeon preferred. The device was particularly well suited to galvanocautery on account of the inclusion of ivory guards to provide a thermal-electrical barrier to prevent electrical arcing and burns.

Extolling the virtues of his instruments Colombat stated:

> *The operator, in using our forceps, has much less occasion to fear laceration, which often results either from tractions made unequally, and in one direction more than in another, or from the fatigue and awkwardness of the assistants. We shall conclude by saying that in operating with the modifications and instruments we have now described, we have no occasion for educated assistants who have frequently witnessed the operation, and who can only be found in the large hospitals of Paris."*

Colombat (1828, as quoted in Ricci, 1990)

Chassaignac's Ecraseur was a more common choice for trachelectomy. Although initially designed for polypectomy, it was sturdy enough for cervical excision and was used for this purpose by a number of nineteenth century surgeons (Fig. 1-14). J. Marion Sims gives the following account of its use in 1861:

> *The patient was etherized and placed on the left side. The speculum was introduced and the chain of the ecraseur was carried around the base of the tumor and worked in the usual manner. An observer reported that with removal of the tumor air was rushing in and out of the vagina. Sims was horrified to find an immense hole of a semi lunar form, in the cul-de-sac of the vagina, through which he observed the peritoneal cavity and its viscera. He approximated the anterior and posterior vagina in such a way as to position the cervical stump within the peritoneal cavity and placed tubes to drain the area."*

Sims (1866)

A trachelectomy operation was described by Theodore Gaillard Thomas (1831–1903) using an instrument identical to Colombat's uterocepts. Thomas took credit for its design and employed it in a cervical amputation procedure using a galvanocaustic apparatus whereby

> *... the wire loop is passed around the neck of the cervix as high up as is deemed safe. Then the current of electricity is made to pass through it, and the loop being slowly tightened, by the turning of the screw by the operator, the cervix is amputated. To accomplish the operation completely, I have devised the forceps shown in [see Fig. 1-13]. By the long sliding screw between the blades, the cervix is drawn into their grasp and fixed by closing them. Then the screw is withdrawn and the cold wire slid over the projecting portions and tightened, and the electric current passing, a red, and not a white heat being established, the cervix is completely removed. By this method immediate hemorrhage is usually controlled, but not so remote hemorrhage. Sometimes on the fifth, sixth, or even tenth day, a most active*

flow takes place in spite of every precaution. For this reason the tampon should be used after such an amputation, and the patient's convalescence be carefully watched."

Thomas (1880)

Early Attempts at Vaginal Hysterectomy

All of the very early operations involving uterine removal were done for prolapse, uterine inversion, or prolapsing tumors and frequently involved a large ligature around the protruding vaginal mass, followed later by sloughing or incision of the distal tissue (Fig. 1-15). Most of these patients died from hemorrhage or sepsis. Surgeons from the early nineteenth century and before were limited by lack of vaginal access (as vaginal specula were only recently developed for surgeries), poor lighting, and poor understanding of hemostasis. Surgeons were also at a disadvantage because they tended to operate only for end-stage cancers and large tumors, often after the woman was already cachetic and anemic.

On April 13, 1812, G.B. Paletta set out to perform a trachelectomy for malignant disease but ultimately performed the first vaginal hysterectomy. Unfortunately, his patient developed peritonitis and died within 3 days of the operation. C.J.M. Langenbeck is frequently credited with the first planned vaginal hysterectomy in 1813 for prolapse and cervical ulceration, a procedure he is reported to have performed with one assistant and without the benefit of anesthesia. Careful review of his account of the operation suggests that the peritoneal cavity was never entered and thus the operation may have been an extraperitoneal enucleation of the uterus. Nonetheless, Langenbeck gave a colorful account of the operation wherein he was left clutching the bleeding organ in one hand and holding one end of the ligature in his teeth while tying the other end with his right hand. The patient survived and the absence of a uterus with a vaginal prolapse and normal tubes and ovaries in the cul-de-sac was documented at autopsy 26 years later.

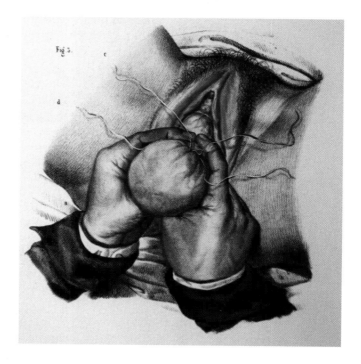

Figure 1-15 Ligature of the prolapsed uterus, either to induce necrosis or as a preparatory step for uterine ablation. (From Bourgery JM: Traite Complet de L'Anatomie de L'Homme Comprenant la Medicine Operatorie. Paris, Guerin, 1866–1868.)

The first planned and successful vaginal hysterectomy to treat a cervical malignancy was performed by J.N. Sauter of Baden, Germany, on January 28, 1822. Sauter's case differs from Langenbeck's in that the uterus was not prolapsed and the peritoneal cavity was opened during the surgery. The patient survived the immediate effects of the surgery but had a large vesicovaginal fistula and died 6 months later. Sauter later made several important recommendations, including emptying the bladder and rectum before the surgery, and suggested sharp dissection with a scalpel close to the cervix and uterus to separate the bladder and rectum. In 1829 Récamier further refined Sauter's techniques by using a specially designed speculum and using ligatures on the uterine arteries.

Of these relatively rare attempts and isolated reports of such operations there were few successes and many failures. Of the first 12 cases of vaginal hysterectomy documented by Senn in 1895, all before 1830, only three recovered, for a mortality rate of 75%. For the most part, gynecologic procedures performed prior to 1850 differed little from those performed during the late eighteenth century. However, a dramatic evolution of gynecologic surgery and instrumentation emerged during the second half of the nineteenth century. With the advent of successful anesthesia in 1846 came the potential for more extensive and carefully executed operations that were often brutal if not impossible in its absence. Techniques of antisepsis introduced by Lister in 1867 and the introduction of a reliable suture material (silk soaked in carbolic acid) paved the way for acceptable outcomes as well as a sense of safety and certainty on the part of both patient and surgeon. Many problems remained and mortality rate was high because most vaginal hysterectomies were for advanced cervical cancer; in such cases eradication of disease was not likely.

The extraordinary range of surgical techniques performed prior to the last quarter of the nineteenth century are beautifully portrayed in the magnificent plates found in Jean-Baptiste Bougery's and Nicolas Henri Jacob's *Traite complet de l'anatomie de l'homme comprenant la medicine operatorie (1831–1854)*. In the entire literature of medicine during the nineteenth century there is nothing that compares with the 749 hand-colored folio-sized lithographs, nearly all of which are in the very realistic style of Nicolas Jacob (see Figs. 1-15 to 1-18).

On January 12, 1861, Samuel Choppin of New Orleans performed the first successful vaginal hysterectomy for prolapse in America. The patient, 38 years of age and the mother of four children, presented with a tumor mass "the size of an infant's head" protruding from her vagina. The patient was given chloroform for anesthesia and the operation commenced as follows:

> The tumor was seized by a pair of vulsellum forceps, dragged down as far as possible. ... and a circular incision made through the vaginal reflection attached to the neck of the uterus. ... I exposed a pedicle made up of the peritoneal attachments of the organ. ... and arrested the haemorrhage, which thus far had been quite profuse. The loop of "Chassaignac's Ecraseur" [see Fig. 1-14] was now thrown around the peritoneal attachments and gradually tightened, during a period of twenty-five minutes, when its division was completed and the uterus, left fallopian tube and ovary were removed. No blood followed the use of the ecraseur. ... Closure of the vagina was effected by means of Sims' clamp suture. The inverted vagina was then reduced and the patient removed to her bed. On the third day suppuration began. ... and continued, profuse at times, for about three weeks, when the wire clamps came away. The patient's general health began to improve rapidly from that moment.
>
> Choppin (1867)

Remarkably, on February 19, 1861 Choppin's patient presented herself before the class of the New Orleans School of Medicine "with her womb

Figure 1-16 A, Circular excision of the neck of the uterus with a scissors. **B,** Conical excision of the neck of the uterus with a knife, employing a vaginal speculum by Paul Segalas, ca. 1830. (From Bourgery JM: Traite Complet de L'Anatomie de L'Homme Comprenant la Medicine Operatorie. Paris, Guerin, 1866–1868.)

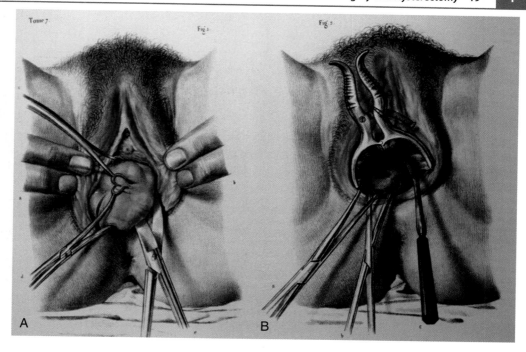

Figure 1-17 Ablation of the uterus via the vagina (low approach). (From Bourgery JM: Traite Complet de L'Anatomie de L'Homme Comprenant la Medicine Operatorie. Paris, Guerin, 1866–1868.)

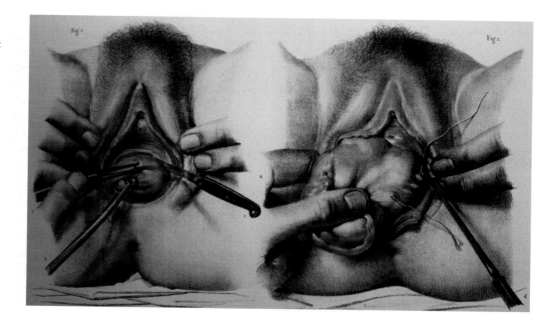

in her hand" to prove that, yes, a patient could indeed survive a vaginal hysterectomy.

From 1850 to 1880 the enthusiasm for vaginal hysterectomy diminished due to improvements in technique of abdominal hysterectomy and to the fact that, since most cases were done for advanced cervical carcinoma, the mortality rate remained very high. After 1880 refinements in technique, and expanded indications for benign diseases, helped lower the mortality rate and popularity of the vaginal approach. In 1881 William A. Freund, after a series of experiments on cadavers, further improved vaginal hysterectomy technique by introducing "compression forceps" (grooved clamps) to be placed on the broad ligaments to control hemorrhage after uterine removal. The clamps were left in place for

Figure 1-18 Ablation (hysterectomy) by hypogastric or subperitoneal approach (high approach). (From Bourgery JM: Traite Complet de L'Anatomie de L'Homme Comprenant la Medicine Operatorie. Paris, Guerin, 1866–1868.)

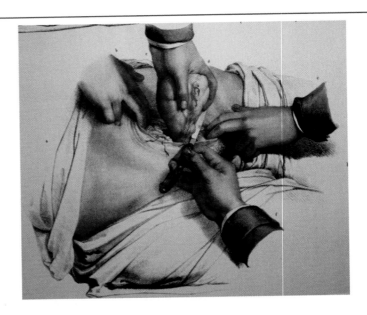

several days, then removed. Freund's work on vaginal and abdominal hysterectomy helped bring these procedures into the modern age.

Karl August Schuchardt (1856–1901) performed his "paravaginal" (mediolateral) incision in November 21, 1893, to facilitate vaginal exposure of a large ulcerating cervical cancer in a 35-year-old mother of eight. It remains a useful adjunct whenever enhanced exposure of the vagina and parametrium is required, as in the radical vaginal hysterectomy for cervical cancer and certain fistula repairs.

Abdominal Hysterectomy

Throughout the greater part of the nineteenth century, prior to asepsis, intra-abdominal uterine surgery was regarded as all but impossible. Although ovariotomy frequently resulted in peritonitis, uterine surgery carried the additional risks of hemorrhage and shock as well. Nearly 90% of attempts to remove a fibroid uterus prior to 1863 were either abandoned or ended with the demise of the patient. An editorial in the London Medico-Chirurgical Review (1825) suggested that extirpation of the uterus abdominally was among the most cruel and unfeasible operations ever executed by the head and hand of man. A review by Palmer in 1880 concluded, "Hysterectomy is indicated when something must be done to relieve suffering and save life; when all other treatment is exhausted."

In 1830 J.M. Delpech did the first abdominovaginal hysterectomy, in which the surgery was started vaginally but a small suprapubic incision was used to sever the upper uterine attachments. Using techniques that had been developed for ovariectomy, the first abdominal hysterectomies were performed in Manchester, England, by Heath in 1842 and by Charles Clay in 1844; the operations were attempted to remove an ovarian mass but hysterectomies (probably supracervical) were done after exploration of the abdomen. Several hundred procedures were performed in Europe after this but mortality rate was probably 50% or higher. The first deliberate supracervical hysterectomy for a myomatous uterus with a correct preoperative diagnosis in America was performed in June 1846 by John Bellinger (1804–1860) of Charleston, South Carolina. Unfortunately, the patient succumbed to peritonitis on the fifth postoperative day.

Subsequently, the first ever successful operation to remove a fibroid uterus was performed by Walter Burnham (1808–1883) on May 25, 1853. However, the procedure was not a deliberate one, the patient having undergone laparotomy for an ovarian cyst. Apparently, at the time of incision the patient vomited and the sarcomatous uterus extruded itself such that it could not be replaced and the necessary surgery was performed.

The first deliberate and successful (the patient survived) abdominal supracervical hysterectomy for a fibroid uterus was performed on September 1, 1853, by Gilman Kimball (1804–1892) of Lowell, Massachusetts. Kimball describes the operation as follows:

> The patient was now put in readiness for the operation by being placed on a properly elevated table, and brought under the influence of chloroform. An incision was made through the linea alba, directly over the most prominent portion of the tumor, exposing it to the extent of about four inches. Another cut of less extent, through the uterine walls brought to view the fibrous mass within. Through this opening, a portion of the diseased mass, thus exposed, was suddenly and forcibly extruded. Attachments rendered this part of the operation rather difficult; but being finally accomplished, and the uterus becoming at once greatly diminished in bulk, it was readily drawn outwards and placed in the hands of an assistant.
>
> A straight, double-armed needle was now passed through the organ in an antero-posterior direction, as low down as the supposed point of its junction with the neck' this part being, of course, left intact due to its relation with the vagina. By this plan of appropriating to each lateral half a separate ligature, there was no great difficulty in making sure against all chance of subsequent hemorrhage.
>
> The remaining part of the operation was very simple and easily accomplished. It consisted of a mere amputation of the diseased structure by a single straight incision carried across from one side to the other ...
>
> The parts having now been made as clean as possible, the wound was brought together, and its edges secured with four sutures, adhesive strips, and a compress wet with warm water and laudanum, completing the dressing.
>
> The operation was somewhat protracted, lasting nearly or quite forty minutes; yet it was not accompanied or followed by any extraordinary or alarming degree of exhaustion. The amount of blood loss did not exceed four ounces.

Kimball (1855)

The first cesarean hysterectomy was performed by Horatio Robinson Storer in Boston on July 21, 1868. Unfortunately, Storer's patient died on the third postoperative day. Storer was also the first American surgeon to teach gynecology as a separate subject and to wear rubber gloves while operating. Eight years would elapse before Edoardo Porro (1842–1902) of Pavia, Italy, performed the operation successfully on May 21, 1876.

On January 30, 1878, after much preparation and cadaver dissection to work out the anatomy and surgical method, Wilhelm A. Freund of Breslau, Germany, performed the first carefully planned total extirpation of the uterus by the abdominal route for uterine cancer. Up to that time no well-defined plan for eradication of uterine disease by abdominal operation had been developed. Moreover, during his procedure he made use of the posture which later was perfected by and is generally credited to Trendelenburg.

His operation, as summarized by Miyazana (1992), consisted of the following steps after the uterine cavity was washed with 10% carbolic acid solution:

1. Perform incision in the linea alba.

2. Pack back the intestines with damp towels.

3. Release uterus from surrounding adhesions.

4. Transfix fundus with a large ligature used as traction.

5. Ligate both broad ligaments with imbricated ligatures in three sections: the upper ligature passed through the substance of the tube above and through that of ovarian ligament below, the middle ligature transfixed the substance of the ovarian ligament above and that of round ligament below, the lower ligature pierced the round ligament above and the lateral vaginal vault below.

6. Excise uterus.

7. Imbricated ligatures were brought down into the vagina and the peritoneum was closed by continuous sutures above the point where the uterus had been excised.

8. Close abdominal wound.

His original technique was later modified by including as little vaginal tissue as possible, but the entire hysterectomy specimen was still secured with three mass ligatures on each side. Great interest in this procedure followed, but most surgeons continued to use vaginal hysterectomy for treatment of carcinoma of the cervix (the most common indication for hysterectomy at that time) because of the high mortality rate from peritonitis. However, as time progressed it became apparent that only 10% to 17% of patients were free of disease 2 years after vaginal hysterectomy, subsequently bringing about the need for reconsideration of the abdominal route.

In 1889 L.A. Stimson of New York proposed and carried out his important contribution to abdominal hysterectomy, namely, preliminary ligation of the ovarian and uterine vessels. He felt that mass ligation was not always efficient protection against hemorrhage and the mass of tissue formed a large stump that caused problems later. He wrote:

> Each artery is sought for at the side of the upper part of the cervix by palpation of the broad ligament between the finger and thumb; after its position has been thus ascertained, a small incision is made through the peritoneum along its course on the front or, preferably, the back of the broad ligament, the artery separated from the veins with a director, and a ligature passed by means of an aneurism needle. The ureter lies to the outer side and is easily avoided. When both uterine arteries have been thus tied, and the ovaries and tubes and the body of the uterus can be removed by a transverse incision just above the clamps and ligatures, and the cut surface will be almost absolutely bloodless.

Stimson (1889)

From the 1880s to 1895 the technique of abdominal hysterectomy continuously improved, especially regarding hemostasis and handling of the cervical stump. This led to a reassessment of abdominal hysterectomy especially for cervical cancer, for which the vaginal route still led to few cancer survivors, although the operative mortality rate was constantly being lessened. In 1895 John Goodrich Clark, while a resident on Howard Kelly's service at the Johns Hopkins Hospital, was aware of the positive margins in a large percentage of the hysterectomy specimens in cervical cancer cases. With this in mind, and noting Halstead's insistence on excising cancerous tissue in one piece, he performed the first radical hysterectomy for invasive cancer of the uterus in April 1895. According to Mathieu (1934) he advised catheterizing the ureters before the operation as suggested by Kelly and then dissected the uterine artery 2.5 cm lateral to the uterus and removed all the tissue of the broad ligaments and a large cuff of the vagina. He drained the pelvis through the vagina with gauze which was then covered with peritoneum.

Continued clarification of pelvic anatomy emerged with the work of Anders Adolf Retzius (1796–1860), who defined the boundaries of the prevesical space (space of Retzius) in 1849, and from the work of Alwin Mackenrodt (1859–

1925), who elegantly described the cause of and cure for uterine prolapse in 1895 and who put forth an accurate description of the pelvic connective tissue including the transverse cervical or cardinal ligaments (Mackenrodt's ligaments).

Renowned physician, William Osler (1849–1919), reflecting on the accomplishments of the nineteenth century in an address to the Johns Hopkins Historical Club in January 1901, stated:

> *In the fullness of time, long expected, long delayed, at last Science emptied upon him from the horn of Amalthea blessings which cannot be enumerated, blessing which have made the century forever memorable; and which have followed each other with a rapidity so bewildering that we know not what to expect next. ... Measure as we may the progress of the world—materially, in the advantages of steam, electricity, and other mechanical appliances; sociologically, in the great many improvements in the conditions of life; intellectually, in the diffusion of education; morally, in a possibly higher standard of ethics—there is no measure which can compare with the decrease in physical suffering in man, women, and child when stricken by disease or accident ... This is the Promethean gift of the century to man.*

The Twentieth Century to the Present

> *"The general surgeon is octopus like, progressively absorbing more and more of the surgical specialties. As soon as one is perfected he takes it over ... The gynecologist was the pioneer as abdominal-pelvic surgery evolved. The general surgeon was his follower."*

H.W. Longyear, President of the American Medical Association, 1907

The momentum established during the latter half of the nineteenth century, related to gynecologic therapy, continued into the twentieth. Howard Kelly's texts—*Operative Gynecology* (1898), *Gynecology and Abdominal Surgery* (with Charles P. Noble, 1907), *Medical Gynecology* (1908), and *Diseases of the Kidneys, Ureters and Bladder* (with Curtis F. Burnam,1914), the latter distinguished by wonderful illustrations by German artist Max Brödel (1870–1941)—all served to define the specialty of modern gynecology and provided the foundation for continued progress well into the century.

Early twentieth century surgeons sought to improve surgical incisions while maintaining exposure. Hermann Johannes Pfannenstiel (1862–1909) described his transverse incision in 1900 and extolled its virtues over the more traditional vertical incision as ensuring better cosmetics and less hernia formation. Alfred Ernst Maylard (1855–1947) sought to enhance exposure over Pfannenstiel's incision by extending the incision through the rectus muscle in an oblique manner so as to leave the more lateral fibers undivided, as he reported in the British Medical Journal in 1907. Finally, Leonid Sergius Cherney (1907–1963), in an effort to maintain strength and cosmetics and to maintain exposure while acknowledging the reluctance to divide the body of the rectus, suggested cutting the rectus muscles at their very insertion into the pubis. Cherney's modified transverse incision was reported in 1941 and proved less bloody and quicker than the Maylard, while providing superior exposure over Pfannenstiel's incision, particularly when access to the space of Retzius was essential.

One of the most renowned gynecologic surgeons of his era, Ernst Wertheim (1864–1920) published his technique for radical hysterectomy in cases of cervical cancer in 1900. Wertheim was said to have performed 1300 such operations with complete follow-up. In his monograph based on 500 cases Wertheim stated:

[O]ne must strive to remove as much as possible of the surrounding tissue together with the primary tumor in order to achieve optimal results as is the case with operative procedures for cancer of other organs. Histological examination of the extirpated organs showed the teaching to be false that cervical cancer transgresses the bounds of the uterus late but rather that in a number of early cases the carcinoma had already sent its offshoots to the parametrium and regional lymph nodes.

Defending the superiority of his abdominal over vaginal approach Wertheim wrote:

Our knowledge of behavior of the regional lymphatics and parametrium, of the mode of spread of the carcinoma, and of what might be expected from a surgical operation, was put on a secure basis for the first time by the extended abdominal operation.

Before becoming chairman of gynecology in Vienna in 1891, Wertheim worked at the German University in Prague as assistant to Friedrich Schauta (1849–1919), who is credited with developing the radical vaginal hysterectomy for carcinoma of the cervix.

Concerning vaginal hysterectomy in cases of complete prolapse, Archibald Donald (1860–1937) developed an operation whereby he performed an anterior and posterior colporrhaphy combined with amputation of the cervix in 1908. Silver suture was employed in his first two cases and catgut for the remainder. Several years later, William Edward Fothergill (1865–1926), a contemporary of Donald's and also from Manchester, England, modified Donald's procedure in 1915 whereby he grasped four points with forceps: one beneath the urethral orifice, two posterolateral to the cervix on each side, and one in the midline of the posterior fornix and superficial to the apex of the pouch of Douglas. These four points (Fothergill's points) were then joined by an incision to begin the operation. Fothergill's stitch involved suturing the stumps of the cardinal ligaments to remaining cervical stump to effectively support the cervix while at the same time anteverting the uterus. Given the relative contributions of both Donald and Fothergill the procedure is referred to as the Manchester Operation.

During the same period (1906), a German surgeon, Albert Siegmund Gustav Döderlein (1860–1941) along with S. Kronig described a vaginal hysterectomy technique which begins with an anterior colpotomy incision through which the fundus of the uterus is delivered and the vasculature of the uterus approached superiorly. In a monograph published in 1915 Mayo described this technique (Fig. 1-19) as being appropriate for women aged 45 to 65 years with third- or fourth-degree prolapse and distention of the vagina.

In 1929 Edward H. Richardson of the Johns Hopkins University Hospital published his simplified technique for abdominal panhysterectomy. It has become the standard extrafascial technique. His procedure (Figs. 1-20 and 1-21) utilized a special vaginal angle suture after removal of the uterus; the stitch is first passed through the anterior vaginal wall 1 cm from the angle, transfixes twice the basal segment of the broad ligament placing a liberal mattress loop, continues through the posterior vaginal wall 1 cm from the angle and then transfixing the stump of the uterosacral ligament (see Fig. 1-21). Richardson claimed that this perfected technique, developed over a period of 4 years, produced minimal rate of mortality and only minor postoperative complications. It has been considered anatomically and surgically sound and relatively simple and the "Richardson stitch" was taught for decades as a technique to help suspend the vaginal vault (and prevent prolapse) after hysterectomy.

Subsequent to Howard Kelly, Richard Wesley TeLinde (1894–1985) held the chair of gynecology at Johns Hopkins for more than 20 years. Appointed in

Figure 1-19 Excision of the uterus and clamping of the broad ligament after the fundus is delivered through the anterior colpotomy. (From Mayo CH: Uterine prolapse with associated pelvic relaxation. Surg Gynecol Obstet 1915;20:253–260.)

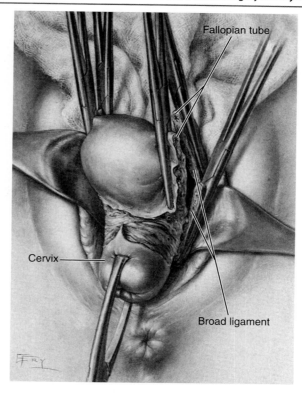

Fallopian tube

Cervix

Broad ligament

Figure 1-20 Richardson technique of abdominal hysterectomy. The uterus has been completely detached and the amputation across the vaginal vault is being completed. Note that the cervix is not being squeezed by any compressing instrument and that it does not come in contact with the field of operation. (From Richardson EH: A simplified technique for abdominal panhysterectomy. Surg Gynecol Obstet 1929;48:248–256; used with permission.)

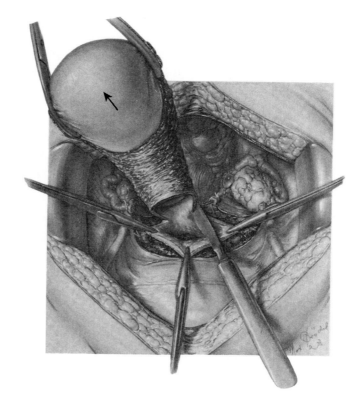

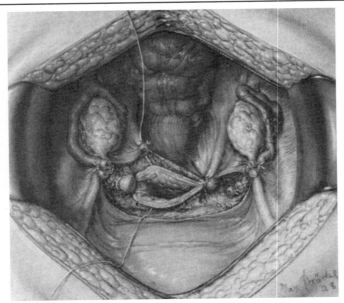

Figure 1-21 Richardson technique of abdominal hysterectomy. The angle stitch is here shown. On the right it can be seen in detail. Note that it is first passed through the anterior vaginal wall 1 cm from the angle; it then twice transfixes the basal segment of the broad ligament, placing within this important structure a liberal mattress loop; it then continues through the posterior vaginal wall 1 cm from the angle and is finally made to transfix the stump of the uterosacral ligament. On the left the suture has been tied, snugly, closing the vaginal angle and approximating to it the two important supporting ligaments. (From Richardson EH: A simplified technique for abdominal panhysterectomy. Surg Gynecol Obstet 1929;48:248–256; used with permission.)

1939, and with a variety of innovations, he is best known for his research regarding carcinoma in situ of the cervix and his comprehensive gynecologic surgical text, *Operative Gynecology,* published in 1946, which was destined to be and has remained the standard American work on the subject under successive authors. TeLinde, in his 1946 textbook *Operative Gynecology,* described that the attitude at Johns Hopkins Hospital up to that time regarding indications for vaginal hysterectomy were conservative. TeLinde recognized Heaney, Danforth, and the Mayo group as excellent vaginal surgeons who were proponents of broader indications for the use of vaginal hysterectomy. TeLinde noted, however, that in their group, when vaginal hysterectomy was applied for cases of prolapse, in 30% of the surgeries the "anatomic results were not good." TeLinde noted that in recent years their group reserved the vaginal hysterectomy for cases of prolapse in which disease of the uterus itself makes its removal "desirable." These indications were small myomas and functional or postmenopausal bleeding. They did not remove the uterus vaginally when carcinoma of the endometrium was present, except in very obese women with pelvic relaxation. TeLinde favored the Watkins interposition or the Manchester procedure for simple cases of uterine prolapse. When a vaginal hysterectomy was done, they favored the Heaney technique.

In 1938 Danforth said in a reading at the American Gynecological Society: "while I do not believe that all excisions of the uterus should be vaginal, I do believe that in many clinics a greater use might be made of this operation." During the 1930s and 1940s, Nobel Sproat Heaney (1880–1955) was among the most influential proponents of vaginal hysterectomy for benign disease. Heaney contended that surgeons were lured to the abdominal approach by a misguided notion that so-called conditions such as chronic appendicitis, prolapse of the cecum, and other questionable conditions were deserving of the gynecologist's surgical attention. Heaney's technique, based on his postgraduate experiences

Figure 1-22 Heaney technique of vaginal hysterectomy. Base of broad ligament with uterine vessels clamped, to be cut at dotted line. (From TeLinde RW: Operative Gynecology. Philadelphia, JB Lippincott, 1946, pp 110–148; used with permission.)

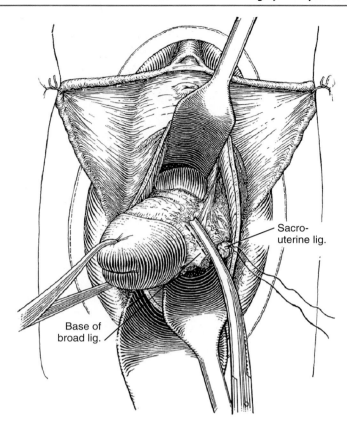

Sacro-uterine lig.

Base of broad lig.

in Nebraska, Germany, and Austria, reported in detail in 1934, continues to receive widespread use with some modifications (Figs. 1-22 to 1-25). He is also remembered eponymously for the Heaney needle holder, retractor, and clamp as well as his pedicle stitch (see Fig. 1-23) which incorporates vessels, peritoneum, and ligaments in a fixation suture.

Few substantive technical changes to the Heaney technique for vaginal hysterectomy and the Richardson technique for benign abdominal hysterectomy have been made even to this day. Most of the clinical improvements were in medicine, blood banking, anesthesia, fluid management, perioperative care, and pain management resulting in substantial decline in mortality and morbidity rates. Siddall and Mack (1947) reported the mortality rate of abdominal hysterectomy at their center declined from 7.3% in 1928 to 1932, to 1.7% from 1933 to 1940, to 0.8% from 1941 to 1945. Mortality rate was slightly lower with supracervical compared to total hysterectomy. By the 1950s, the reported mortality rate from hysterectomy was down to 0% to 0.2%. The increasing safety of abdominal surgery and the drawbacks of leaving the cervix (cancer and bleeding) led to almost universal abandonment of supracervical hysterectomy by 1955.

Postoperative infection and abscesses continued to be a problem leading to numerous methods of vaginal cuff closure, with and without the use of drains. Prophylactic antibiotics, both as intraoperative irrigants and as single or multiple perioperative doses, were shown in the 1970s to significantly reduce vaginal cuff cellulitis and pelvic abscess after both vaginal and abdominal hysterectomy. The common use of midline abdominal incisions for benign hysterectomies was gradually replaced by the Pfannenstiel incision for appropriate cases, yielding better cosmesis and fewer hernias.

Figure 1-23 Heaney technique of vaginal hysterectomy. Transfixion of sacrouterine ligament: the "Heaney stitch." (From TeLinde RW: Operative Gynecology. Philadelphia, JB Lippincott, 1946, pp 110–148; used with permission.)

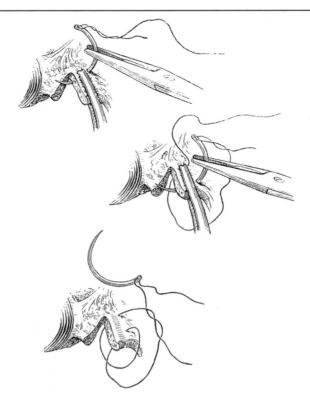

Figure 1-24 Heaney technique of vaginal hysterectomy. Upper portion of broad ligament, including tube, ovarian ligament and round ligament, clamped. (From TeLinde RW: Operative Gynecology. Philadelphia, JB Lippincott, 1946, pp 110–148; used with permission.)

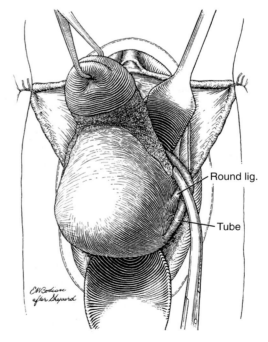

Laparoscopic hysterectomy was first reported by Reich and coworkers in 1989. Intense interest in this approach was fueled by the development of operative laparoscopy techniques, enhanced optics and lighting, and improved energy delivery. Several variations of total and supracervical laparoscopic hysterectomy have been developed over the last 20 years, yielding even better cosmetic results, quicker patient recovery, and less pain. Technological innovations, such as the addition of robotic assistance and single-port access, may

Figure 1-25 Heaney technique of vaginal hysterectomy, showing cut surface of broad and sacrouterine ligaments. The ovary is examined. (From TeLinde RW: Operative Gynecology. Philadelphia, JB Lippincott, 1946, pp 110–148; used with permission.)

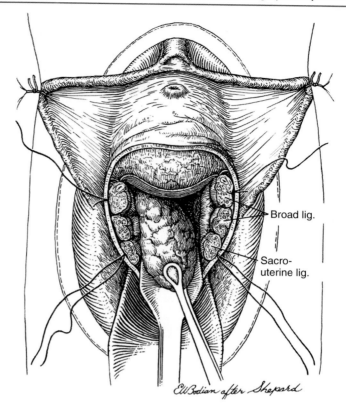

further decrease the number of laparotomies needed to perform hysterectomies, and lessen the morbidity and pain in affected women.

Selected Readings

Allen JL, Rampone JF, Wheeless CR: Use of a prophylactic antibiotic in elective major gynecologic operations. Obstet Gynecol 1972;39:218–224.

The American Armamentarium Chirurgicum Catalog of Surgical Instruments. Chicago, George Tiemann & Co, 1889.

Baskett TF: On the shoulders of giants: Eponyms and names in obstetrics and gynecology. London, RCOG Press, 1998.

Baskett TF: Hysterectomy: Evolution and trends. Best Pract Res Clin Obstet Gynecol 2005;19: 295–305.

Bennion E: Antique Medical Instruments. Berkeley, University of California Press, 1986.

Benrubi GI: History of hysterectomy. J Fla Med Assoc 1988;75:533–538.

Brill AI: Hysterectomy in the 21st century: Different approaches, different challenges. Clin Obstet Gynecol 2006;49:722–735.

Burch JC, Lavely HT: Hysterectomy. Ann Surg 1952;136:720–731.

Choppin S: Removal of the uterus and its appendages in a case of procidentia uteri, by means of the ecraseur. S J Med Sci 1867;I:624.

Choulant JL: Bibliotheca Medico-Historica. Leipzig, Germany, W Englemann Publisher, 1842.

Colombat de L'Isere M: Sur l'amputation du col de la matrice dans les affections cancéreuses, suivant un nouveau procédé. Rev Med Francais et Etranger 1828;30:194.

Danforth WC: The place of vaginal hysterectomy in present-day gynecology. Am J Obstet Gynecol 1938;36:787–797.

Fothergill WE: Anterior colporrhaphy and its combination with amputation of the cervix as a single operation. J Obstet gynaecol Br Emp 1915;27:146.

Garrison FH, Morton LT: Morton's Medical Bibliography, 5th ed. Adtershot, England, Scholar Press, 1991.

Greenspan RE: Medicine: Perspectives in History and Art. Alexandria, VA, Ponteverde Press, 2006.

Heaney NS: A report of 565 vaginal hysterectomies performed for benign pelvic disease. Am J Obstet Gynecol 1934;28:751–755.

Johnson TH (transl): The Works of Ambroise Paré. London, 1678.

Kimball G: Successful case of extirpation of the uterus. Boston Med Surg J 1855;52:249–255.

Lash AF: A method for reducing the size of the uterus in vaginal hysterectomy. Am J Obstet Gynecol 1942;42:452–459.

Lever JCW: A Practical Treatise on Organic Diseases of the Uterus. London, 1843.

Mathieu A: The history of hysterectomy. West J Surg Obstet Gynecol 1934;42:1–13.

Mayo CH: Uterine prolapse with associated pelvic relaxation. Surg Gynecol Obstet 1915;20:253–260.

Miyazawa K: Technique for total abdominal hysterectomy: Historical and clinical perspective. Obstet Gynecol Surv 1992;47:433–447.

Palmer CD: Laparotomy and laparo-hysterectomy their indications and statistics, for fibroid tumors of the uterus. Trans Am Gynecol Soc 1880;5:361–383.

Ricci JV: The Development of Gynaecological Surgery and Instruments. San Francisco, Norman Publishing, 1990.

Richardson EH: A simplified technique for abdominal panhysterectomy. Surg Gynecol Obstet 1929;47:248–256.

Saffron MH: Thomas Rowlandson: Medical caricatures. New York, Editions Medicina Rara, 1971.

Senn N: The early history of vaginal hysterectomy. JAMA 1895;25:476–482.

Siddall RS, Mack HC: Improvement in hysterectomy mortality. Surg Gynecol Obstet 1947;85:176–184.

Sims JM: Clinical Notes on Uterine Surgery. London, Robert Hardwicke, 1866.

Speert H: Obstetrics and Gynecology: A History and Iconography. San Francisco, Norman Publishing, 1973.

Speert H: Obstetric and Gynecologic Milestones Illustrated. New York, Parthenon Publishing Group, 1996.

Stimson LA: On some modifications in the technique of abdominal surgery, limiting the use of the ligature en masse. Trans Am Surg Assoc 1889;7:65–72.

Strachan JB: Am J Med Sci 1829;5:307–309.

Stromayr C: Die Handschrift des Schnitt-und Augenarztes Caspar Stromayr, Lindau Manuscript, 1559, edited by W. von Brunn, Berlin, 1925.

TeLinde RW: Operative Gynecology, 1st ed. Philadelphia, JB Lippincott, 1946.

Temkin O (transl): Soranus' Gynecology. Baltimore, The Johns Hopkins University Press, 1956.

Thomas TG: A Practical Treatise on the Diseases of Women. Philadelphia, Lea, 1880.

Vesalius: On the Fabric of the Human Body, vol. I to VI. San Francisco, Norman Publishing, 1998.

Wertheim E: Zur frage der radical operation beim uteruskrebs. Arch Gynakol 1900;61:627.

Anatomy of the Uterus and Its Surgical Removal

2

Amy J. Park M.D.
Matthew D. Barber M.D., M.H.S.

 Video Clips on DVD

2-1 Anterior Abdominal Wall
2-2 Anatomy of the Uterus and Adnexa
2-3 Vasculature
2-4 Lower Urinary Tract
2-5 Avascular Planes of the Pelvis

The removal of the uterus may be performed through a variety of approaches: abdominal, laparoscopic, and vaginal. In order to effectively perform a hysterectomy, the surgeon should have an intimate knowledge of the anatomy of the anterior abdominal wall and the pelvis in order to safely attain access, maximize exposure, secure vascular pedicles, and avoid injury to the surrounding vasculature, nerves, and viscera. This chapter will discuss the surgical anatomy of the pelvis focusing specifically on the anatomic relationships necessary for the surgical removal of the uterus.

Surgical Anatomy

Anterior Abdominal Wall

The most common approach to hysterectomy in the United States is the abdominal one, although the laparoscopic approach is also gaining in popularity. For these approaches, the surgeon must access the intra-abdominal cavity via the anterior abdominal wall, which is primarily accessed below or at the level of the umbilicus.

Surface anatomy and bony landmarks can aid the surgeon to identify underlying structures and appropriately plan surgical incisions or laparoscopic trocar placement. The umbilicus marks the approximate location of where the aorta bifurcates into the right and left common iliac arteries. The anterior superior iliac spines are where the inguinal ligaments originate, and the pubic symphysis is where the inguinal ligaments as well as the rectus abdominis muscles insert (Fig. 2-1).

From superficial to deep, the abdominal wall consists of skin, subcutaneous fat, Camper's fascia, Scarpa's fascia, rectus sheath, rectus muscles, and parietal peritoneum. Camper's fascia consists of a fatty layer that is not easily appreciated, while Scarpa's fascia presents as a thin fibrous layer that may be fused with the rectus fascial sheath. The rectus sheath is composed of the aponeuro-

Figure 2-1 Surface anatomy of the anterior abdominal wall. (Reprinted from Drake RL, Vogl AW, Mitchell AWM, et al: Gray's Atlas of Anatomy. Philadelphia, Elsevier, 2008, p 200.)

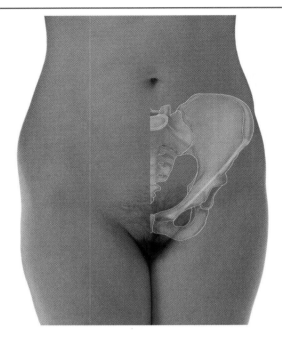

ses of the external oblique, internal oblique, and transversus abdominis (or transversalis) muscles. Above the arcuate line (located approximately one half of the distance between the umbilicus and the pubic symphysis), the rectus sheath divides into an anterior and posterior sheath. The anterior sheath is located anterior to the rectus muscles and consists of the aponeuroses of the external oblique, and the anterior layer of the internal oblique, and the posterior sheath consists of the aponeuroses of transversus abdominis muscle and the posterior layer of the internal oblique and is located posterior to the rectus muscles. Below the arcuate line, all layers of the rectus sheath are fused and located anterior to the rectus muscles (Fig. 2-2). The rectus fascia is the most important layer for closure of the anterior abdominal wall. Successful closure of this layer prevents herniation, incarceration, or evisceration of the abdominal contents. Because of the primarily transverse orientation of the abdominal wall muscle fibers, reapproximation of a vertical suture line in the rectus fascia is under more tension compared to transverse incisions, making vertical incisions more prone to dehiscence. The rectus muscles fuse in the midline at the linea alba. The pyramidalis muscle arises from the pubic bone, is located anterior to the rectus muscles, and inserts into the linea alba several centimeters above the pubic symphysis.

The inguinal ligament is the anatomic boundary between the abdomen and the thigh. The round ligament travels through the inguinal canal and terminates at the labia majora. Additionally, the ilioinguinal nerve and the genital branch of the genitofemoral nerve pass through the inguinal canal. As the external iliac vessels cross underneath the inguinal ligament, they become the femoral artery and vein. The inferior epigastric artery originates off the external iliac artery just before it becomes the femoral artery and travels through the transversalis fascia into a space between the rectus muscle and posterior sheath. The inferior epigastric vessels travel from their lateral origins obliquely toward a more medial location as they approach the umbilicus (Fig. 2-3). The superficial epigastric vessels originate from the femoral vessels and branch extensively as they approach the umbilicus. These superficial vessels can be transilluminated through the anterior abdominal wall during laparoscopy but

Figure 2-2 Cross-section of anterior abdominal wall above/below arcuate line. The rectus sheath is shown above and below the arcuate line (located approximately one half the distance from the umbilicus to the pubic symphysis). The anterior sheath consists of the aponeuroses of the external oblique and the anterior layer of the internal oblique, while the posterior sheath consists of the aponeuroses of transversus abdominis muscle and the posterior layer of the internal oblique. Below the arcuate line, all layers of the rectus sheath are fused and located anterior to the rectus muscles.

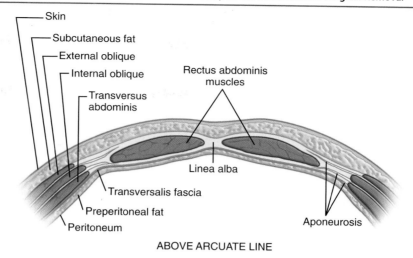

- Skin
- Subcutaneous fat
- External oblique
- Internal oblique
- Transversus abdominis
- Rectus abdominis muscles
- Linea alba
- Transversalis fascia
- Preperitoneal fat
- Peritoneum
- Aponeurosis

ABOVE ARCUATE LINE

BELOW ARCUATE LINE

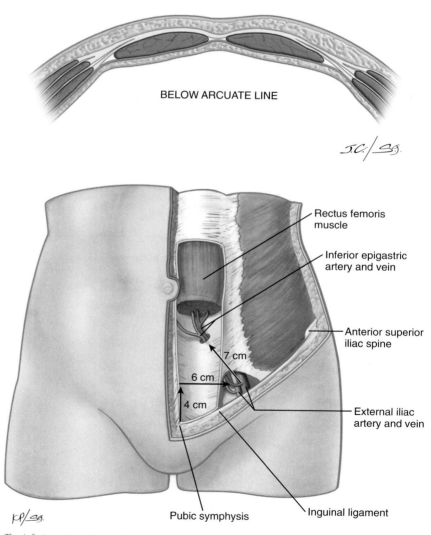

- Rectus femoris muscle
- Inferior epigastric artery and vein
- Anterior superior iliac spine
- External iliac artery and vein
- Inguinal ligament
- Pubic symphysis
- 7 cm
- 6 cm
- 4 cm

Figure 2-3 The inferior epigastric vessels are important landmarks on the anterior abdominal wall as they present a significant risk for injury and subsequent hematoma during laparoscopic port insertion. The lower abdominal trocars should be placed laterally to the vessels after the vessels are identified. The inferior epigastric artery originates off the external iliac artery just before it becomes the femoral artery and travels through the transversalis fascia into a space between the rectus muscle and posterior sheath. The inferior epigastric vessels travel from their lateral origins obliquely toward a more medial location as they approach the umbilicus. If one travels approximately 4 cm above the pubic symphysis in the midline, then 6 to 7 cm from this point laterally, this point demarcates where the inferior epigastric vessels penetrate the fascia of the transversus abdominis muscle. The vessels then travel another 7 cm obliquely to enter the posterior rectus sheath. The inferior epigastric vein flows into the external iliac vein just before it becomes the femoral vein, cephalad to the inguinal ligament.

the inferior epigastric vessels must be visualized intra-abdominally where they run lateral to the medial umbilical ligaments. (See DVD Video 2-1 for video demonstration of the anatomy of the anterior abdominal wall. 📷)

Of the incisions commonly used in gynecologic surgery, the vertical midline incision affords the best visualization and most rapid entry, but at the cost of increased postoperative pain and risk of wound dehiscence and ventral hernias. It usually extends from just below the umbilicus to the pubic symphysis, but can be extended cephalad to the xiphoid process if exposure to the upper abdomen is required. After incising through the skin, subcutaneous fat, and Scarpa's fascia, the rectus sheath is opened in a vertical fashion and the rectus muscles are then divided and the posterior rectus sheath (above the arcuate line) and peritoneum are opened in order to access the intraperitoneal contents (Fig. 2-4).

Figure 2-4 The vertical midline incision affords the best visualization and most rapid entry **(A)**. It usually extends from just below the umbilicus to the pubic symphysis. It avoids the inferior epigastric vessels. After incising through the skin, subcutaneous fat, and Scarpa's fascia, the rectus sheath is opened in a vertical fashion and the rectus muscles are then divided and the posterior rectus sheath (above the arcuate line) is opened in order to access the intraperitoneal contents **(B)**. The peritoneum is opened in the midline, taking care to avoid the underlying bowel **(C)**.

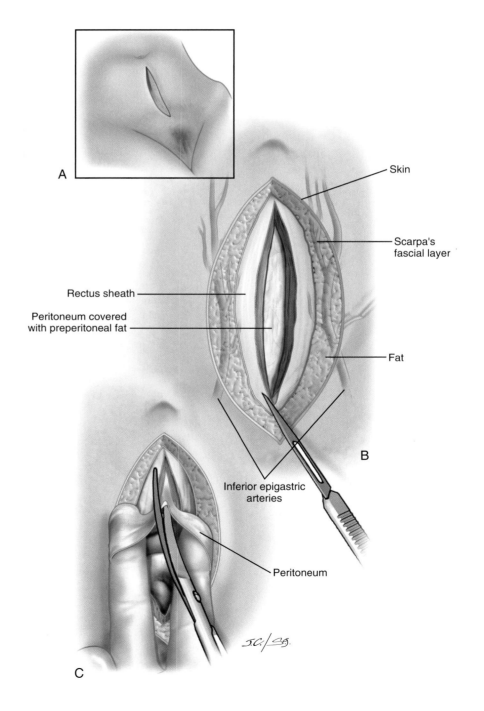

The transverse incisions used in gynecologic surgery are the Pfannenstiel, Maylard, and Cherney incisions. Compared to vertical incisions, these transverse incisions have the advantages of improved cosmesis and wound healing and less postoperative pain. These incisions can be categorized into muscle-sparing (Pfannenstiel) and muscle-splitting (Maylard and Cherney) incisions. The Pfannenstiel and Maylard incisions are made approximately two fingerbreadths above the pubic symphysis (Fig. 2-5). For the Pfannenstiel incision, the skin, subcutaneous fat, Camper's and Scarpa's fasciae, and rectus sheath are transected in a transverse fashion; then the rectus fascia are dissected off the underlying rectus muscles and muscles are separated vertically in the midline (i.e., muscle sparing) in order to gain access to the peritoneum and intra-abdominal cavity. In order to perform the Maylard incision, after making a transverse incision in the rectus fascia the surgeon incises the rectus muscles in a transverse fashion (i.e., muscle splitting) starting from the midline and working laterally without dissecting the rectus muscles off the overlying rectus sheath. The inferior epigastric vessels must be identified (usually around 6 to 7 cm lateral from the midline) and ligated prior to transecting the rectus muscles laterally (Fig. 2-6). The Maylard incision affords better visualization and access than the Pfannenstiel incision, but at the cost of increased postoperative pain and discomfort. In contrast to the Maylard and Pfannenstiel incisions, the Cherney incision is performed 1 cm above the pubic symphysis, but is performed in a similar fashion until the rectus muscles are reached. The rectus muscles are then dissected off their insertion on the pubic symphysis and are reflected cephalad after ligating the inferior epigastric vessels as they enter the rectus muscles obliquely (Fig. 2-7). This incision is most often used for retropubic procedures (e.g., the Burch urethropexy or paravaginal defect repair).

The iliohypogastric and ilioinguinal nerves are sensory nerves that may be damaged with low transverse incisions and lower abdominal laparoscopic trocar placement. Such an injury can result in neuropathic chronic pain syndromes consisting of burning pain and altered skin sensitivity in the affected region. The iliohypogastric nerve innervates the skin of the suprapubic area, while the ilioinguinal nerve innervates the groin area, upper labial majora, and upper medial thigh. The iliohypogastric nerve enters the abdominal wall approximately 2 cm medial and 1 cm inferior to the anterior superior iliac spine and travels obliquely, terminating 3.7 cm lateral to the midline and 5 cm above the pubic symphysis. The ilioinguinal nerve enters the abdominal wall 3 cm medial and 3.7 cm inferior to the anterior superior iliac spine, traveling obliquely to terminate 2.7 cm lateral to the midline and 1.7 cm above the pubic symphysis. Injuries to these nerves may be averted during laparoscopy by placing the lower abdominal trocars 2 cm medial and superior to the anterior superior iliac spines (Fig. 2-8). Nerve entrapment may also occur during the lateral closure of transverse incisions as the paths of these nerves unavoidably traverse the lateral aspect of these incisions. Patients who complain of burning pain in the lower abdomen, pelvic area, and upper medial thigh that increases with Valsalva maneuver and that is not relieved with narcotics but improves with hip flexion and forward leaning of the trunk should undergo a diagnostic and therapeutic trial of local anesthetic injection at a site approximately 3 cm medial to the anterior superior iliac spine where the nerves originate.

The parietal peritoneum is often covered by preperitoneal fat, and is located just below the rectus muscles. The median umbilical ligament is caused by the presence of the urachus, and is a vertical structure located in the midline. The medial umbilical ligaments are paired structures consisting of the obliterated

Figure 2-5 The Pfannenstiel and Maylard incisions are made approximately 2 fingerbreadths above the pubic symphysis in a curvilinear fashion. The incision is made through the skin, subcutaneous fat, Scarpa's fascia, and rectus sheath (**A** and **B**). The cranial portion of the fascial flap is sharply dissected upward off the underlying rectus muscles. The peritoneum is entered in the midline between the rectus muscles (**C**).

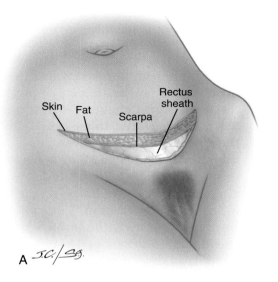

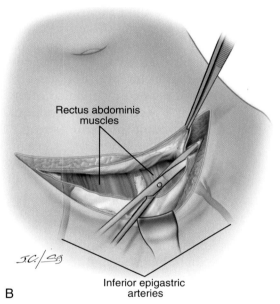

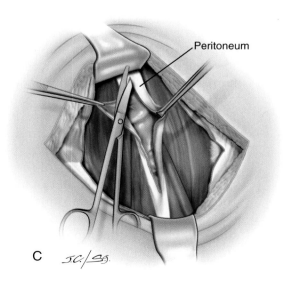

Figure 2-6 Maylard incision. **A,** The inferior epigastric vessels have been ligated, and the rectus muscles are then divided transversely. **B,** The peritoneum is entered sharply. The inferior epigastric vessels have been spared in this case.

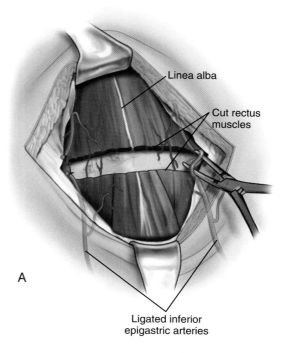

Linea alba

Cut rectus muscles

A

Ligated inferior epigastric arteries

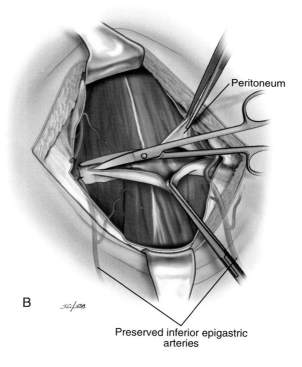

Peritoneum

B

Preserved inferior epigastric arteries

Figure 2-7 A, The Cherney incision is made just above the pubic symphysis. Once the rectus sheath is reached, it is divided transversely *(dotted line),* and the inferior epigastric vessels are ligated and transected, if desired. The insertion of the rectus muscle is reflected off the pubic symphysis cranially, and the rectus muscle is dissected off the underlying peritoneum. **B,** The peritoneum is then opened transversely in order to provide excellent pelvic exposure.

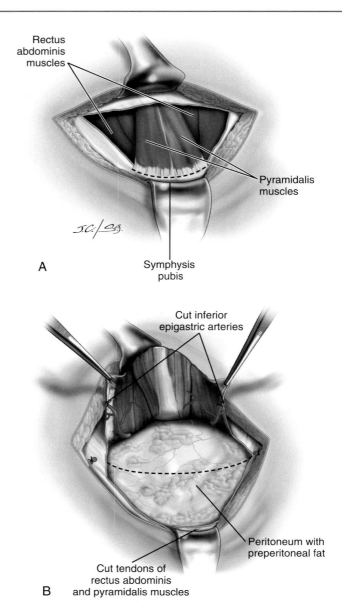

umbilical arteries, which connect the internal iliac vessels to the umbilical cord, and are located laterally to the median umbilical ligament (Fig. 2-9). The medial umbilical ligaments are an important landmark in locating the inferior epigastric vessels during the placement of lower abdominal ports during laparoscopy, as the vessels are located laterally to the medial umbilical ligaments. During laparoscopy, after the umbilical trocar is placed, the anterior superior iliac spine (ASIS) is palpated and the lower abdominal trocar should be inserted two fingerbreadths medial and superior to the ASIS, lateral to the medial umbilical ligaments and the inferior epigastric vessels (Fig. 2-10). The medial umbilical ligaments also form the boundaries of the dome of the bladder, which is contiguous with the parietal peritoneum and located cephalad to the pubic symphysis. Entry into the abdominal cavity necessitates caution as one travels caudally, and initial entry should be performed cephalad toward the umbilicus and the peritoneum and then taken down in layers as one approaches the pubic symphysis in order to avoid bladder injury. Because the apex of the bladder is triangular in shape, and is highest in the midline, incising the peritoneum

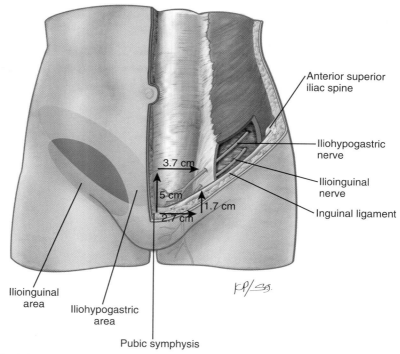

Figure 2-8 The iliohypogastric and ilioinguinal nerves are sensory nerves that may be damaged with low transverse incisions and lower abdominal laparoscopic trocar placement, leading to neuropathic chronic pain syndromes. The iliohypogastric nerve innervates the skin of the suprapubic area, and the ilioinguinal nerve innervates the groin area, upper labial majora, and upper medial thigh. The iliohypogastric nerve enters the abdominal wall approximately 2 cm medial and 1 cm inferior the anterior superior iliac spine and travels obliquely, terminating 3.7 cm lateral to the midline and 5 cm above the pubic symphysis. The ilioinguinal nerve enters the abdominal wall 3 cm medial and 3.7 cm inferior to the anterior superior iliac spine, traveling obliquely to terminate 2.7 cm lateral to the midline and 1.7 cm above the pubic symphysis. Injuries to these nerves may be averted during laparoscopy by placing the lower abdominal trocars 2 cm medial and superior to the anterior superior iliac spines.

Figure 2-9 The left inferior epigastric vessels are visualized lateral to the obliterated umbilical ligament.

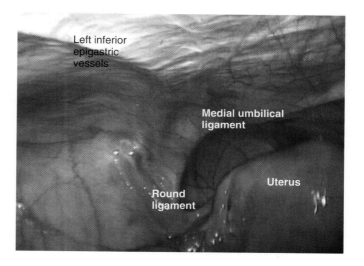

laterally as you approach the pubic symphysis is less likely to result in visceral injury.

Uterus and Adnexa

The uterus consists of the uterine corpus and the cervix. The corpus, or body of the uterus, consists of an inverted triangular endometrial cavity surrounded

Figure 2-10 Laparoscopic port placement is usually safe 2 fingerbreadths medial and superior to the anterior superior iliac spines in order to avoid injury to the inferior epigastric vessels and the ilioinguinal and iliohypogastric nerves.

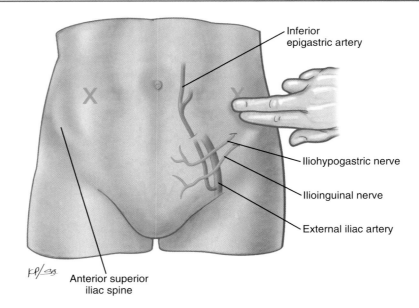

Inferior epigastric artery

Iliohypogastric nerve

Ilioinguinal nerve

External iliac artery

Anterior superior iliac spine

by the myometrium and serosa (Fig. 2-11). The portion of the uterus superior to the endometrial cavity is called the fundus of the uterus. The cervix is the conduit between the endometrial cavity and the vagina. In the reproductive-aged female, the corpus is much larger than the cervix, while in prepubertal and postmenopausal females, their relative length is similar. However, the overall size of the uterus can vary considerably, depending on hormonal levels, previous parturition, or the presence of fibroids or adenomyosis.

The myometrium consists of muscle fibers that crisscross diagonally with those of the other side. The endometrium lines the uterine cavity, with a superficial layer that consists of columnar epithelium and stroma that changes with the menstrual cycle, which is supplied by spiral arteries that spasm and cause the shedding of this layer with each menses. A deeper basal layer, supplied by different arteries, regenerates a new layer after each menstrual cycle.

The cervix is composed of dense fibrous connective tissue with a minimal amount of smooth muscle located on the periphery that connects the myometrium to the muscle in the vaginal wall. This smooth muscle layer surrounds the cervix, and is where the cardinal and uterosacral ligaments insert. The internal os is the opening of the endocervical canal into the endometrial cavity, while the external os is the opening of the canal on the vaginal side. At the external os the columnar epithelium that extends from the endocervical canal transforms into stratified squamous epithelium upon exposure to the acidic environment of the vagina that occurs with the onset of puberty and the effects of estrogen. This area is known as the transition zone and is susceptible to dysplastic and malignant transformation.

The broad ligament covers the lateral uterine corpus and upper cervix, and extends superiorly to the round ligaments and posteriorly to the infundibulo-pelvic ligaments. It consists of anterior and posterior leafs, and is composed of visceral and parietal peritoneal layers containing smooth muscle, vessels, and connective tissue, and is not the type of ligament associated with skeletal joints. The cardinal and uterosacral ligaments lie below the broad ligament, while the round ligaments, tubes, and ovaries lie at its upper margins. Various portions of the broad ligament are named for nearby structures, for example, the meso-salpinx (located near the fallopian tubes) and the mesovarium (located near the ovary) (Fig. 2-12).

Figure 2-11 A, Diagram of a sagittal view of the uterus, cervix, and vagina. **B,** A view of the pelvis, with the uterus, tubes, and ovaries.

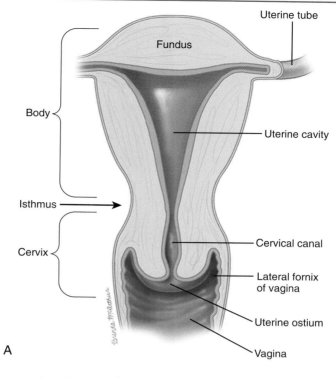

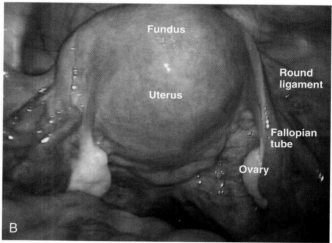

The round ligaments are extensions of the uterine musculature. They begin at the anterior lateral aspects of the fundus, travel through the retroperitoneum, then enter the inguinal canal and terminate at the labia majora (Fig. 2-13). The male homologue is the gubernaculum testis.

The uterine adnexa consist of the fallopian tubes and ovaries. The fallopian tubes connect the endometrial cavity to the intra-abdominal cavity. They arise from the uterine corpus posterior to the round ligaments. Each tube is divided into four distinct areas: the *interstitial* portion, where the tube passes through the cornu; the *isthmus*, with a narrow lumen and thick muscular wall; the *ampulla*, with a larger lumen and mucosal folds; and the *fimbria*, located at the end of the tube with frondlike projections that increase the surface area for ovum pick-up. The outer muscularis layer of the tube consists of longitudinal fibers and the inner layer consists of circular fibers.

Figure 2-12 A closer view of the uterus, broad ligament, tubes, and ovaries. (Reprinted from Drake RL, Vogl AW, Mitchell AWM, et al: Gray's Atlas of Anatomy. Philadelphia, Elsevier, 2008, p 229.)

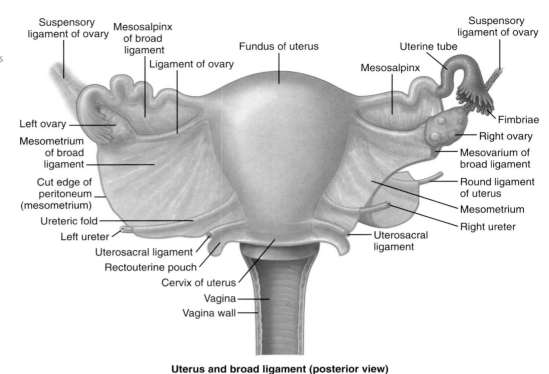

Figure 2-12 A closer view of the uterus, broad ligament, tubes, and ovaries. (Reprinted from Drake RL, Vogl AW, Mitchell AWM, et al: Gray's Atlas of Anatomy. Philadelphia, Elsevier, 2008, p 229.)

Uterus and broad ligament (posterior view)

The ovary is connected medially to the uterus through the utero-ovarian ligament; laterally it is connected to the pelvic sidewall through the infundibulopelvic ligament (also known as the suspensory ligament of the ovary) through which the ovarian vessels travel (Fig. 2-14). It is also attached to the broad ligament through the mesovarium. The ovary consists of an outer cortex, where the ova and follicles are located, and medulla, where the blood vessels and connective tissue compose a fibromuscular tissue layer. (See DVD Video 2-2 for video demonstration of the anatomy of the uterus and adnexa.)

Uterine Support Structures

The pelvic viscera are covered by endopelvic fascia, a connective tissue layer that provides support to the pelvic organs, yet allows for their mobility to permit storage of urine and stool, coitus, parturition, and defecation. Histologically, it is composed of collagen, elastin, adipose tissue, nerves, vessels, lymph channels, and smooth muscle. Several areas of the endopelvic fascia (and its associated peritoneum) have been named by anatomists. These are really condensations of the endopelvic fascia and not true ligaments: uterosacral ligament, cardinal ligament, broad ligament, mesovarium, mesosalpinx, and the round ligament. The principal connective tissue support structures for the uterus are the cardinal ligaments and the uterosacral ligaments. These two structures are intimately related and together form an intricate three-dimensional connective tissue structure that originates at the cervix and upper vagina and inserts at the pelvic sidewall and sacrum and is sometimes called the uterosacral/cardinal complex. The broad ligament, mesovarium, mesosalpinx, and round ligament do not play a role in support of the pelvic organs.

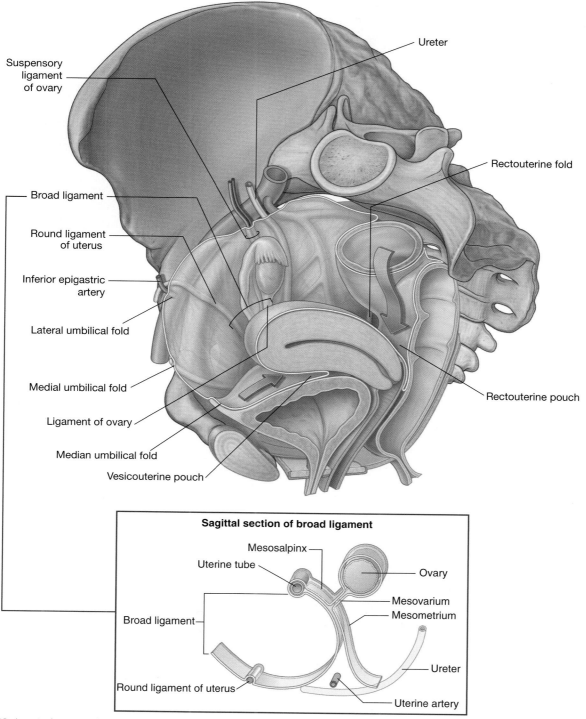

Figure 2-13 A sagittal section of the pelvis. The round ligament enters the deep inguinal ring, travels through the inguinal canal, and exits through the superficial inguinal ring. The ureter lies in close proximity to the uterine vessels and the ovarian vessels in the retroperitoneal space. (Reprinted from Drake RL, Vogl W, Mitchell AWM: Gray's Anatomy for Students. Philadelphia, Elsevier, 2005, p 416, Fig. 5-58A.)

Three levels of connective tissue supports of the uterus and vagina have been described (Fig. 2-15). The uterosacral/cardinal ligament complex provides level I support. The uterosacral/cardinal ligament complex suspends the uterus and upper vagina in its normal orientation. It serves to maintain vaginal length and keep the vaginal axis nearly horizontal in a standing woman so that it can be supported by the levator ani muscles. Loss of level I support contributes to

Figure 2-14 The right ovarian vessels travel through the infundibulopelvic ligament to supply the right ovary and tube.

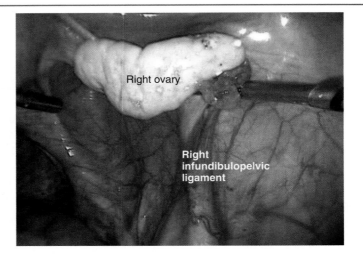

Right ovary

Right infundibulopelvic ligament

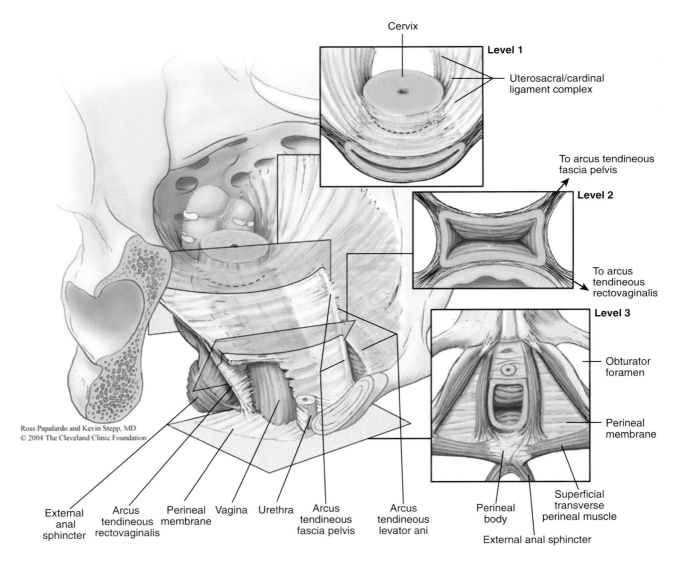

Ross Papalardo and Kevin Stepp, MD
© 2004 The Cleveland Clinic Foundation

Cervix

Level 1

Uterosacral/cardinal ligament complex

To arcus tendineous fascia pelvis

Level 2

To arcus tendineous rectovaginalis

Level 3

Obturator foramen

Perineal membrane

External anal sphincter   Arcus tendineous rectovaginalis   Perineal membrane   Vagina   Urethra   Arcus tendineous fascia pelvis   Arcus tendineous levator ani   Perineal body   Superficial transverse perineal muscle

External anal sphincter

Figure 2-15 Integrated levels of uterovaginal support as seen in a standing woman. The three levels of support of the vagina and uterus showing the continuity of supportive structures throughout the entire length of the genital tract. In level 1, the uterosacral/cardinal ligament complex suspends the uterus, cervix, and upper vagina from the lateral pelvic walls. Fibers of level I extend both vertically and posteriorly toward the sacrum. Fibers of level II provide lateral support and attach the midportion of the vagina to the arcus tendineus fascia pelvis and to the arcus tendineus rectovaginalis. Level III support is the most distal component, consisting of the fusion of the vagina anteriorly to the urethra, posteriorly to the perineal membrane and perineal body, and laterally to the levator ani muscles. (Reprinted with permission of The Cleveland Clinic Center for Medical Art & Photography, copyright 2009. All rights reserved.)

Figure 2-16 The retropubic or prevesical space. The endopelvic fascia connects laterally to the aponeurosis of the levator ani muscles at the arcus tendineus fasciae pelvis, providing level II support. Defects in these lateral attachments are called paravaginal defects and lead to anterior or posterior compartment defects, e.g., cystoceles and rectoceles. The iliopectineal line, or Cooper's ligament, runs along the superior border of the ischiopubic rami bilaterally and is where Burch urethropexy sutures are anchored.

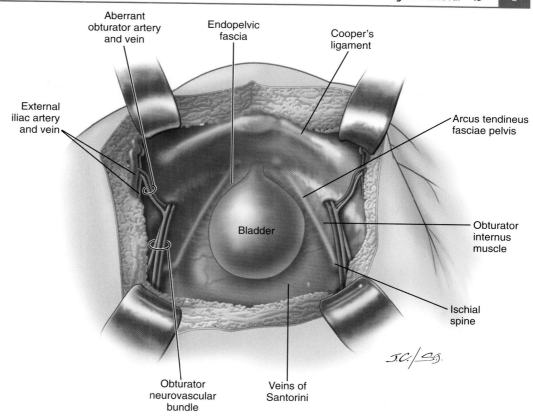

prolapse of the uterus. At the time of hysterectomy, care should be taken to incorporate the detached uterosacral/cardinal ligament remnants into the vaginal cuff repair in an attempt to preserve apical support of the vagina and subsequent prolapse. Any symptomatic vaginal support defects should also be addressed at the time of hysterectomy.

Contiguous with the uterosacral/cardinal ligament complex at the location of the ischial spine is level II support—the paravaginal attachments. The anterior vaginal is suspended laterally to the arcus tendineus fasciae pelvis (ATFP) or "white line" which is a thickened condensation of fascia overlying the iliococcygeus muscle (Fig. 2-16). The ATFP originates on the ischial spine and inserts on the inferior aspect of the pubic symphysis. The posterior vaginal wall is suspended laterally by a similar structure, the arcus tendineous rectovaginalis. Defects at this level result in anterior or posterior compartment defects (e.g., cystoceles and rectoceles). Level III support is the most distal component, consisting of the fusion of the vagina anteriorly to the urethra, posteriorly to the perineal membrane and perineal body, and laterally to the levator ani muscles. A defect in this level posteriorly results in perineal body descent and can contribute to defecatory dysfunction, or anteriorly can cause urethral hypermobility and stress incontinence. Level II and level III support structures are important for maintaining support and function of the vagina, bladder, and rectum, but their contribution to uterine support is minimal.

Vasculature

The aorta provides the blood supply to the pelvic structures. It bifurcates at approximately L4-L5 into the right and left common iliac arteries. The inferior vena cava, where the right and common iliac veins return their blood flow, is located to the right of the aortic bifurcation. The left common iliac vein travels anterior to the sacrum medial to the aortic bifurcation and joins the right common iliac vein posterior to the right common iliac artery. The common iliac arteries then divide into the external iliac and internal iliac (or hypogastric) arteries. The external iliac artery is located medial to the psoas muscle, but the external iliac vein is much larger and lies posterior and medial to the artery. The external iliac vein also covers the obturator fossa, where the obturator neurovascular bundle and lymph nodes are located medial to the obturator internus muscle. The internal iliac artery branches into the anterior and posterior divisions. The posterior division travels toward the ischial spine, branching into the lateral sacral, iliolumbar, and superior gluteal arteries. The anterior division of the internal iliac artery branches into the obliterated umbilical, uterine, superior vesical, obturator, vaginal, and inferior gluteal and internal pudendal arteries (Fig. 2-17A and B). In order to identify and access any of these major pelvic vessels, a retroperitoneal dissection must be performed and the ureter must be identified prior to the cauterization or ligation of any of the vessels. Ligation of the hypogastric artery is a useful surgical technique in the setting of massive pelvic hemorrhage. Collateral flow from the aortic branches (i.e., lumbar and middle sacral artery) or through the inferior mesenteric branches (i.e., superior hemorrhoidal vessels) prevents ischemia of the pelvic organs.

The uterus, tubes, and ovaries are supplied by the uterine and vaginal branches from the anterior division of the internal iliac arteries and from the ovarian arteries from the aorta. The uterine, vaginal, and ovarian vessels form an arterial cascade where collateral flow can supply the uterus, adnexa, and vagina (Fig. 2-18). The uterine artery originates from the internal iliac artery in the retroperitoneum. It may share a common origin with the obliterated umbilical artery, internal pudendal, and vaginal artery. In fact, the obliterated umbilical artery can serve as a useful landmark during abdominal or laparoscopic surgery, as tugging on the obliterated umbilical artery can often help identify the uterine artery in cases of distorted pelvic anatomy. The uterine artery travels through the cardinal ligament and passes over the ureter, which is located approximately 1.5 cm lateral to the cervix. It then joins the uterus at the junction between the cervix and the uterine corpus at approximately the level of the internal cervical os and provides blood flow upward toward the corpus and downward toward the cervix (Fig. 2-19). It also sends a branch to the cervicovaginal junction at the lateral aspect of the vagina. The vagina also receives its blood supply from this uterine branch as well as from a vaginal branch of the internal iliac artery, which anastomose along the vagina laterally at the 3 o'clock and 9 o'clock positions.

The ovarian arteries arise from the abdominal aorta. The right ovarian vein returns to the inferior vena cava while the left ovarian vein returns to the left renal vein. They travel in close proximity to the ureter, along the medial aspect of the psoas muscle, and supply the ovaries through the infundibulopelvic ligament (or suspensory ligament of the ovary) (see Fig. 2-14). (See DVD Video 2-3 for demonstration of the vasculature of the pelvis. 🎥)

Because of the collateral blood supply of the uterus, achieving hemostasis during hysterectomy requires securing the three main arterial supplies: the uterine artery, collateral flow from the ovarian vessels that is supplied via the utero-ovarian ligament, and collateral flow inferiorly from the vaginal arteries. Because of the close proximity of the ureters to each of these vessels, many of the fundamental steps of a hysterectomy revolve around securing this collateral

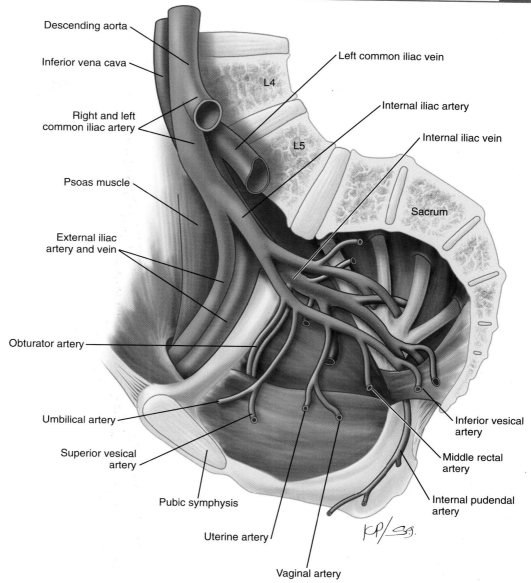

Figure 2-17 The aorta provides the blood supply to the pelvic structures. It bifurcates at approximately L4-L5 into the right and left common iliac arteries. The inferior vena cava, where the right and common iliac veins return their blood flow, is located to the right of the aortic bifurcation. The left common iliac vein travels anterior to the sacrum medial to the aortic bifurcation and joins the right common iliac vein posterior to the right common iliac artery. The common iliac arteries then divide into the external iliac and internal iliac (or hypogastric) arteries. The external iliac artery is located medial to the psoas muscle, and the external iliac vein is much larger and lies posterior and medial to the artery. The external iliac vein also covers the obturator fossa, where the obturator neurovascular bundle and lymph nodes are located medial to the obturator internus muscle. The internal iliac, or hypogastric, artery branches into the anterior and posterior divisions. The posterior division travels toward the ischial spine, branching into the lateral sacral, iliolumbar, and superior gluteal arteries. The anterior division of the internal iliac artery branches into the obliterated umbilical, uterine, superior vesical, obturator, vaginal, and inferior gluteal and internal pudendal arteries.

blood flow while avoiding ureteral injury. During the abdominal or laparoscopic approaches, the first step in this process typically involves entering the retro-peritoneal space where the ovarian vessels, uterine vessels, and the ureters are located. The next step is to secure the collateral blood flow supply from the ovarian vessels via the utero-ovarian ligament in the case of hysterectomy alone, or the infundibulopelvic ligament when performing a concomitant salpingo-oophorectomy. Because the close proximity, the ureter should be

Figure 2-18 Blood supply of the uterus. The uterus, tubes, and ovaries are supplied by the uterine and vaginal branches from the anterior division of the internal iliac arteries and from the ovarian arteries from the aorta. These vessels form an arterial cascade where collateral flow can supply the uterus, adnexa, and vagina. The uterine artery travels through the cardinal ligament and passes over the ureter, which is located approximately 1.5 cm lateral to the cervix. It then joins the uterus at the junction between the cervix and the uterine body.

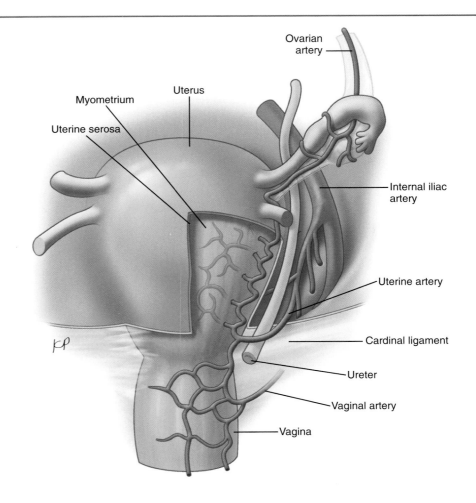

identified in the retroperitoneum prior to ligating or cauterizing the infundibulopelvic ligament. Dissection of the bladder off the uterus and cervix, skeletonization of the uterine artery, and traction of the uterus cephalad aids in taking the ureter away from the uterine artery during clamping or ligating or cauterizing of this vessel. As the uterine artery enters the uterus at approximately the cervicouterine junction, ligation of this vessel starts by placing a clamp at this level. Many small perforating vessels are given off as the uterine artery spirals up and down the lateral length of the uterus and cervix. Because of this, securing the uterine vessels and the anastomosing vaginal vessels requires a sequential series of clamping and suture ligation down the side of the cervix on each side until the vagina is entered. Each clamp is placed medial to the previous one in order to avoid ureteral injury; with each sequential ligation, the ureter is deflected more laterally.

Lower Urinary Tract

The structures of the urinary system located within the pelvis include the bladder, urethra, and distal segment of the ureters. The bladder is quite distensible and its borders span the lower anterior abdominal wall anteriorly, the pubic bones and levator ani and obturator internus muscles laterally, and the cervix and vagina posteriorly. It can be divided into two main portions: the dome and the base. The dome of the bladder is contiguous with the parietal peritoneum of the anterior abdominal wall, its upper boundaries roughly correspond to the obliterated umbilical ligaments and urachus, and its lower

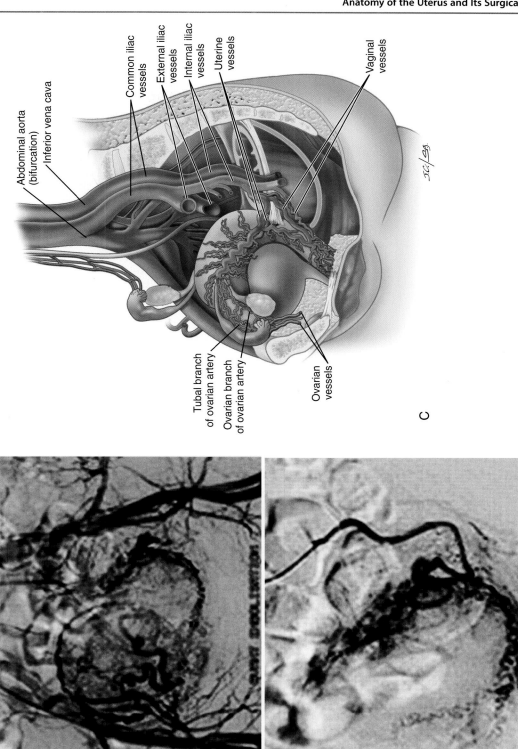

Abdominal aorta (bifurcation)
Inferior vena cava
Common iliac vessels
External iliac vessels
Internal iliac vessels
Uterine vessels
Vaginal vessels
Tubal branch of ovarian artery
Ovarian branch of ovarian artery
Ovarian vessels

A

B

C

Figure 2-19 A, Angiogram of the uterus and its blood supply prior to performing a uterine artery embolization. The uterine artery is seen branching off the internal iliac artery, entering the uterus, and then branching into several spiral arteries lateral to and within the body of the uterus. The concentration of enlarged spiraling arteries seen to the left of midline represents the blood supply to the uterine fibroid. **B,** A sagittal view of the uterine artery as it branches off from the internal iliac artery and anastomoses with the vaginal artery. **C,** A schematic representation of B. The uterine artery and vein is located just lateral to the uterosacral ligament insertion into the uterus. The anastomosis between the uterine and vaginal vessels is seen here.

Figure 2-20 Abdominal view of the inside of the bladder. The base of the bladder consists primarily of the trigone. The trigone is a triangular area of smooth muscle with the boundaries of the two ureteral orifices and the bladder neck/urethra. The trigone lies on the upper vagina. The urethra connects the bladder to the vagina, averaging 2 to 3 cm in length.

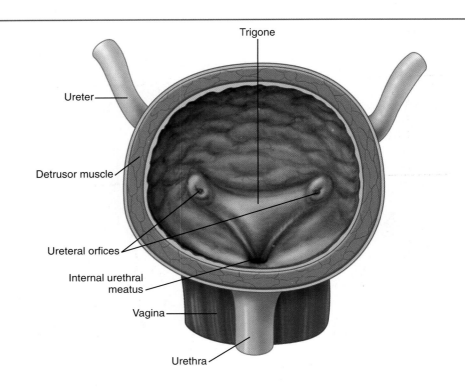

Trigone

Ureter

Detrusor muscle

Ureteral orfices

Internal urethral meatus

Vagina

Urethra

boundary is the lower uterine segment and anterior cervix. The bladder is separated from the pubic bone by a potential space, the prevesical or retropubic space, which contains the venous plexus of Santorini. When empty, the bladder is pyramid-shaped, with the apex pointed toward the pubic bone. When full, the bladder is spherical, with normal capacities ranging from 300 to 700 mL, and can transform from being a pelvic organ to an abdominal one, rising above the pubic bone. When the bladder is distended, the musculature of the dome can become relatively thin, and therefore, prior to initiating the surgical procedure, decompression of the bladder through Foley catheter drainage can help avoid injury. The base of the bladder consists of the trigone and a thickening of the detrusor muscle known as the detrusor loop, whose thickness, unlike the dome, does not vary with filling of the bladder. The trigone is a triangular area of smooth muscle and its boundaries are the two ureteral orifices and the bladder neck/urethra. The trigone lies anterior to the upper vagina. The bladder is supplied by the superior vesical artery or the obliterated umbilical artery, and the inferior vesical artery, which can either arise from the internal pudendal artery or the vaginal artery. Histologically, the bladder is lined by the urothelium, which is covered by the crisscrossing smooth muscle fibers of the detrusor muscle, and the outer adventitial serosal layer (Fig. 2-20).

Bladder injury can occur at the dome during peritoneal entry during an open procedure, or suprapubic port placement during a laparoscopic case. It also can occur during the dissection of the bladder off the lower uterine segment and cervix, with the bladder defect most commonly occurring in the midline just superior to the intraureteric ridge (i.e., supratrigonal). Risk factors for this type of injury include previous cesarean sections, prior pelvic infection, endometriosis, distorted anatomy from fibroids or malignancy, or prior bladder surgery such as anterior colporrhaphy.

The urethra connects the bladder to the vagina. It averages about 2 to 3 cm in length and 6 mm in diameter. It connects to the base of the bladder, which is termed the bladder neck, or vesical neck, then continues fused to the vagina in its distal two thirds, and terminates with the external urethral meatus in the vestibule directly above the vaginal opening. Its blood supply consists of the extensions of the pudendal vessels and the inferior vesical vessels.

The ureters are approximately 25 to 30 cm in length from the renal pelvis to the trigone of the bladder, and are located retroperitoneally along their entire length. They are divided into the abdominal and pelvic segments by the pelvic brim, each of which is approximately 12 to 15 cm in length. The ureters are most easily identified at the pelvic brim, where they cross the bifurcation of the common iliac into the external and internal iliac vessels (Fig. 2-21). The left ureter is often obscured by the sigmoid colon, and visualization can be facilitated by sharply incising the sigmoid colon attachments to the left pelvic sidewall. The ureter travels into the pelvis along with the ovarian vessels, making the identification of the ureter imperative prior to performing an oophorectomy. The ureter usually lies medial to the infundibulopelvic ligament, but when it lies in close proximity to the ovarian vessels, it may be necessary to open the retroperitoneal space lateral to the infundibulopelvic ligament and create a window between the ovarian vessels and the ureter in order to safely secure the ovarian vascular pedicle. In the case of concomitant salpingo-oophorectomy at the time of hysterectomy, opening the broad ligament between the round ligament and the infundibulopelvic ligament provides excellent retroperitoneal access and the opportunity to identify the ureter.

The course of the pelvic ureter is similar on each side. It travels medially to the internal iliac artery and its anterior division. It then dives medially in a deep trajectory to enter the parametrium and course below the uterine artery ("water under the bridge"), approximately 1.5 cm lateral to the internal cervical os. The ureter passes through the cardinal ligament/anterior bladder pillar (i.e., tunnel of Wertheim), then travels medially and anteriorly over the vaginal fornix to enter the trigone of the bladder.

The ureter is supplied by the blood vessels it crosses, namely, the ovarian, internal iliac, superior vesical, and inferior vesical arteries. Above the pelvic brim, the blood supply enters from the medial side, and below the pelvic brim, the blood supply enters laterally. During ureterolysis, the surgeon can avoid ischemic injuries by staying outside the adventitial sheath surrounding the ureter, although this may be difficult to do in the setting of malignancy, or significant scarring or fibrosis as a result of endometriosis or prior pelvic radiation.

In 1% of the population, the ureter is duplicated. Duplications may be partial or complete. Partial duplications result in joining of the duplicate ureters before entering the bladder. The ureters arise from the wolffian ducts embryologically; those ureters that originate from a normal position on the wolffian duct have normally positioned ureteral orifices and upper urinary tracts. However, the ureters arising from an abnormal position on the wolffian ducts are associated with ectopic insertions, renal dysplasia, and related complications. Therefore, the appearance of the upper tract usually predicts the site of insertion—in other words, a normal pelvicaliceal system is usually related to a normally positioned ureteral orifice. Similarly, an extremely ectopic ureteral orifice will usually subtend a dysplastic, poorly functioning segment. The existence of a urinary tract anomaly may not even be known prior to undertaking a hysterectomy, but every effort should be made to identify the ureter in the normal location. If the patient has a history of a müllerian or urinary tract anomaly (e.g., a solitary kidney), preoperative imaging with an intravenous pyelogram may prepare the surgeon's expectations of what or where the surgeon may find the ureters intraoperatively.

Ureteral injury most commonly occurs during simple abdominal hysterectomy, and at the following sites: the pelvic brim near the infundibulopelvic

Figure 2-21 Pelvic course of the ureter. **A,** The ureters are most easily identified at the pelvic brim, where they cross the bifurcation of the common iliac into the external and internal iliac vessels. The uterus is rotated to stretch the ureter and uterine vessels. The ureter crosses over the bifurcation of the common iliac vessels at the pelvic brim in close proximity to the ovarian vessels, then travels through the retroperitoneal space and the broad ligament under the uterine vessels to insert into the bladder. **B,** Diagram of the course of the left ureter during clamping of the left uterine vessels at hysterectomy.

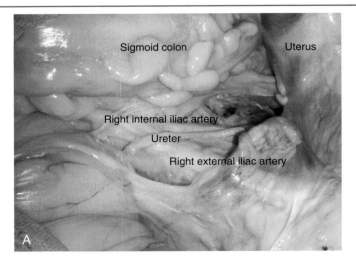

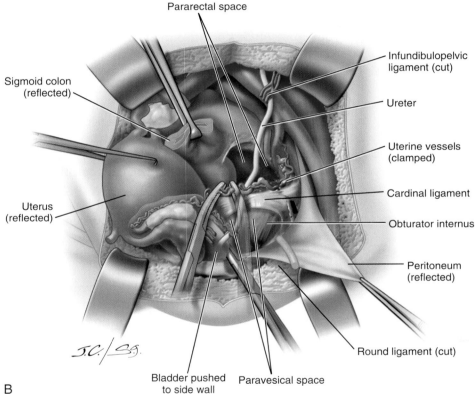

ligament (while securing the ovarian vessels), the cardinal ligament where the ureter crosses under the uterine artery (while securing the uterine vessels), the vaginal cuff (securing the lateral angles), and lateral pelvic sidewall above the uterosacral ligaments (obtaining hemostasis, performing a concomitant culdoplasty or excision of endometriosis) (Fig. 2-22). As discussed earlier, traction of the uterus cephalad and dissection of the broad ligament in order to skeletonize the uterine arteries before ligation or cauterization can help avoid injury. During laparoscopic hysterectomy, pushing the uterine manipulator and cervical cup into the pelvis and anteverting the uterus can deflect the ureters down and laterally at the level of the uterine arteries and at the vaginal cuff prior to securing these pedicles. Vaginal hysterectomy is rarely associated with ureteral injury. The combination of downward traction on the cervix and

Figure 2-22 Course of the ureter. Common sites of ureteral injury during hysterectomy are noted (*dotted circles*).

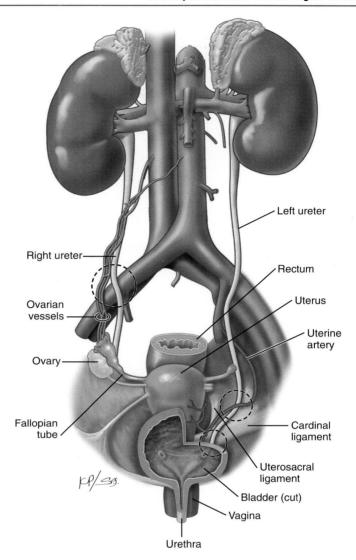

Left ureter

Right ureter

Rectum

Ovarian vessels

Uterus

Uterine artery

Ovary

Fallopian tube

Cardinal ligament

Uterosacral ligament

Bladder (cut)

Vagina

Urethra

anterior retraction of the bladder through the anterior peritoneal opening lifts the ureter an additional 1 cm away, so that it lies more than 2 cm away from the parametrium during the hysterectomy (Fig. 2-23). The diagnosis of ureteral injury can easily be made through performing a cystoscopy after the injection of intravenous indigo carmine dye and identifying a lack of spillage from one of the ureteral orifices. (See DVD Video 2-4 for video demonstration of the anatomy of the lower urinary tract. 📹)

Sigmoid Colon and Rectum

The sigmoid colon descends into the pelvis curving from the left (descending) colon slightly to the left of the midline and sacrum and is extraperitoneal, unlike much of the colon. It is attached to a distinct mesentery in its midportion, which can be traumatized during packing of the bowel out of the pelvis and cause some bleeding. Its blood supply derives from the sigmoid arteries, branches of the inferior mesenteric artery. It is characterized by the presence of three taeniae coli and appendiceal epiploicae. There are often physiologic attachments of the sigmoid colon epiploicae to the left pelvic sidewall that may need to be dissected in order to adequately visualize the left infundibulopelvic

Figure 2-23 Ureter anatomy in relation to the uterus at total vaginal hysterectomy. Upward traction of the bladder during vaginal hysterectomy increases the distance of the ureter away from the area of clamp placement.

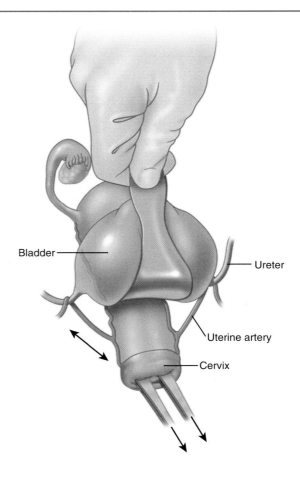

ligament or left ureter at the time of left salpingo-oophorectomy. Care should be taken to avoid injury to the genitofemoral nerve, which runs on the surface of the psoas muscle during this dissection.

Once the sigmoid colon is in the pelvis, its course straightens and it enters the retroperitoneum at the posterior cul-de-sac, becoming the rectum. The rectum is approximately 15 to 20 cm in length and is characterized by the absence of appendiceal epiploicae, lack of a true mesentery and divergence of the three taeniae coli. Once retroperitoneal, it expands into the rectal ampulla, an area of stool storage, then bends downward to an almost 90-degree angle to become the anus. There are a series of anal valves to assist in the prevention of gas and stool leakage. The anus is surrounded by the internal anal sphincter and external anal sphincter. The internal anal sphincter consists of a thicker layer of the circular involuntary smooth muscle fibers, which provides 80% of the resting tone of the sphincter; the external anal sphincter consists of some voluntary skeletal muscle fibers and is attached to the coccyx. The rectum and anus rest on the sacrum and levator ani muscles and the vagina lies anterior to the rectum. The blood supply to the rectum and anus consists of an anastomotic arcade of vessels from the superior rectal (hemorrhoidal) branch of the inferior mesenteric artery, and the middle and inferior rectal (hemorrhoidal) branches of the internal pudendal artery.

Spaces and Avascular Planes of the Pelvis

The pelvis contains several potential spaces and connective tissue planes that allow the urinary, reproductive, and gastrointestinal systems to function

Figure 2-24 Sagittal view of the anterior and posterior cul-de-sacs. The anterior cul-de-sac is also known as the vesicouterine pouch, and refers to the space between the dome of the bladder and the anterior surface of the uterus. The posterior cul-de-sac, rectouterine pouch, or pouch of Douglas refers to the space between the uterus and rectum.

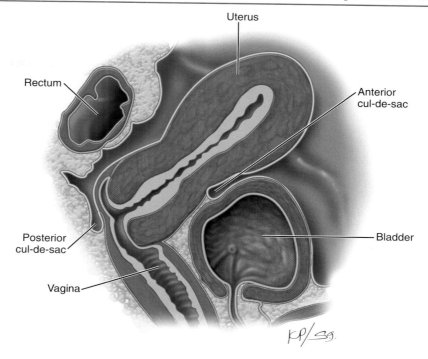

independently of each other. Two intraperitoneal potential spaces within the pelvis that the gynecologic surgeon should be familiar with are the anterior and posterior cul-de-sacs. The anterior and posterior cul-de-sacs separate the uterus from the bladder and rectum, respectively (Fig. 2-24). The anterior cul-de-sac is also known as the vesicouterine pouch, and refers to the space between the dome of the bladder and the anterior surface of the uterus. The peritoneum overlying the dome of the bladder is loose and allows the bladder to expand. This loose peritoneal fold is called the vesicouterine fold, which is dissected during abdominal hysterectomy in order to create the bladder flap, access the vesicovaginal space, and dissect the bladder off the lower uterine segment and anterior cervix. During vaginal hysterectomy, the vesicovaginal space is dissected in order to access the vesicouterine fold, which is visualized, grasped, and incised in order to enter the anterior cul-de-sac.

The posterior cul-de-sac, rectouterine pouch, or pouch of Douglas refers to the space between the uterus and rectum. Its borders are the vagina anteriorly, the rectosigmoid posteriorly, and the uterosacral ligaments laterally. Because the rectum is not directly adjacent to the posterior cervix colpotomy via the posterior cul-de-sac is generally the safest and easiest route of initial peritoneal entry during vaginal hysterectomy.

A number of avascular planes or spaces exist retroperitoneally within the pelvis that can be valuable to the pelvic surgeon. These spaces lack blood vessels and nerves and are filled with loose areolar tissue, allowing blunt dissection of these avascular planes. The surgeon should be thoroughly familiar with these spaces, as well as their relationships with each other, in order to avoid injury to the viscera and vasculature, restore normal anatomic relationships in the case of distorted anatomy, to perform pelvic reconstruction, and to resect pelvic disease such as endometriosis or cancer. Knowledge of these spaces is fundamental for most major gynecologic surgery. These spaces include the vesicovaginal, paravesical, pararectal, rectovaginal, prevesical (or retropubic), and presacral spaces (Fig. 2-25). (See DVD Video 2-5 for demonstration of the avascular planes of the pelvis. 📷)

Figure 2-25 *Axial view of the pelvis illustrating the avascular spaces within the pelvis.*

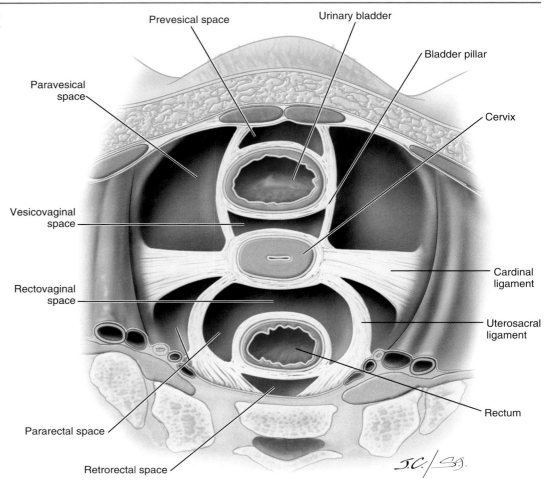

Vesicovaginal Space

The vesicovaginal space is located in the midline between the bladder and anterior vagina. Its boundaries are the bladder anteriorly, the bladder pillars laterally, and the anterior vaginal adventitia posteriorly. The bladder pillars contain veins from the vesical plexus and the ureter, some cervical branches of the uterine artery anteriorly into the sides of the bladder base, and some extensions of the stronger connective tissue portions of the cardinal ligament. The vesciovaginal space is developed in order to dissect the bladder off the lower uterine segment and anterior cervix during hysterectomy. Dissection anterior to the cervix in the midline between the bladder pillars will reveal a loose areolar avascular layer when in the proper plane. Veering laterally can result in bleeding from the bladder pillars and obscure visualization during this dissection.

Paravesical Space

The paravesical spaces are paired spaces that lie inferior to the cardinal ligaments. Their boundaries are the bladder pillars and retropubic space medially, the obturator internus muscle and the pelvic sidewalls laterally, and the cardinal ligaments superiorly. The anterior leaf of the broad ligament forms the roof of the paravesical space while the levator ani is the floor. This space is developed by opening the anterior leaf of the broad ligament and first identifying the external iliac artery and vein. Gentle traction of the adipose and areolar tissue located between the superior vesical/obliterated umbilical artery and the external iliac vessels toward the bladder medially will expose this space (Fig.

Figure 2-26 Development of the paravesical and pararectal spaces.

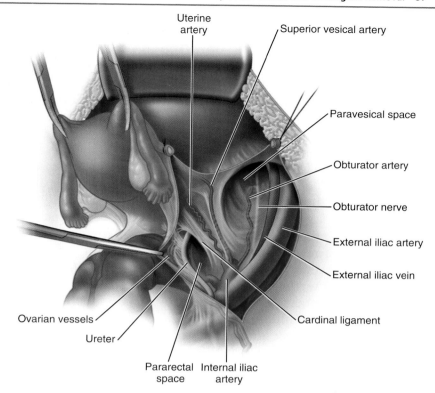

Uterine artery

Superior vesical artery

Paravesical space

Obturator artery

Obturator nerve

External iliac artery

External iliac vein

Cardinal ligament

Ovarian vessels

Ureter

Pararectal space   Internal iliac artery

2-26). Development of the paravesical space is an essential step in the performance of a radical hysterectomy or pelvic lymphadenectomy. It also facilitates identification of the course of the distal ureter between the cardinal ligament and the bladder, which may be valuable for benign hysterectomies when the anatomy is distorted, as in the case of a cervical or broad ligament fibroid.

Pararectal Space

The pararectal spaces lie in the retroperitoneum bilaterally just superior to the cardinal ligament. Its borders are formed inferiorly by the cardinal ligament; medially by the uterosacral ligament, rectal pillar, ureter, and ovarian vessels; laterally by the internal iliac vessels and piriformis muscles; and posteriorly by the levator ani muscles and coccygeus muscle/sacrospinous ligament. This space is developed by incising the broad ligament in a cephalic direction lateral to the ovarian vessels (infundibulopelvic ligament). The ovarian vessels and the ureter are adherent to the medial leaf of the broad ligament. Blunt dissection lateral to these structures and medial to the internal iliac vessels allows the development of the pararectal space, which can be carried all the way down to the levator ani muscles (see Fig. 2-26). An alternative approach, often useful during laparoscopic surgery, is to incise the medial leaf of the broad ligament inferior to the ovarian vessels and above the ureter. The lower edge of the incised peritoneum with the accompanying ureter is retracted medially while blunt dissection is performed retroperitoneally between the medial leaf of the broad ligament and the internal iliac vessels to develop the lower portion of the pararectal space. Development of the pararectal space is useful for mobilizing the ureter, particularly in cases of distorted anatomy like an obliterated posterior cul-de-sac from endometriosis. If both the pararectal and paravesical spaces are developed, the tissue in between is the cardinal ligament (parametrium). Isolating the cardinal ligament by developing these spaces facilitates identification of the uterine artery along its course from the internal iliac to the uterus and the distal ureter as it passes through the parametrium below the uterine artery, which may be valuable in cases of distorted uterine or pelvic anatomy (e.g., broad ligament fibroid, severe endometriosis). From the vaginal approach, the pararectal space can be entered by dissecting the posterior vaginal epithelium off the underlying rectum, then bluntly dissecting lateral to the rectum to develop the space. This approach is useful for accessing the sacrospinous ligament when needed for vaginal vault suspension.

Rectovaginal Space

The rectovaginal space starts caudally at the superior margin of the perineal body (2–3 cm above the hymenal ring) and extends superiorly between the posterior vagina and the rectum through the posterior cul-de-sac. Its most cephalad border is the posterior cul-de-sac just inferior to the cervix. It contains loose areolar tissue that can be dissected bluntly. Its lateral boundaries are the rectal pillars, which are fibers from the cardinal-uterosacral ligament complex that connect to the lateral rectum and then to the sacrum. They divide the rectovaginal space from the pararectal spaces. Occasionally the surgeon may need to enter the rectovaginal space during a hysterectomy when the patient has altered anatomy due to an obliterated cul-de-sac from pelvic inflammatory disease or endometriosis or due to the presence of a posterior lower uterine segment, broad ligament, or cervical fibroid. Vaginal surgeons access the rectovaginal space when performing a posterior colporraphy.

Prevesical or Retropubic Space

The prevesical or retropubic space is a potential space between the bladder and the pubic bone. This space is also often referred to as the space of Retzius. It is bounded by the pubic bone, the peritoneum, and muscles of the anterior abdominal wall. Its lateral borders are the arcus tendineus fascia pelvis and the ischial spines. Within this space lie the dorsal clitoral neurovascular bundle, located in the midline, and the obturator neurovascular bundle, located laterally as it enters the obturator canal. An accessory obturator artery can arise from the external iliac artery and run along the pubic bone. The space lateral to the bladder neck and urethra contain nerves innervating the bladder and urethra as well as a venous plexus (venous plexus of Santorini) that can ooze with the placement of sutures, for instance, while performing a Burch urethropexy. These Burch sutures are anchored into the iliopectineal line, or Cooper's ligament, which runs along the superior border of the ischiopubic rami bilaterally (see Fig. 2-16).

Presacral Space

The presacral space is located between the sacrum posteriorly and the rectum anteriorly. Its upper boundary is the bifurcation of the aorta and it is bounded laterally by the internal iliac arteries. It is unlikely that entry of the presacral space would be necessary in the performance of a hysterectomy, but a number of procedures that might be performed concomitantly with a hysterectomy may require access to the presacral space including presacral neurectomy, sacral colpopexy, and rectal resection.

Nerves of the Pelvic Cavity

The autonomic nervous system innervates the pelvis through the superior hypogastric plexus, a ganglionic plexus that receives sympathetic input from the thoracic and lumbar splanchnic nerves and afferent pain input from the pelvic viscera. It lies over the bifurcation of the aorta in the presacral space that splits into two hypogastric nerves that run along the internal iliac vessels. These nerves connect to the inferior hypogastric plexus, a plexus of nerves and ganglia located lateral to the pelvic viscera. Parasympathetic input derives from S2-S4 via the pelvic splanchnic nerves that travel to join the hypogastric plexuses through the lateral pelvic wall.

The inferior hypogastric plexus consists of three areas: the vesical plexus, uterovaginal plexus, and the middle rectal plexus. The uterovaginal plexus lies on the medial side of the uterine vessels, lateral to the uterosacral ligaments' attachment to the uterus, and continues cephalad along the uterus and caudally along the vagina. These caudal fibers innervate the vestibule and clitoris, and travel in the parametrial tissue lateral to the uterine artery and uterosacral and cardinal ligament pedicles, but within the tissue that is taken during a radical hysterectomy. It receives sympathetic input from T10-L1 and parasympathetic input from S2-S4. Because of the dissection in the parametrial tissues during hysterectomy, patients may have short-term voiding dysfunction and urinary retention postoperatively.

The ovary and tubes are innervated by a nerve plexus that originates in the renal plexus with fibers from T10 and parasympathetic fibers from the vagus nerve that run along the ovarian vessels.

The lumbar and sacral plexuses are formed from the intervertebral and sacral foramina. The lumbar plexus lies within the psoas muscle, and the sacral plexus lies on the piriformis muscle. The femoral nerve is the major branch of the lumbar plexus, supplying sensory and motor function to the thigh. Its genito-femoral branch (L1-L2) lies on the surface of the psoas muscle and can be damaged from pressure from a retractor blade and lead to anesthesia in the medial thigh and lateral labia. The femorocutaneous nerve (L2-L3) may be compressed from a retractor placed lateral to the psoas muscle or from hyperflexion of the hip in lithotomy position, leading to numbness or altered sensation in the anterior thigh. The major branch of the sacral plexus, the sciatic nerve, exits the pelvis through the inferior portion of the greater sciatic foramen to innervate the muscles of the hip, pelvic diaphragm, perineum, and lower leg (Fig. 2-27).

Cases of Distorted Anatomy

Case 1: Cervical Fibroid

A 49-year-old female gravida 3, para 3 presents with irregular vaginal bleeding which started 6 months ago and is heavier than usual. Previously she had regular menstrual cycles every 28 to 30 days. She also complains of pelvic pressure and some dyspareunia at the vaginal apex. Speculum examination reveals an enlarged cervix with the cervical os displaced anteriorly. Bimanual examination reveals an enlarged irregularly shaped cervix measuring 5 cm that protrudes into the left parametrium. Cervical cytologic examination and endocervical curettage are normal. Magnetic resonance imaging (MRI) of the pelvis reveals a smooth mass measuring 4 × 6 × 4.3 cm in the posterior aspect of the cervix extending to the left pelvic sidewall consistent with a cervical fibroid (Fig. 2-28).

Discussion
The location of this fibroid presents a challenge to the gynecologic surgeon because of the close proximity of the ureters to the fibroid and the uterine vessels at the cardinal ligaments. The ureters are usually 1.5 to 2 cm away from the surgical clamps during suture ligation but may be closer when this scenario occurs. The uterine artery originates from the internal iliac artery and penetrates the uterus at the cervicouterine junction. With a laterally expanding cervical fibroid, such as the one in this case, the course of the uterine artery is distorted so that it is more lateral and anterior and considerably closer to the cervix. Similarly, the course of the ureter is displaced anterolaterally and abuts the expanded cervix as it passes under the uterine artery (Fig. 2-29). The bladder is displaced toward the pubic bone and the vaginal fornices are expanded to accommodate the enlarged cervix. In the case of a uterine fibroid(s) that expands laterally into the parametrium, whether from the cervix or the uterine body, the surgeon will need to identify the altered course of the ureter and the uterine artery prior to securing the uterine vessels. This

Figure 2-27 The pelvic viscera are innervated by the autonomic nervous system. The sympathetic nerve fibers originate in the thoracic and lumbar spinal cord and travel to the pelvic viscera via the hypogastric plexus. The superior, middle, and inferior hypogastric plexuses are seen here. The parasympathetic nerve fibers join the inferior hypogastric plexus via the pelvic nerves (sacral nerve roots 2, 3, 4). The pelvic nerves and inferior hypogastric plexus are shown joining the right uterine plexus.

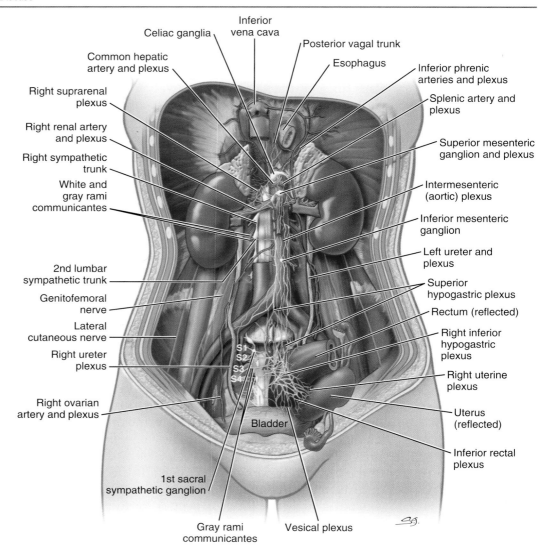

Figure 2-28 Case 1. Sagittal T₂-weighted image shows large, smooth mass (M) measuring 4 × 6 × 4.3 cm with heterogeneous signal intensity in posterior cervix consistent with a cervical fibroid. Note anterior displacement of external os (*arrowhead*). (Reprinted with permission from Brown MA, Mattrey RF, Stamato S, et al: MRI of the female pelvis using vaginal gel. AJR 2005;185:1221–1227.)

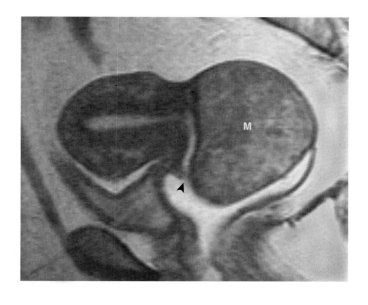

Figure 2-29 Case 1 and 2. Uterus with cervical fibroid (*right*) and broad ligament fibroid (*left*) resulting in displacement of the ureter and uterine blood supply.

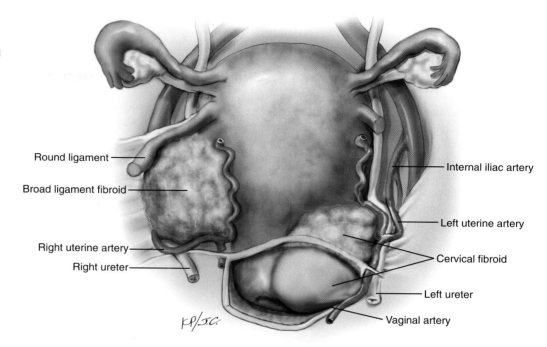

Round ligament

Broad ligament fibroid

Right uterine artery

Right ureter

Internal iliac artery

Left uterine artery

Cervical fibroid

Left ureter

Vaginal artery

Case 1: Cervical Fibroid—cont'd

is facilitated by entering the retroperitoneum and developing the pararectal, paravesical, and vesicovaginal spaces as outlined in this chapter. Within the pararectal space, the ureter can be identified as it enters the pelvis over the pelvic brim and follows its course toward the cardinal ligament where it is seen coursing underneath the uterine artery. Developing the paravesical and vesicovaginal spaces helps to expose the distal course of the ureter and mobilize the bladder off the fibroid and uterus in order to secure the uterine vessels safely and facilitate the remainder of the hysterectomy. Of note, this extensive dissection of the parametrium is essentially the same as when performing a radical hysterectomy for cervical cancer. In some instances a lateral fibroid may distort the retroperitoneal anatomy so much that the surgeon may consider performing a myomectomy in order to provide some restoration of normal anatomy so that the uterine vessels can be identified and secured while avoiding ureteral or bladder injury. Gynecologic and urologic surgeons should be prepared for a higher risk of hemorrhage and ureteral injury in difficult cases such as this. See Chapter 6 for further details on the surgical techniques that can be used in the case of an abdonimal hysterectomy complicated by distorted anatomy resulting from uterine fibroids.

Case 2: Broad Ligament Fibroid

A 42-year-old female gravida 2, para 2 presents with dysmenorrhea, urinary frequency, and menorrhagia. She has tried depot-medroxyprogesterone acetate, which did not relieve her symptoms. Bimanual examination reveals a bulky irregular 12-week-sized uterus with a firm mass that extends into the right parametrium. Pelvic ultrasound reveals a 6 × 5 × 5.5 cm uterine fibroid on the right extending from the lateral uterus to the pelvic sidewall. The uterine body is displaced to the left. She now desires a hysterectomy.

Discussion

This case is similar to that of the cervical fibroid seen in Case 1 in that the patient has a fibroid that protrudes laterally from the uterine body. It extends into the parametrium endangering the ureter by bringing the ureter in close proximity to the uterine blood supply. If the fibroid extends laterally from the lower portion of uterine body so that it is retroperitoneal and within the broad ligament, it is often called a "broad ligament fibroid." In contrast to Case 1, a large fibroid that protrudes laterally from the uterine body rather than the cervix may displace the course of the uterine artery and ureter both laterally and posteriorly so that it is deeper in the pelvis. From an abdominal or laparoscopic perspective the entry of the uterine artery into the uterus and the distal course of the ureter is often hidden below the laterally expanding fibroid, making safe ligation of the uterine vessels a challenge.

Case 2: Broad Ligament Fibroid—cont'd

Figure 2-29 illustrates the displacement of the course of the ureter and uterine artery in the case of a cervical fibroid and a large broad ligament fibroid. In either of these cases, if the fibroid is large enough, the entire uterine body can be displaced contralaterally. In the case of a broad ligament fibroid, the broad ligament will be expanded outward to accommodate the uterine fibroid, and the course of the round ligament is often distorted. As with Case 1, the surgeon will need to expose the course of the ureter and the uterine artery by developing the pararectal and paravesical spaces. This can be accomplished by entering the retroperitoneum above and lateral to the fibroid to develop these avascular spaces as previously described. The course of the ureter should be identified as should the uterine artery as it originates from the internal iliac vessels. The ureter can then be mobilized laterally away from the fibroid so that the uterine artery can be ligated safely, usually close to its origin. In some circumstances, it may be necessary to perform a myomectomy to remove the broad ligament fibroid in order to gain appropriate visualization of the ureter and uterine blood supply. See Chapter 6 for further discussion of the surgical techniques at abdominal hysterectomy that may be valuable in cases of distorted anatomy.

Case 3: Endometriosis with Obliterated Posterior Cul-de-sac

A 40-year-old female gravida 1, para 1 presents with long-standing dyspareunia, dysmenorrhea, and dyschezia refractory to management with oral contraceptive pills. She denies rectal bleeding. She had a previous laparoscopy at an outside hospital consistent with endometriosis, and responded to a trial of depo-leuprolide acetate but disliked the side effects. She now desires definitive surgical management with hysterectomy. Bimanual examination reveals a nonmobile retroverted, 8-week-sized uterus, and rectovaginal examination reveals irregular nodularity in the upper rectovaginal septum. At the time of laparoscopic hysterectomy, severe endometriosis with an obliterated posterior cul-de-sac is noted (Fig. 2-30).

Discussion

Common sites of endometriosis in the pelvis include the fallopian tubes, ovaries, anterior and posterior cul-de-sacs, the broad ligament, and uterosacral ligaments. Histologically, endometriosis is characterized by the presence of endometrial glands and stroma outside the endometrial cavity and uterine musculature. Other important histologic features include fibrin deposition secondary to inflammatory reactions, neovasularization resulting from the production of angiogenic factors, and fibrosis. The fibrosis and inflammation associated with endometriotic implants can result in a significant adhesion formation and distortion of pelvic anatomy. In this case, endometriosis and associated fibrosis and inflammation have obliterated the posterior cul-de-sac via adhesions from the anterior rectum to the posterior cervix and vagina. Additionally, adhesions from the uterosacral ligaments and broad ligament to the back of the uterine fundus are seen. It is not uncommon in cases of endometriosis that have obliterated the posterior cul-de-sac to find endometriotic nodules that have infiltrated retroperitoneally into the rectovaginal space. The finding of nodularity on rectovaginal examination in this case suggests that this may have occurred. In rare cases, infiltration can extend into or through the rectal wall. In cases of endometriosis and an obliterated posterior cul-de-sac it can be expected that the associated fibrosis of the uterosacral ligaments and medial broad ligament will result in medial deviation of one or both ureters. In order to avoid injury to the rectum or ureters at the time of hysterectomy, extensive dissection of the posterior cul-de-sac and rectovaginal space is required. The dissection plane should be close to the uterus and cervix to help avoid accidental proctotomy. Additionally, the pararectal spaces should be developed bilaterally and the ureters mobilized laterally off the medial broad ligament.

Figure 2-30 Case 3. This patient has extensive adhesions of the rectum to the posterior cervix and vagina due to severe endometriosis.

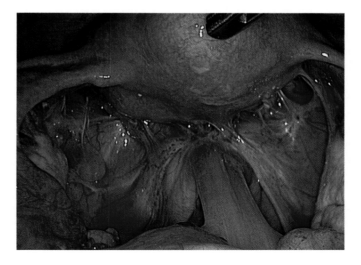

Case 4: Uterovaginal Prolapse

A 67-year-old female gravida 3, para 3 presents with a 6-month history of "something bulging through her vagina." The bulging sensation has gradually worsened over the last several months and now she sees and feels a bulge that protrudes "several inches" beyond the vaginal opening. She also reports increased urinary frequency, nocturia, and feeling of incomplete bladder emptying. She has a 10-year history of mild stress urinary incontinence symptoms which resolved approximately 4 months ago. On physical examination, she is noted to have complete uterovaginal prolapse (stage 4) with the cervix protruding 6 cm beyond the hymen. She desires surgical correction of her pelvic organ prolapse.

Discussion

Pelvic organ prolapse is downward descent of the pelvic organs that results in a protrusion of the vagina, uterus, or both. It can affect the anterior vaginal wall, posterior vaginal wall, and uterus or apex of the vagina, usually in some combination. Loss of vaginal or uterine support in women presenting for routine gynecologic care is seen in 43% to 76% of patients, with 3% to 6% having descent beyond the hymen. As noted earlier in this chapter, the principal connective tissue support structures for the uterus are the cardinal/uterosacral ligament complex or level I support. (See section "Uterine Support Structures" and Fig. 2-15.) Loss of the integrity of these supports, often in conjunction with impairment of pelvic floor muscle function, can result in uterine prolapse. In this case of complete uterovaginal prolapse, defects in lateral vaginal attachments (level II support) and the perineum (level III support) are also likely. In cases of complete uterovaginal prolapse, the uterus, with the cervix as its leading edge, protrudes through the vaginal opening and the anterior and posterior vaginal walls completely evert (Fig. 2-31). Along with the uterus and vagina, the bladder, distal rectum, and anterior and posterior cul-de-sacs are displaced caudad. With prolapse of the anterior vaginal wall, the bladder base and the portion of the bladder dome superior to the trigone (i.e., supratrigonal region) prolapse while the anterior aspect of the bladder, which lies adjacent to the pubic bone and anterior abdominal wall, often remains tethered in place. In cases of uterovaginal prolapse, the distal reflection of the bladder is typically 2 to 3 cm proximal to the cervix. Eversion of the bladder trigone displaces the ureteral orifices distally so that they are approximately at the level of the distal bladder reflection. The course of the distal ureters is also significantly altered (Fig. 2-32). Anterior vaginal prolapse can also result in urethral kinking and associated voiding dysfunction. In this patient's history, the consequences of progressive urethral kinking are noted by the resolution of stress urinary incontinence symptoms, the development of irritative voiding symptoms such as frequency and nocturia, and the feeling of incomplete bladder emptying. Posteriorly, the distal rectum often prolapses with the uterus and vagina, but not to the same degree as the bladder. Typically, the posterior cul-de-sac, which may contain prolapsing small intestine (i.e., enterocele), lies behind the upper half or so of the posterior vaginal wall while the distal rectum lies behind the distal posterior vaginal wall. As such, entry into the posterior cul-de-sac during hysterectomy in cases of uterovaginal prolapse is often easily accomplished, although anterior entry can be more challenging. See Chapter 8 for details of the surgical technique of hysterectomy for uterovaginal prolapse.

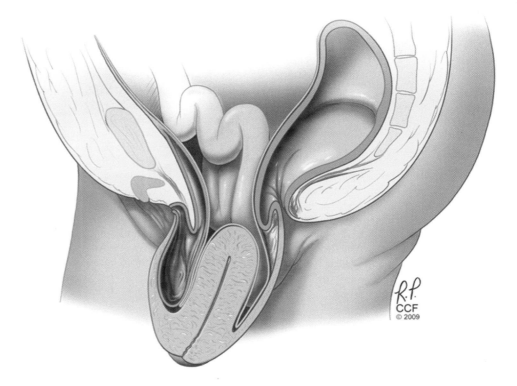

Figure 2-31 Case 4. Complete uterovaginal prolapse. (Reprinted with permission from The Cleveland Clinic Center for Medical Art & Photography, copyright 2009. All rights reserved.)

Figure 2-32 Case 4. Uterovaginal prolapse. The displaced location of the bladder and ureters are demonstrated. The distal bladder reflection is marked a horizontal line 2 to 3 cm above the anterior cervix. Ureteral catheters have been placed bilaterally allowing palpation of the distal ureter course which is also marked. The ureteral orifices are located just above the distal bladder reflection. (Photograph provided by W. Allen Addison, M.D. Duke University Medical Center.)

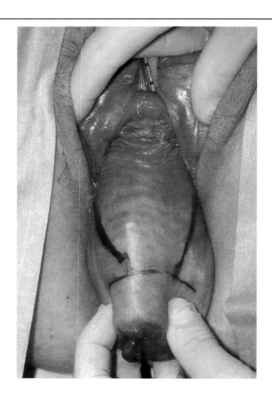

Suggested Readings

Baggish MS, Karram MM (eds): Atlas of Pelvic Anatomy and Gynecologic Surgery, 2nd ed. Philadelphia, Elsevier, 2006.

Balzer K, Witte H, Recknage S, et al: Anatomic guidelines for the prevention of abdominal wall hematoma induced by trocar placement. Surg Radiol Anat 1999;21:87–89.

Barber MD: Contemporary views on female pelvic anatomy. Cleveland Clin J Med 2005;72:S3–11.

DeLancey JOL: Anatomic aspects of vaginal eversion after hysterectomy. Am J Obstet Gynecol 1992;166:1717–1724.

Falcone T, Drake RL, Hurd WW: Surgical anatomy of the abdomen and pelvis. In Falcone T, Hurd WW (eds): Clinical Reproductive Medicine and Surgery. Philadelphia, Mosby, 2007.

Fernbach SK, Feinstein KA, Spencer K, Lindstrom CA: Ureteral duplication and its complications. Radiographics 1997;17:109–127.

Hemmings R, Falcone T: Endometriosis. In Falcone T, Hurd WW (eds): Clinical Reproductive Medicine and Surgery. Philadelphia, Mosby, 2007.

Hofmeister FJ, Wolfgram RC: Methods of demonstrating measurement relationships between vaginal hysterectomy ligatures and the ureters. Am J Obstet Gynecol 1962;83:938–948.

Hurd WW, Bude RO, DeLancey JOL, et al: The location of abdominal wall blood vessels in relationship to abdominal landmarks apparent at laparoscopy. Am J Obstet Gynecol 1994;171:642–646.

Jelovsek JE, Maher C, Barber MD: Seminar on pelvic organ prolapse. Lancet 2007;369:1027–1038.

Nichols DH, Clarke-Pearson DL: Gynecologic, Obstetric and Related Surgery, 2nd ed. Philadelphia, Mosby, 2000.

Rahn DD, Bleich AT, Wai CY, et al: Anatomic relationships of the distal third of the pelvic ureter, trigone, and urethra in unembalmed female cadavers. Am J Obstet Gynecol 2007;197:668.e1–4.

Rock JA, Jones HW (eds): Te Linde's Operative Gynecology, 9th ed. Philadelphia, Lippincott, 2003.

Stepp K, Barber M: Genital anatomic correlates of the pelvic floor. In Davila GW, Ghoniem G, Wexner S (eds): Pelvic Floor Dysfunction: A Multidisciplinary Approach. New York, Springer-Verlag, 2006.

Whiteside JL, Barber MD, Walters MD, Falcone T: Anatomy of ilioinguinal and iliohypogastric nerves in relation to trocar placement and low transverse incisions. Am J Obstet Gynecol 2003;189;1574–1578.

Epidemiology and Indications of Hysterectomy: Changing Trends

Matthew D. Barber M.D., M.H.S.

Today, hysterectomy is the second most frequent major operation performed on women in the United States, following only cesarean section. Over 600,000 hysterectomies are performed each year in the United States with an estimated annual cost of over $5 billion. The hysterectomy rate of the United States is among the highest in the developed world and approximately 23% of U.S. women have had a hysterectomy. Over the past several decades, new developments have been made in the surgical approaches to hysterectomy and in alternatives to hysterectomy for benign gynecologic conditions. This chapter will discuss the epidemiology of hysterectomy including the trends in hysterectomy rates over the last four decades and factors that influence these rates including both patient and physician factors. This chapter will also discuss the current indications for hysterectomy and their changing trends.

Epidemiology

There has been a steady decline in the annual incidence of hysterectomy over the last four decades from a peak of about 10.4 per 1000 women in 1975 to 6.0 per 1000 in 1997 to approximately 5.4 per 1000 between 2000 and 2004 according to national estimates. From 1997 through 2005, U.S. hysterectomy rates have decreased approximately 1.9% per year. Decreasing rates have been highest in women 45 years and older and in the Northeast and South regions. A recent population-based study from Olmsted County, Minnesota noted that the overall rate of hysterectomy declined by 36% from 1965 to 2002; however, unlike national trends the decline was most pronounced among women aged 25 to 34 years. The explanation for the decline in hysterectomy rates over the last several decades is likely multifactorial including changing patient and physician attitudes toward hysterectomy and an increase in the number and effectiveness of alternative therapies for benign gynecologic conditions.

The estimated rate of hysterectomy and distribution of surgical approach in the United States from 2000 to 2004 is shown in Table 3-1. Approximately two thirds of hysterectomies are performed abdominally in the United States and this has changed little over the last two decades in spite of clear benefits for the vaginal and laparoscopic approaches in terms of hospital stay, recovery

Table 3-1 Estimated Rate of Hysterectomy and Distribution of Surgical Approaches: United States, 2000–2004

Year	Number of Procedures*	Rate per 1000 Woman-Years†	Abdominal (%)	Vaginal (%)	LAVH (%)
2000	620,000	5.4	68.3	22.3	9.4
2001	637,000	5.5	66.6	22.2	11.2
2002	659,000	5.6	68.9	20.6	10.5
2003	606,000	5.1	67.9	22.0	10.6
2004	610,000	5.1	67.8	22.1	10.1
2000–2004: total/average	3,131,000	5.4	67.9	21.7	10.4

*Estimates rounded to the nearest thousand.
†Per 1000 female civilian residents 15 years or older.
LAVH, laparoscopically assisted vaginal hysterectomy.
Adapted from Whiteman MK, Hillis SD, Jamieson DJ, et al: Inpatient hysterectomy surveillance in the United States, 2000–2004. Am J Obstet Gynecol 2008;198:34.

time, and cost. The rate of laparoscopic hysterectomy has increased from approximately 0.3% in 1990 to 11.8% in 2003 largely at the expense of fewer vaginal hysterectomies. In approximately 5.5% of hysterectomies, the cervix is preserved (subtotal hysterectomy). For more details about the trends, benefits, and alternatives of the different routes of hysterectomy please refer to Chapter 4.

Factors Influencing Hysterectomy Rate

Factors associated with increased risk of hysterectomy beyond medical indication include increasing parity, poor health, younger age at menarche, high body mass index, smoking, lower socioeconomic status, geography, and physician factors. Age also plays a considerable role in rates of hysterectomy. Although some studies have suggested racial differences in hysterectomy rates, the most recent Centers for Disease Control (CDC) data demonstrate no overall difference in hysterectomy rates between black and white women. However, black women do have significantly higher rates than white women between the ages of 35 and 44, with lower rates at other ages. This is likely explained by the increased prevalence of uterine leiomyoma seen in black women. Some studies suggest that Hispanic women have lower rates of hysterectomy compared to non-Hispanic white women. The reason for this is unclear.

Although the true relationship between the rate of hysterectomy and many of the preceding risk factors is unclear, a few warrant further consideration including age, geography, socioeconomic factors, and physician factors.

Age

The prevalence of hysterectomy in the United States increases over much of the life span, peaking around age 75, then slightly decreasing (Fig. 3-1). By the end of the reproductive period (age 18–44), 18% of women will have undergone a hysterectomy. By age 75, the rate is approximately 48%. Women age 40 to 44 have the highest incidence of hysterectomy (11.7/1000 woman-years) with 64% of all hysterectomies being performed on those between ages 35 and 54.

Figure 3-1 Hysterectomy incidence and prevalence in the United States according to age and calendar year. (Redrawn from Merrill RM: Hysterectomy surveillance in the United States, 1997–2005. Med Sci Monit 2008;14:CR26.)

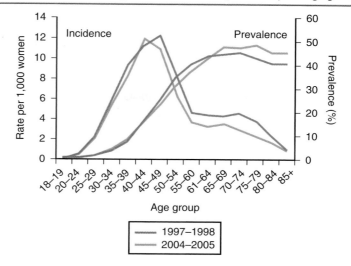

Incidence and prevalence based on weighted data.
Data sources: Behavior Risk Factor Surveillance System, National Hospital Discharge Survey.

Figure 3-2 Comparison of published hysterectomy rates from different countries. USA, United States of America; UK, United Kingdom; NSW, New South Wales. (Adapted from Spilsbury K, Semmens JB, Hammond I, Bolck A: Persistent high rates of hysterectomy in Western Australia: A population-based study of 83,000 procedures over 23 years. Br J Obstet Gynaecol 2006;113:806.)

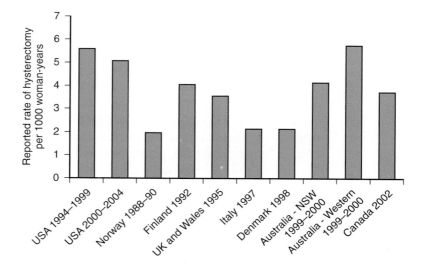

At age 35, a woman has a 12.9% probability of undergoing a hysterectomy in the next 10 years. At age 45, the probability is 11.7%. All age groups have noted a decline in the rate of hysterectomy over the last two decades with the greatest decline noted in those age 45 to 64 (−3%) and ages 65 and older (−5%). A recent survey of almost 300,000 insurance claims in New York demonstrated that women who undergo hysterectomy are approximately 4 years older on average than women with similar diagnoses receiving nonhysterectomy alternatives (49.7 versus 46 years). Age also has a significant influence on indications for hysterectomy and this topic will be discussed further later in the chapter.

Geographic Variation

Rates of hysterectomy vary considerably between and within countries. Figure 3-2 compares the rates of hysterectomy across various countries. Rates of hysterectomy are highest in the United States and Australia, which have rates

Figure 3-3 Comparison of proportion of hysterectomies performed by the abdominal route across published studies from different countries. . USA, United States of America; UK, United Kingdom; NSW, New South Wales. (Adapted from Spilsbury K, Semmens JB, Hammond I, Bolck A: Persistent high rates of hysterectomy in Western Australia: A population-based study of 83,000 procedures over 23 years. Br J Obstet Gynaecol 2006;113:806.)

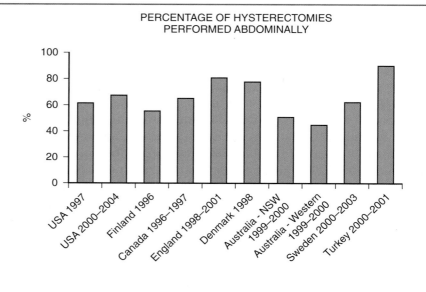

almost double those of Norway, Denmark, and Italy. There are also wide variations between countries in the route by which hysterectomy is performed. The proportion of hysterectomies performed by the abdominal route is lowest in Australia (46%–52%) whereas over 80% of hysterectomies in England are performed abdominally and over 90% of those performed in Turkey are by the abdominal route (Fig. 3-3). Reasons for these geographic variations are unclear but are thought to be due to a combination of differing patient perceptions and demands, clinician preferences, and health care systems.

Within the United States, geographic region also appears to influence hysterectomy rates. Rates for women living in the South (6.5/1000) are significantly higher than for those in the West (4.8/1000) and Northeast (4.3/1000). Similarly, the average age at the time of hysterectomy is significantly younger for women living in the South than for those living in the Northeast (44 versus 49 years old). As previously noted, the South is among the regions with the greatest decline in hysterectomy rates over the last two decades; however, it still remains the region with the highest hysterectomy rate. The availability of gynecologists, the numbers of hospital beds per capita, the types of health care insurance available, and regional variations in patient and physician attitudes toward hysterectomy are thought to contribute to geographic variation within the United States.

Socioeconomic Factors

Lower socioeconomic status has been associated with increased rates of hysterectomy in several studies. Similarly, level of education has also been found to be inversely related to hysterectomy rates. Additionally, obesity and smoking are factors associated with increased hysterectomy rates and are also associated with lower socioeconomic status. Socioeconomic status and education may influence risk of hysterectomy through their impact on health choices, access to medical care and alternative medical treatments, and other life circumstances.

Two recent studies suggest that the relationship between socioeconomic status and hysterectomy risk is complex, however. A comparison of three British cohorts found that hysterectomy risk and socioeconomic status was associated with childhood socioeconomic status but not adult economic circumstances (Cooper et al, 2005). Moreover, they found that among British women born in the 1940s and 1950s, those of lower socioeconomic status had a greater risk of hysterectomy than those of higher socioeconomic class. However, in an older cohort of British women, born in the 1920s and 1930s, the converse was found and women from more deprived socioeconomic backgrounds had a reduced risk of hysterectomy compared with those from less deprived backgrounds. A second study comparing cohorts in Britain and Australia confirmed these findings by noting an inverse association between indicators of socioeconomic status and hysterectomy in both Australian and British women born in 1946 or later (Cooper et al, 2008). In women born in the 1920s and 1930s there was no evidence of a relationship between adult socioeconomic status and rate of hysterectomy. This suggests that socioeconomic differentials in hysterectomy may be dynamic, varying over time. Further, it suggests that the socioeconomic impact on hysterectomy may be influenced by changes over time in access to medical care, women's and doctors' treatment preferences, the availability of alternative treatments, and trends in characteristics such as fertility, oral contraceptive use, and obesity.

Physician Factors

A number of "physician factors" have been suggested to influence rates of hysterectomy including physician gender, practice type, and years in practice. Physician gender has been implicated as a factor influencing the hysterectomy rates in a number of studies, but the results have been conflicting, with some studies suggesting male gynecologists overutilize hysterectomy and others suggesting female gynecologists have higher hysterectomy rates. In 1994, a survey of practice patterns of surgeons in North Carolina found that male physicians with a primarily rural practice reported that they were more likely to perform hysterectomy ($P < .001$) than other groups (Bickell et al, 1994). In contrast, a 1996 study of 3-year hospital discharge data from Arizona reported that female gynecologists were more likely than males to perform hysterectomy on patients hospitalized with a hysterectomy-associated diagnosis (Geller et al, 1996). More recently, a survey of over 300,000 insurance claims from New York over a 4-year period found no gender difference in the utilization of hysterectomy or in the type of hysterectomy performed (Gretz et al, 2008a). This survey did find differences in hysterectomy utilization by practice type, however. Gynecologic oncologists were more likely than physicians with a gynecology-only or a general obstetrics and gynecology practice to perform hysterectomies than alternatives to hysterectomies. Additionally, gynecologic oncologists and gynecology-only physicians were more likely to perform a laparoscopic hysterectomy than obstetrician-gynecologists. A number of studies suggest that greater years in practice are associated with higher hysterectomy rates; however, it is unclear if this is the result of changing referral patterns and patient mix as a physician's practice matures or changing attitudes toward hysterectomy. A survey in the 1990s found that gynecologists were more likely to perform hysterectomy at higher rates if they were further from their training, practiced in areas with fewer gynecologists, or had more patients with abnormal bleeding or cancer. In a 2006 survey of the fellows of the American College of Obstetricians and Gynecologists, younger age of the physician and being in an academic practice were significantly associated with decreased choice of hysterectomy for their patients. Other physician factors that may influence hysterectomy rates include training, regional practice patterns, and local insurance mix, although these factors are less well studied.

Indications for Hysterectomy

Broadly speaking, the vast majority of hysterectomies are performed to relieve the symptoms of pain, bleeding, or both. According to current estimates, uterine leiomyomas, uterine prolapse, and endometriosis are the most frequent indications, accounting for as many as 70% of all hysterectomies (Table 3-2). Approximately 10% of hysterectomies in the United States are performed for malignancy. A list of common disease processes for which hysterectomy is appropriate can be found in Table 3-3. As mentioned, age has an important influence on the relative frequency of these indications. In reproductive age women, uterine fibroids and menstrual irregularities are the most common indications. In postmenopausal women, uterine prolapse and premalignant or malignant disease are the most frequent indications. Figure 3-4 demonstrates the cumulative risk of hysterectomy by indication over a woman's lifespan. The rate of hysterectomy by indication has changed somewhat over the last

Table 3-2 Estimated Percentage of Hysterectomies by Diagnosis: United States, 2000–2004

Year	Diagnosis					
	Cancer	**Endometrial Hyperplasia**	**Uterine Leiomyoma**	**Endometriosis**	**Uterine Prolapse**	**Other***
2000	8.9	2.3	44.2	15.3	15.5	13.6
2001	9.2	2.4	39.0	20.1	15.1	14.2
2002	9.2	2.6	41.6	17.8	13.5	15.4
2003	9.2	3.1	39.8	18.3	14.0	15.7
2004	9.4	3.0	38.7	17.1	14.5	17.3
2000–2004: average	9.2	2.7	40.7	17.7	14.5	15.2

*Includes cervical dysplasia and menstrual disorders.
Adapted from Whiteman MK, Hillis SD, Jamieson DJ, et al: Inpatient hysterectomy surveillance in the United States, 2000–2004. Am J Obstet Gynecol 2008;198:34.

Table 3-3 Indications for Hysterectomy

Benign Disease	Malignant Disease
Uterine leiomyomas	Cervical cancer
Excessive menstrual bleeding	Endometrial cancer
Pelvic organ prolapse	Ovarian cancer
Endometriosis	Fallopian tube cancer
Adenomyosis	Gestational trophoblastic tumors
Pelvic inflammatory disease*	Rectal or bladder cancer with uterine involvement
Chronic pelvic pain	
Dysmenorrhea	
Obstetric indications†	
Cervical intraepithelial neoplasia (CIN)‡	
Atypical endometrial hyperplasia	

*Hysterectomy may be indicated in some cases of pelvic inflammatory disease that is refractory to medical management, or for a ruptured or persistent tubo-ovarian abscess. In patients who desire future fertility, unilateral adnexectomy is often adequate, however.
†Hysterectomy may be required for obstetric emergencies such as uterine rupture, hemorrhage, placenta accreta, or endometritis unresponsive to medical management. Hysterectomy also may be necessary in some cases of cornual or cervical ectopic pregnancy and for complications from therapeutic or septic abortions.
‡In general, CIN is treated conservatively, with high success rate. Rarely, hysterectomy may be indicated for cases of CIN III that cannot be completely removed with cervical conization.

Figure 3-4 Prevalence-corrected probability of hysterectomy across the age span in Utah by cause, 1995–1997. (Redrawn from Merrill RM: Prevalence corrected hysterectomy rates and probabilities in Utah. Ann Epidemiol 2001;11:127–135.)

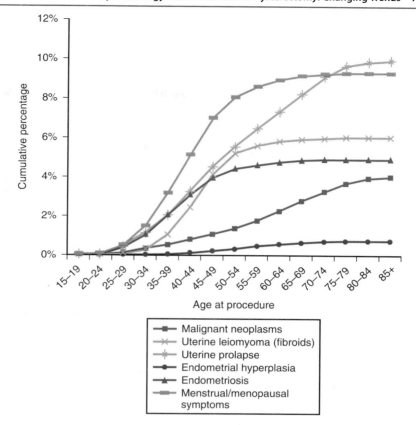

decade. From 1997 to 2005 the rate of hysterectomy for uterine leiomyomas has decreased but the rate for menstrual bleeding, endometriosis, and pain has increased. The decline in the rate of hysterectomy for uterine leiomyomas is likely the result of an increase in nonhysterectomy alternatives for this indication, including uterine fibroid embolization and minimally invasive approaches for myomectomy. It is unclear why there has been an increase in hysterectomies for bleeding, endometriosis, and pain, however.

In general, the following criteria should be met before considering a hysterectomy for benign disease:

1. The patient should have completed childbearing.
2. An adequate trial of medical or nonsurgical management has been attempted, if such a therapy exists.
3. A workup has been performed to rule out nonuterine causes of the patient's symptoms or causes for which a hysterectomy would be inappropriate.
4. If indicated, a workup has been performed to rule out gynecologic malignancy.
5. An appropriate informed consent process has been undertaken that includes a detailed discussion of risks and benefits of hysterectomy and a balanced discussion of hysterectomy alternatives.

A detailed review of each of the indications listed in Table 3-3 is beyond the scope of this chapter; however, certain indications bear further discussion.

Uterine Leiomyomas

Uterine leiomyomas or fibroids are one of the most common conditions affecting women of reproductive age. They account for approximately a third of all hysterectomies. Symptoms attributable to uterine leiomyomas include excessive menstrual bleeding, dysmenorrhea, pelvic pain, and so-called "bulk symptoms," or symptoms related to pressure on adjacent organs such as ureteral obstruction, urinary frequency and urgency, rectal pressure, pelvic pressure, and increasing abdominal girth. Uterine leiomyomas are very common, with some studies estimating that as many as 60% to 80% of women are affected. However, most of affected women never develop symptoms and are unaware of their presence. The development of fibroid symptoms largely depends upon their size, number, and location. Fibroid growth is associated with the presence of estrogen so that they stop growing and often shrink after menopause. One of the few identified risk factors for uterine fibroids is race. The incidence of uterine fibroids among black women is approximately three times that among white women. In addition, uterine fibroids are diagnosed earlier in black women, who are more likely to undergo both hysterectomy and myomectomy for fibroids. Other known risk factors include obesity and low parity. Smoking appears to decrease the risk (presumably from decreased estrogen levels).

In general, hysterectomy should be reserved for those women with symptomatic fibroids who no longer desire fertility. In the past, gynecologists frequently performed hysterectomies on women with fibroids whose uterine size was greater than 12 weeks, even if asymptomatic. The rationale for this choice included avoidance of future symptoms, concern about increased operative morbidity if the uterus continued to enlarge, and the inability to assess the ovaries during routine pelvic examination if an enlarged uterus was present. Evidence to support this rationale is lacking. Today, hysterectomy in asymptomatic women with uterine fibroids is rarely indicated regardless of uterine size. Exceptions include ureteral obstruction and signs suggesting the possibility of uterine leiomyosarcoma, such as rapid uterine growth or growth after menopause. In postmenopausal women not taking exogenous estrogen, uterine enlargement suggests the possibility of malignancy and hysterectomy is often indicated. In premenopausal women, leiomyosarcoma is exceedingly rare, even in the presence of rapid uterine growth. In one study of women undergoing hysterectomy for rapid uterine growth, the incidence of uterine sarcoma was only 0.27%, bringing this indication for hysterectomy into question (Parker et al, 1994).

Hysterectomy should be considered in a woman with symptomatic uterine fibroids who no longer desires fertility, particularly if the severity of symptoms is such that they interfere with her daily life. Prior to proceeding with a hysterectomy, other sources for the patient's symptoms should be ruled out. Women with excessive or irregular menstrual bleeding should be evaluated with endometrial sampling, hysteroscopy, or ultrasound. In those with fibroids and pelvic pain, other sources of the pain should be ruled out, including other gynecologic diseases and urologic, gastrointestinal, and musculoskeletal disorders. Although many advocate a trial of medical management before proceeding with hysterectomy, the evidence supporting this requirement is lacking in women with uterine fibroids. In spite of this, a trial of medical management is often prudent prior to considering hysterectomy because of hysterectomy's definitive nature and associated risks.

Alternatives to hysterectomy that should be discussed in women with symptomatic fibroids include myomectomy, which can be performed hysteroscopically, laparoscopically, and abdominally, and uterine fibroid embolization (see Chapter 12 for detailed discussion). The need for subsequent hysterectomy after myomectomy because of persistent or recurrent symptoms is 0.5% to 12%, and the need for subsequent medical therapy ranges from 4% to 76%, depending upon the technique and length of follow-up. Myomectomy has the obvious advantage of allowing future fertility. Uterine embolization for fibroids was first reported in 1995. A recent study comparing uterine fibroid embolization to hysterectomy found marked improvement in symptoms and quality of life in both groups. Even though hysterectomy resulted in an elimination of bleeding symptoms, those who underwent embolization noted a 61% reduction in bleeding and 48% reduction in uterine size (Volkers et al, 2007). Hysterectomy also demonstrated an advantage in improving pelvic pain, but had a higher long-term complication rate. Uterine fibroid embolization is not recommended for those who desire future fertility. The use of gonadotropin-releasing hormone (GnRH) agonists is not a viable long-term treatment option for uterine fibroids in most women because of fibroid regrowth after treatment cessation and the long-term risks of estrogen deficiency. However, the use of GnRH agonists in perimenopausal women with symptomatic fibroids until they reach menopause has been effective.

Excessive Uterine Bleeding

Excessive uterine bleeding accounts for approximately 20% of hysterectomies. This condition can be broadly classified into *menorrhagia*, or heavy menses that is cyclic and presumed to be ovulatory, and *metrorrhagia*, or intermenstrual bleeding that is noncyclic and presumed to be associated with an ovulatory disturbance. The term "dysfunctional uterine bleeding" refers to abnormal uterine bleeding in which anatomic causes have been ruled out. This term has largely fallen out of favor because of its nonspecificity. Common causes of menorrhagia include leiomyomas, adenomyosis, and coagulaopathy. Menorrhagia without an anatomic abnormality such as a fibroid or polyp may be related to local production of vasoactive prostanoids; nonsteroidal anti-inflammatory agents have been shown to be effective therapy. Common causes of metrorrhagia include anovulation, endometrial polyps, and leiomyomas. Other causes of abnormal uterine bleeding include pregnancy, gynecologic malignancy, pelvic infection, endometrial hyperplasia, and trauma. In the evaluation of excessive bleeding, underlying causes are sought by endometrial sampling, hysteroscopy, and/or ultrasound. Evaluation for coagulopathy should also be considered. Treatment is indicated when anemia is present or the bleeding interferes with the patient's quality of life. In cases in which the uterine cavity is normal and malignancy has been ruled out, medical management consisting of oral contraceptives, cyclic progestins, a levonorgesterel-releasing intrauterine system, or cyclic nonsteroidal anti-inflammatory drugs is usually effective. Hysterectomy is indicated only in women who do not desire fertility and have failed medical management. Endometrial ablation is an alternative to hysterectomy in this situation and is effective in reducing excessive bleeding in 70% to 90% of patients. However, amenorrhea occurs in only 45% and recurrent excessive bleeding occurs in 15% to 25% of cases. Approximately 9% to 34% of patients who receive endometrial ablation will undergo subsequent hysterectomy.

Pelvic Organ Prolapse

Surgical management of pelvic organ prolapse (POP) accounts for approximately 15% to 18% of hysterectomies in the United States. Symptoms associated with POP include pelvic pressure, vaginal bulging, urinary incontinence, voiding dysfunction, fecal incontinence, defecatory dysfunction, and sexual dysfunction. Surgery is considered in patients with symptomatic prolapse who will not use or have failed in using a pessary. In patients who are asymptomatic or are minimally bothered, surgery is rarely indicated regardless of the extent of the prolapse. The annual incidence of surgery for POP is between 1.5 and 4.9 cases per 1000 women-years. A women's lifetime risk of surgery for prolapse by age 80 years is approximately 7%. The peak incidence of POP surgery occurs in women aged 60 to 69 years (42.1 per 10,000 women). However, almost 58% of procedures are performed in women under the age of 60 years.

Generally, a hysterectomy is indicated at the time of surgical correction of prolapse when uterine prolapse is present. However, there are an increasing number of options for uterine preservation in women with uterovaginal prolapse. Uterine prolapse is typically not an isolated event and is often associated with other pelvic support defects. A hysterectomy alone is almost never adequate treatment for prolapse; typically, associated surgical repairs are necessary. Even in the rare cases of isolated uterine prolapse, a vaginal vault suspension of some type is required. In cases of isolated anterior or posterior vaginal wall prolapse when the uterus is well supported, a hysterectomy is often unnecessary. Studies have also demonstrated that a hysterectomy is unnecessary at the time of Burch colposuspension for treatment of stress urinary incontinence, unless uterine prolapse is also present. In patients with symptomatic uterine prolapse who still desire fertility or otherwise desire uterine preservation, options include use of a pessary or a uterine suspension procedure such as sacral hysteropexy, sacrospinous hysteropexy, or one of several commercially available vaginal mesh procedures.

Chronic Pelvic Pain

Chronic pelvic pain is a complex condition with multiple causes. The evaluation of chronic pelvic pain should include an evaluation for urologic, gastrointestinal, musculoskeletal, psychological, and gynecologic sources of the pain. Depression is common in these patients regardless of the cause. The prevalence of sexual abuse in this population maybe as high as 60%. A multidisciplinary approach to management is necessary for these patients, addressing somatic, psychological, and social issues as well as sleep disturbance and other factors. Hysterectomy should be performed only for chronic pelvic pain in those patients whose pain is of uterine origin and does not respond to nonsurgical management. See Chapter 5 for further discussion of the indications and outcomes of hysterectomy for treatment of chronic pelvic pain.

Endometriosis

Endometriosis is a common gynecologic source of chronic pelvic pain, dysmenorrhea, and dyspareunia. Diagnostic laparoscopy is necessary to diagnose endometriosis; however, some advocate a trial of medical management in those patients with pelvic pain suspected of having endometriosis without definitive laparoscopic diagnosis. Effective medical treatments for pelvic pain resulting from endometriosis include oral contraceptive pills, oral or depot progestins, the levonorgesterel-releasing intrauterine system, danazol, and GnRH agonists. Conservative surgical treatment of endometriosis involves excision or ablation of endometriotic implants, typically by laparoscopy. Hysterectomy should be considered in patients with pelvic pain from endometriosis only if fertility is no longer desired and medical and conservative surgical therapy has proved inadequate. An oophorectomy is often recommended at the time of hysterectomy for endometriosis. Approximately 20% of hysterectomies in reproductive age women are performed for pelvic pain resulting from endometriosis. See Chapter 5 for the expected outcomes after hysterectomy for endometriosis. Further discussion of the role of oophorectomy in these patients is found in Chapter 9.

Dysmenorrhea

Dysmenorrhea, or painful menses, can be idiopathic (primary dysmenorrhea) or the result of an identified underlying condition (secondary dysmenorrhea.) Conditions known to cause secondary dysmenorrhea include endometriosis, adenomyosis, and uterine leiomyomas. Typically, dysmenorrhea can be adequately treated with nonsteroidal anti-inflammatory drugs alone or in combination with oral contraceptives or other hormonal agents such as cyclic progestins and the levonorgesterel-releasing intrauterine system. A hysterectomy is indicated for intractable dysmenorrhea refractory to medical management only in patients who no longer desire fertility.

SUMMARY: Over the last four decades, the rate of hysterectomy in the United States has slowly declined. In spite of this, it still remains the second most common major surgical operation performed on women. This decline in hysterectomy rates is likely due to changing patient and physician attitudes toward hysterectomy and to an increasing number of effective nonhysterectomy alternatives. However, hysterectomy remains a highly effective treatment for many gynecologic conditions when alternatives have failed. The most common indications for hysterectomy in premenopausal women are uterine leiomyomas and menstrual disturbances, although the rates of hysterectomy for leiomyomas have declined somewhat. In postmenopausal women, uterine prolapse and premalignant or malignant disease are the most frequent indications. There is wide variation in rates of hysterectomy between and within countries and a number of nonmedical factors appear to affect hysterectomy rates, including patient socioeconomic and physician factors. More research is necessary to fully understand the cause of these variations.

Suggested Reading

Babalola EO, Bharucha AE, Schleck CD, et al: Decreasing utilization of hysterectomy: A population-based study in Olmsted county, Minnesota, 1965–2002. Am J Obstet Gynecol 2007;196:214.

Bickell NA, Earp JA, Garrett JM, et al: Gynecologists' sex, clinical beliefs and hysterectomy rates. Am J Public Health 1994;84:1649–1652.

Carlson KJ, Nichols DH, Schiff I: Current concepts: Indications for hysterectomy. N Engl J Med 1993;328:856–860.

Cooper R, Lawlor DA, Hardy R: Socio-economic position across the life course and hysterectomy in three British cohorts: A cross-cohort comparative study. Br J Obstet Gynaecol 2005;112(8): 1126–1133.

Cooper R, Lucke J, Lawlor DA, et al: Socioeconomic position and hysterectomy: A cross-cohort comparison of women in Australia and Great Britain. J Epidemiol Community Health 2008;62(12): 1057–1063.

Geller SE, Burns LR, Brailer DJ: The impact of nonclinical factors on practice variations: case of hysterectomies. Health Serv Res 1996;30:729–750.

Gretz H, Bradley WH, Zakashansky K, et al: Effect of physician gender and specialty on utilization of hysterectomy in New York, 2001–2005. Am J Obstet Gynecol 2008a;199:347.

Gretz H, Bradley WH, Zakashansky K, et al: Patient clinical factors influencing use of hysterectomy in New York, 2001–2005. Am J Obstet Gynecol 2008b;199:349.

Jacobson GF, Shaber RE, Armstrong MA, Hung Y: Hysterectomy rates for benign indications. Obstet Gynecol 2006;107:1278–1283.

Jelvosek JE, Maher C, Barber MD: Seminar on pelvic organ prolapse. Lancet 2007;369:1027–1038.

Merrill RM: Prevalence corrected hysterectomy rates and probabilities in Utah. Ann Epidemiol 2001;11:127–135.

Merrill RM: Hysterectomy surveillance in the United States, 1997 through 2005. Med Sci Monit 2008;14:CR24–CR31.

Myers ER, Barber MD, Couchman GM, et al: Management of Uterine Fibroids. Evidence Report/ Technology Assessment. (Prepared by Duke University under Contract No. 290-97-0014., Task Order 4.) Agency for Healthcare Research and Quality, 2001.

Parker WH, Fu YS, Berek JS: Uterine sarcoma in patients operated on for presumed leiomyoma and rapidly growing leiomyoma. Obstet Gynecol 1994;83:414–418.

Spilsbury K, Semens JB, Hammond I, Bolck A: Persistent high rates of hysterectomy in Western Australia: A population-based study of 83,000 procedures over 23 years. Br J Obstet Gynaecol 2006;113:804–809.

Volkers NA, Hehenkamp WJK, Birnie E, et al: Uterine artery embolization versus hysterectomy in the treatment of uterine fibroids: 2 year's outcomes from the randomized EMMY trial. Am J Obstet Gynecol 2007;196:519e.1–519e.11.

Whiteman MK, Hillis SD, Jamieson DJ, et al: Inpatient hysterectomy surveillance in the United States, 2000–2004. Am J Obstet Gynecol 2008;198:34.

Wu JM, Wechter ME, Geller EJ, et al: Hysterectomy rates in the United States, 2003. Obstet Gynecol 2007;110:1091–1095.

Preoperative and Perioperative Considerations and Choosing the Route of Hysterectomy

Mark D. Walters M.D.
Tommaso Falcone M.D.

The indications for hysterectomy for benign disease in 2005 changed little over the past decade, with uterine leiomyomata (33%) and menstrual disorders (17%) being the most common, followed by uterine prolapse (13%) and endometriosis (9%) (www.hcupnet.ahrq.gov, 2007). Alternatives to hysterectomy are generally available and should be discussed with the patient. However, once the decision to perform a hysterectomy has been made, the type and route of hysterectomy must be chosen, and efforts must be made to accomplish the surgery as safely as possible. Hysterectomy can be performed vaginally, abdominally, or with laparoscopic or robotic assistance. The Nationwide In-Patient Sample of the Healthcare Cost and Utilization Project reported 538,722 hysterectomies for benign disease in 2003 (www.hcupnet.ahrq.gov, 2007; Wu et al, 2007). An analysis of these United States data showed that abdominal (total and subtotal) hysterectomy was performed in 66.1% of cases, followed by vaginal route in 21.8% of cases and laparoscopic route in 11.8% (Wu et al, 2007). By region of the country, the South has the highest hysterectomy rate and the Northeast has the lowest. The percentage of laparoscopic procedures is similar across all regions (Wu et al, 2007).

This chapter will review considerations in the pre- and perioperative assessment and planning of hysterectomy and will discuss the issues and evidence for choosing the best route of hysterectomy for the patient.

General Preoperative Considerations

Preoperative Health Assessment

Preoperative health assessment is critical for optimal surgical outcome. The preoperative health assessment for hysterectomy should include a complete evaluation of the patient's health status by a complete history and physical examination. There is no routinely recommended imaging, blood tests, or other tests such as electrocardiogram (ECG). These tests should be ordered on the basis of the patient's underlying medical problem. This choice might include ordering a serum creatinine in patients with diabetes or hypertension or an ECG in patients with a history of heart disease. In certain cases, the preoperative evaluation identifies medical conditions that are unstable enough to adversely affect the postoperative outcome, and appropriate referral for medical management can be made (Johnson and Porter, 2008). Individual hospitals may have their own requirements for assessment before surgical intervention that may be age-adjusted.

Careful assessment of prescription and nonprescription drugs is important. Nonsteroidal anti-inflammatory drugs (NSAIDs), including aspirin, have antiplatelet effects due to inhibition of cyclooxygenase with decreased thromboxane A_2 production. These drugs should be discontinued before surgery by at least 7 days, or four to five times the drug half-life to diminish the risk of intraoperative bleeding. Vitamin E should be discontinued 10 to 14 days before surgery, also because of concern for the risks of bleeding. If iron deficiency anemia is diagnosed before surgery, intraoperative or postoperative blood product use can be minimized with preoperative treatment with iron supplementation or use of menstrual cycle suppressive therapy, such as continuous oral contraceptives or gonadotropin-releasing hormone (GnRH) agonists, that help restore normal hemoglobin levels. The use of GnRH agonists should also be considered if their use will convert an abdominal procedure to a vaginal or laparoscopic one. The potential for blood transfusion or use of blood products should be discussed with the patient and their refusal documented. If excessive blood loss is expected, intraoperative blood salvage techniques and autologous blood donation should be considered.

Women taking contraceptives or hormone replacement therapy are at increased risk for venous thromboembolic events after hysterectomy. In general, contraceptives should be stopped 4 to 6 weeks before hysterectomy, although this may be difficult in women with anemia and severe menorrhagia (ACOG Practice Bulletin No. 84, 2007). There are no studies on the possible reduction of thromboembolic events with discontinuation of hormone replacement therapy before hysterectomy. This decision to discontinue hormone replacement therapy should then be based on the overall risk to the patient for a venous thromboembolic event. Stress dose steroids may be necessary for patients on chronic corticosteroids. Some medications, such as β-blockers, should be continued on the day of surgery.

Preoperative Testing

A recent normal Papanicolaou (Pap) smear should be documented before hysterectomy. Sampling of the endometrium or pelvic ultrasound should be considered in patients who are at risk for a malignancy, such as women with postmenopausal bleeding and polycystic ovary syndrome. Based on age alone, it is generally recommended that women over 39 years of age with persistent anovulatory bleeding have an endometrial assessment after excluding pregnancy. Some guidelines suggest this cutoff should be age 35 (ACOG Practice Bulletin No. 14, 2000). Pelvic pain should be thoroughly investigated before hysterectomy is considered; alternative treatments should be discussed that include a wide range of medical suppressive therapy, physical therapy, and possible assessment by pain management specialists. If a pelvic mass is palpated on pelvic examination, a transvaginal ultrasound examination should be performed. No other imaging has been shown to be superior (ACOG Practice Bulletin No. 83, 2007). If there is a suspicious mass on transvaginal ultrasound examination, appropriate consultation with a gynecologic oncologist is recommended before surgery. Uterine prolapse is often accompanied by other pelvic floor disorders, such as urinary and fecal incontinence. These problems need

Table 4-1 Preoperative Evaluation and Documentation before Hysterectomy

- Obtain informed consent regarding options, risks, benefits, outcomes, and personnel involved
- Document completion of childbearing
- Document that an adequate trial of medical or nonsurgical management has been offered and attempted or refused (informed refusal)
- Document explanation to patient of risks and benefits of prophylactic oophorectomy
- Ascertain health status of the patient
- Determine need for imaging or testing
- Assess need for medical consultation
- Estimate potential blood loss and assess need for correction of preoperative anemia
- Assess need for autologous blood products or other intraoperative measures
- Review most recent cervical cytology findings and need for further gynecologic investigation such as endometrial assessment

Table 4-2 Perioperative Measures

Prophylactic antibiotics initiated within 1 hour before incision
Use of first- or second-generation cephalosporin
Discontinuing prophylactic antibiotics within 24 hours after surgery
Prophylaxis for venous thromboembolic events
Potential maintenance of β-blocker regimen
Strict glycemic control
Surgical time-out

to be assessed preoperatively and, if appropriate, corrected at the time of hysterectomy.

Informed Consent

Informed consent for hysterectomy should be methodical; it is a process rather than a single event. Multiple factors need to be documented in the medical record, including whether the patient has completed childbearing (Table 4-1). The route of hysterectomy should be discussed with the general concept that conversion from a laparoscopic or vaginal approach to laparotomy, if necessary, may be required to safely carry out the intended procedure.

Perioperative Considerations

Pregnancy should be ruled out in all reproductive-aged women on the day of surgery. Attention to perioperative details (Table 4-2) such as prophylactic antibiotics and prevention of venous thromboembolic events are important to ensure a safe outcome. The most important perioperative management protocols involve the use and timing of prophylactic antibiotics to decrease the risk of surgical site infections and treatments or maneuvers for the prevention of venous thromboembolic events. Other factors, such as maintenance of β-blockade and glycemic control are important (Mahid et al, 2008). A careful general medical risk assessment should be done. Mahid and associates found that, in addition to factors in Table 4-2, impaired functional status, American Society of Anesthesiologists (ASA) class 4 or 5, and hypothermia ($<96°$ C) on arrival to the postanesthesia care unit (PACU) were statistically of clinical importance in predicting risks of morbidity and mortality. Smoking cessation should be urged in all patients ideally 6 to 8 weeks before surgery.

Prophylactic Antibiotics

The time of administration of the antibiotic is critical to lowering the frequency of surgical site infection (Classen et al, 1992; Bratzler and Houck, 2004). The antibiotic should be given preoperatively to achieve minimal inhibitory concentrations (MICs) in the skin and tissues by the time the incision is made. This typically means an intravenous injection within 60 minutes of incision with a first- (cefazolin) or second- (cefoxitin) generation cephalosporin (Bratzler and Houck, 2004). These antibiotics were chosen because the likely site infection pathogens for hysterectomies are gram-negative bacilli, enterococci, group B streptococci, and anaerobes. If the patient is allergic to cephalosporins, metronidazole 500 mg intravenously is recommended. These guidelines also recommend discontinuing prophylactic antibiotics within 24 hours after the operation. Longer procedures require re-dosing; the recommending interval for cefazolin is 3 to 5 hours and for cefoxitin 2 to 3 hours (Bratzler and Houck, 2004).

Recent guidelines from the American Heart Association have recommended that administration of antibiotics solely to prevent endocarditis in patients undergoing a genitourinary procedure be abandoned except in the most severe circumstances (Wilson et al, 2007).

Prevention for Venous Thromboembolic Events

It is important to assess the patient for her risk of venous thromboembolic events before surgery. Conditions that place a patient at higher risk are listed in Table 4-3.

Postoperative bed rest in the hospital or at home places the patient at increased risk of venous thromboembolic event. In general, all patients undergoing hysterectomy require a prevention strategy and, by definition, are at moderate risk (ACOG Practice Bulletin No. 84, 2007). In these patients, low-dose unfractionated heparin (5000 units every 12 hours) or low-molecular-weight heparin (e.g., enoxaparin 40 mg or 2500 units of dalteparin daily) or intermittent pneumatic compression device is recommended. Either form of heparin should be started 2 hours before surgery, and the compression stockings are placed on the patient in the operating room before incision. These

Table 4-3 Risk Factors for Venous Thromboembolic Events after Hysterectomy

Increasing age
Immobility, paresis
Underlying diagnosis for hysterectomy
    Cancer
    Cancer treatment (hormonal therapies, chemotherapy, radiotherapy)
Medical history or illness
    Cardiac or pulmonary failure
    Previous venous thromboembolic event
    Inherited or acquired thrombophilias
    Nephrotic syndrome
    Myeloproliferative disorders
    Other medical disorders
Lifestyle and related factors
    Obesity
    Smoking
Varicose veins
Medication
    Estrogen or selective estrogen receptor modulators
    Oral contraceptives
    Hormone replacement therapy

treatment approaches should be continued until the patient is ambulatory. Patients over 40 years of age and those under 40 years of age who have risk factors (such as obesity) require a similar approach, with some modification in the unfractionated heparin (5000 units every 8 hours) or low-molecular-weight heparin (5000 units dalteparin or similar enoxaparin 40 mg daily). In patients who are over 60 years of age and have significant risk factors, such as previous venous thromboembolic event, malignancy, or hypercoagulable state, unfractionated heparin (5000 units every 8 hours) or low-molecular-weight heparin (5000 units dalteparin or enoxaparin 40 mg daily) and intermittent pneumatic compression devices should be used. Patients on oral contraceptives up to the time of hysterectomy should be considered for heparin therapy (ACOG Practice Bulletin No. 84, 2007). In high-risk patients, prophylaxis may be needed after discharge for several weeks.

Other Preventive Strategies

The surgical time-out is a useful process for determination of correct procedure and site. Its observation is an accepted quality parameter for surgery (Altpeter et al, 2007).

The value of a mechanical bowel preparation for prevention of infectious complications of an intraoperative bowel leak or for reducing the rates of anastomotic leak if bowel surgery is performed has been challenged in a meta-analysis (Guenaga et al, 2003). Therefore, it does not seem necessary to "bowel prep" all patients undergoing a hysterectomy for benign disease solely in case of an inadvertent enterotomy.

Choosing the Route of Hysterectomy

The choice of hysterectomy route should be individualized to the patient and the indication of surgery. Important factors in this choice are the extent of gynecologic disease and the need to perform concomitant procedures; relative risks and benefits of each type of hysterectomy; patient preferences; and the surgeon's competence, preference, and available support facilities. In choosing the route of hysterectomy, the surgeon should consider the following questions:

What is the best access to appropriately treat the disease that requires the hysterectomy?

What is the safest route for the patient? Which technique is associated with the lowest risk of complication?

Do concurrent or special procedures need to be performed, and what is the best access for them?

What technique will allow the patient the fastest recovery from surgery?

Does the informed patient have a preference for hysterectomy approach?

Gynecologic Factors That Influence the Route of Hysterectomy

The route of uterine removal should largely be determined by factors shown in Table 4-4. Because of its well-documented advantages and relatively lower complication rates, vaginal hysterectomy should be the approach of choice when feasible. Factors that impair vaginal access to the uterus and make vaginal hysterectomy difficult include a narrow pubic arch (angle < 90 degrees),

Table 4-4 Factors Influencing Choice of Route of Hysterectomy for Benign Disease

Vaginal shape and accessibility to the uterus
Uterine size and shape
Extent of extrauterine disease, need for concurrent procedures, and other clinical factors*
Surgeon competence and available support facilities
Preference of the informed patient

*Examples are accessibility of laparoscopy or laparotomy, as with previous abdominoplasty or hernia repair; anesthesia issues; and morbid obesity.

a narrow vagina (narrower than two fingerbreadths, especially at the apex), and an undescended immobile uterus. When one or more of these factors are present, the laparoscopic or abdominal route should be considered. In spite of its frequent mention, nulliparity and previous cesarean sections in and of themselves are not contraindications to the vaginal route. Many nulliparous women and women who have not delivered vaginally have adequate vaginal caliber to allow successful completion of the vaginal hysterectomy (Le Tohic et al, 2008). Even in the case of minimal uterine descent, if the upper vagina allows adequate access for transection of the uterosacral and cardinal ligaments, uterine mobility will improve, making the remainder of the vaginal hysterectomy easier to accomplish. For such borderline cases, the surgeon should pay careful attention to patient positioning, lighting, and surgical assistance to optimize the chance of a successful vaginal hysterectomy. The patient should be counseled that a laparotomy or laparoscopy may be necessary to complete the hysterectomy if vaginal removal is not possible.

When vaginal access is adequate and the uterus is enlarged, vaginal hysterectomy can often be accomplished safely using uterine size reduction techniques such as wedge morcellation, uterine bisection, and intramyometrial coring. A randomized trial comparing the vaginal to the abdominal route for women with enlarged uteri (200 to 1300 g) demonstrated decreased operating time, febrile morbidity, postoperative narcotic use, and hospital stay for those who receive vaginal hysterectomy (with or without morcellation) compared to total abdominal hysterectomy (Benassi et al, 2002). When considering whether to perform a vaginal hysterectomy in a woman with an enlarged uterus, uterine shape is often more important than actual size. Before beginning any morcellation procedure the uterine vessels must be ligated bilaterally and the peritoneal cavity should be entered both anteriorly and posteriorly. If the cervix or lower uterine segment is enlarged or contains fibroids that prevent uterine artery ligation or entry into the peritoneal cavity, then the procedure should not be performed vaginally, regardless of size. In contrast, if the lower uterine segment is accessible surgically, then even very large uteri (up to 20-week size) can be removed transvaginally by an appropriately skilled surgeon. Although the upper limit of uterine size for which a vaginal hysterectomy should be done has not been established, most surgeons would consider 16- to 18-week size as a reasonable and practical upper limit.

Dorsey et al (1995) observed that the practice style and personal preferences of surgeons probably play a significant role in selection of hysterectomy type. Thus, it is possible that, with appropriate evidence-based treatment guidelines and adequate surgical education and skill, the proportion of hysterectomies performed vaginally can be increased (Davies et al, 1998; Kovac, 2000). Kovac and associates (2002) studied the effect of adopting published guidelines for choosing the route of hysterectomy in a resident clinic population. They found that resident physicians who followed the guidelines increased the proportion

Figure 4-1 Algorithm for determining the route of hysterectomy. (Adapted from Kovac SR: Clinical opinion: Guidelines for hysterectomy. Am J Obstet Gynecol 2004;191:635–640.)

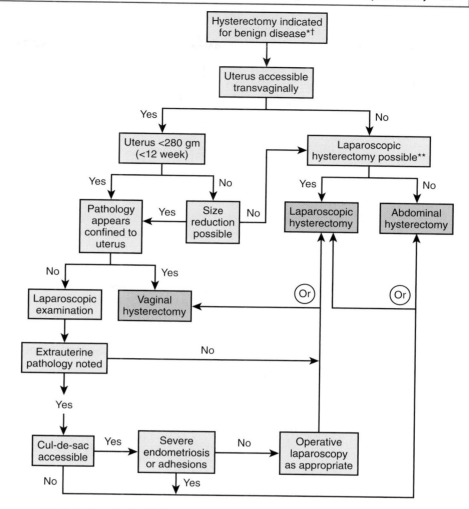

* Failed all medical and alternative options.
† Assumption is made that any prophylactic oophorectomy for normal ovaries will follow the route of hysterectomy.
** Surgeon skill, equipment, facilities available; abdomen accessible for laparoscopic access; general anesthesia possible.

of hysterectomies performed vaginally to over 90% and reduced the ratio of abdominal to vaginal hysterectomy from 3:1 to 1:11. Use of uterine morcellation and other sophisticated, uterine-size-reduction techniques were necessary in only 11% of cases (Kovac et al, 2002). Kovac (2000) has shown that application of evidence-based guidelines on route of hysterectomy could increase the percentage of vaginal hysterectomies done, and thus would lower the rate of complications and be cost-saving. Figure 4-1 illustrates a proposed clinical algorithm to help determine the most appropriate route of hysterectomy.

The presence of disease outside the uterus, such as adnexal disease, obliterated cul-de-sac, severe endometriosis, or severe pelvic adhesions, usually precludes vaginal hysterectomy. In these cases, the abdominal or laparoscopic approach is preferred. When visualization of the pelvis or abdomen is required for diagnosis, such as with ovarian masses or chronic pelvic pain, the vaginal route may not be appropriate initially. However, such cases might benefit from a diagnostic or operative laparoscopy followed by a vaginal hysterectomy. In 1990, Stovall and associates reported on 46 patients in whom intraoperative laparoscopy was used to evaluate pelvic pain and disease after they had been advised to have an abdominal hysterectomy. The authors found that, in general, uterine size and adnexal disease had been overestimated and uterine mobility underestimated. In 91% of patients, vaginal hysterectomy was performed successfully at the same setting as the laparoscopy (Stovall et al, 1990).

Operative laparoscopy to complete all or part of the hysterectomy is used in approximately 12% of hysterectomies in the United States today (Wu et al, 2007). There still remains considerable debate about the appropriate indications for the various types of laparoscopic hysterectomies. Randomized trials have demonstrated that, compared with vaginal hysterectomy, laparoscopic hysterectomy has a longer operating time and greater cost with similar complication rates and postoperative recovery (Garry et al, 2004). Therefore, unless unique circumstances dictate the use of a laparoscope, laparoscopic hysterectomy has no advantages over vaginal hysterectomy. It should instead be considered an alternative to abdominal hysterectomy for those patients in whom a vaginal hysterectomy is not indicated or is deemed not feasible. Randomized trials comparing laparoscopic hysterectomy to abdominal hysterectomy generally demonstrate a longer operating time and perhaps slightly higher risk of lower urinary tract injury, but less blood loss, fewer wound infections, fewer febrile episodes, a more rapid postoperative recovery, and an earlier return to work for those who receive the laparoscopic surgery (Johnson et al, 2006). Circumstances in which the laparoscopic approach may be helpful include hysterectomy in a patient with documented endometriosis, chronic pelvic pain, known pelvic adhesive disease, or a concurrent benign adnexal mass that requires removal. Laparoscopic hysterectomy is particularly useful in patients with limited vaginal access and in those women who desire a subtotal (supracervical) hysterectomy. For enlarged uteri, no studies have yet compared the use of laparoscopic hysterectomy with morcellation compared to vaginal hysterectomy with morcellation.

Experience with the surgical robot to assist in hysterectomy is limited at this time. Surgical times are generally longer and costs greater than with conventional hysterectomies, and a significant learning curve exists. More data are necessary to determine its actual place in the performance of hysterectomy. This topic is discussed in greater depth in Chapter 10.

Complication Rates and Cost Considerations

The choice of hysterectomy route should be strongly influenced by complication rates as reported in the literature. In 1982, the Centers for Disease Control (CDC) published one of the largest studies evaluating differences in complications between vaginal and abdominal hysterectomies. The study included 1851 patients aged 15 to 44 years in whom hysterectomy was performed for benign gynecologic disorders. In this study, the odds of one or more complication after abdominal hysterectomy was 1.7 times that of vaginal hysterectomy. The rate of febrile morbidity was 1.9 times higher and the risk of transfusion was 2.1 times higher for the abdominal than the vaginal route (Dicker et al, 1982).

In 2004, the eVALuate study consisted of two parallel randomized trials, one comparing laparoscopic with abdominal hysterectomy, the other comparing laparoscopic with vaginal hysterectomy (Garry et al, 2004). This study showed that, compared with abdominal hysterectomy, laparoscopic hysterectomy took longer to perform, but was associated with less pain, quicker recovery, and better short-term quality of life. In addition, laparoscopic hysterectomy was associated with a significantly higher rate of major complications compared with abdominal hysterectomy. In the trial comparing vaginal hysterectomy

Table 4-5 Comparison of Different Approaches to Hysterectomy

Vaginal Hysterectomy		Laparoscopic Hysterectomy
Versus Abdominal Hysterectomy	**Versus Laparoscopic Hysterectomy**	**Versus Abdominal Hysterectomy**
Shorter duration of hospital stay Faster return to normal activity Decreased postoperative febrile morbidity	Shorter operating time	Faster postoperative recovery and return to normal activity Shorter duration of hospital stay Lower intraoperative blood loss/smaller drop in hemoglobin level Decreased postoperative febrile morbidity Fewer wound or abdominal wall infections Longer operating time Higher rate of lower urinary tract (bladder and ureter) injuries

Adapted from Johnson N, Barlow D, Lethaby, et al: Surgical approach to hysterectomy for benign gynecological disease. Cochrane Database Syst Rev 2006;CD003677.

with laparoscopic hysterectomy, vaginal hysterectomy took less time, but had a similar overall rate of complications. All three procedures were associated with improvements in physical and mental quality-of-life measures, body image scale, and aspects of sexual activity at 4 and 12 months after hysterectomy, with few differences among routes of hysterectomy (Garry et al, 2004).

A recent Cochrane review validated the perception that vaginal hysterectomy is the surgical route of choice for hysterectomy (Johnson et al, 2006). This review included 3643 patients from 27 randomized trials. It compared abdominal hysterectomy with vaginal hysterectomy and three types of laparoscopic hysterectomies. Laparoscopic hysterectomy was reported on the basis of how much of the procedure is done laparoscopically: (1) uterine artery ligated laparoscopically and vaginal cuff closed laparoscopically, (2) uterine artery ligated laparoscopically but vaginal vault sutured vaginally, and (3) uterine artery ligated vaginally and vaginal cuff sutured vaginally. Table 4-5 lists the observations of the systematic review (Johnson et al, 2006). The report concluded that there are improved outcomes with vaginal hysterectomy and, when vaginal access is not possible, laparoscopic hysterectomy has advantages over abdominal hysterectomy in certain clinical situations, but with higher rates of some complications.

Cost analysis trials consistently demonstrate that vaginal hysterectomy is the most cost-effective route (Dorsey et al, 1996; Schulpher et al, 2004). Laparoscopic hysterectomy can be cost-effective relative to abdominal procedure (Falcone et al, 1999), but the difference is more finely balanced and may vary somewhat among different surgeons, health systems, and countries and depend on the perspective (e.g., societal vs. institutional) used in analysis (Schulpher et al, 2004). The main cost determinants are the length of hospital stay, operating room time, and the use of disposal surgical devices (Dorsey et al, 1996).

Prophylactic Oophorectomy and Other Considerations during Hysterectomy

The choice of when to perform prophylactic oophorectomy at the time of hysterectomy should be based on patient age, risk factors, and her informed wishes rather than the route of hysterectomy (ACOG Practice Bulletin No. 89, 2008). However, in practice, Keshavarz and associates (2002) showed that the rate of prophylactic oophorectomy was four times higher with an abdominal approach compared with a vaginal one. Ideally, the same factors should influence the decision of whether an oophorectomy is appropriate or not independent of whether the hysterectomy is abdominal, laparoscopic, or vaginal. Surgeons also ideally would be able to perform oophorectomy with equal facility by any approach. One standard proved technique of vaginal oophorectomy that is applicable in most cases was described by Ballard and Walters (1996). Patients who are candidates for vaginal hysterectomy and who desire prophylactic oophorectomy based on their risk profile and informed wishes should be counseled that vaginal oophorectomy is possible in a majority of cases (Ballard and Walters, 1996) but that laparoscopy or mini-laparotomy may be necessary to complete the oophorectomy. A randomized trial of vaginal hysterectomy with bilateral oophorectomy versus laparoscopic-assisted vaginal hysterectomy with bilateral oophorectomy (LAVHO) for women having vaginal hysterectomy and prophylactic oophorectomy showed more complications and longer operating time in the LAVHO group without an offsetting advantage in rate of oophorectomy (Agostini et al, 2006). Thus, the *routine* use of laparoscopic assistance at vaginal hysterectomy for this indication is not supported by evidence, but occasionally may be necessary based on patient characteristics and the surgeon's skill level and familiarity with vaginal oophorectomy. This issue is discussed in more detail in Chapter 9.

Special surgical considerations related to the patient's pathology or preferences occasionally influence the route of hysterectomy. An example of this includes the patient's or surgeon's choice of supracervical hysterectomy dictating that an abdominal or laparoscopic/robotic route be chosen, even when a vaginal hysterectomy technically could have been done. Finally, informed patients may request a certain type and route of hysterectomy, even when several options exist (ACOG Committee Opinion No. 395).

Selected Readings

ACOG Practice Bulletin No. 14. Management of anovulatory bleeding. The American College of Obstetricians and Gynecologists, March, 2000.

ACOG Practice Bulletin No. 83. Management of adnexal masses. The American College of Obstetricians and Gynecologists. Obstet Gynecol 2007;110:201–214.

ACOG Practice Bulletin No. 84. Prevention of deep vein thrombosis and pulmonary embolism. The American College of Obstetricians and Gynecologists. Obstet Gynecol 2007;110:429–440.

ACOG Practice Bulletin No. 89. Elective and risk reducing salpingo-oophorectomy. The American College of Obstetricians and Gynecologists, Obstet Gynecol 2008;111:231–241.

ACOG Committee Opinion No. 395. Surgery and patient choice. The American College of Obstetricians and Gynecologists. Obstet Gynecol 2008;111:243–247.

Agostini A, Vejux N, Bretelle F, et al: Value of laparoscopic assistance for vaginal hysterectomy with prophylactic bilateral oophorectomy. Am J Obstet Gynecol 2006;194:351–354.

Altpeter T, Luckhardt K, Lewis JN, et al: Expanded surgical time-out: A key to real-time data collection and quality improvement. J Am Coll Surg 2007;204:527–532.

Ballard LA, Walters MD: Transvaginal mobilization and removal of ovaries and fallopian tubes after vaginal hysterectomy. Obstet Gynecol 1996;87:356–389.

Benassi L, Rossi T, Kaihura CT, et al: Abdominal or vaginal hysterectomy for enlarged uteri: A randomized clinical trial. Am J Obstet Gynecol 2002;187:1561–1565.

Bratzler DW, Houck PM (for the Surgical Infection Prevention Guidelines Writers Workgroup): Antimicrobial prophylaxis for surgery: An advisory statement from the National Surgical Infection Prevention Project. Clin Infect Dis 2004;38:1706–1715.

Classen DC, Evans RS, Pestotnik SL, et al: The timing of prophylactic administration of antibiotics and the risk of surgical-wound infection. N Engl J Med 1992;326:281–286.

Davies A, Vizza E, Bournas N, et al: How to increase the proportion of hysterectomies performed vaginally. Am J Obstet Gynecol 1998;179:1008–1012.

Dicker RC, Greenspan JR, Strauss LT, et al: Complications of abdominal and vaginal hysterectomy among women of reproductive age in the United States: The collaborative review of sterilization. Am J Obstet Gynecol 1982;144:841–848.

Dorsey JH, Steinberg EP, Holtz PM: Clinical indications for hysterectomy route: Patient characteristics or physician preference? Am J Obstet Gynecol 1995;173:1452–1460.

Dorsey JH, Holtz PM, Griffiths RI, et al: Costs and charges associated with three alternative techniques of hysterectomy. N Engl J Med 1996;335:476–482.

Falcone T, Paraiso MF, Mascha E: Prospective randomized clinical trial of laparoscopically assisted vaginal hysterectomy versus total abdominal hysterectomy. Am J Obstet Gynecol 1999;180: 955–962.

Garry R, Fountain J, Mason S, et al: The eVALuate study: Two parallel randomised trials, one comparing laparoscopic with abdominal hysterectomy, the other comparing laparoscopic with vaginal hysterectomy. BMJ 2004;328:129:1–7. Erratum in BMJ 2004;328:494.

Guenaga KF, Matos D, Castro AA, et al: Mechanical bowel preparation for elective colorectal surgery. Cochrane Database Syst Rev 2003;Issue 2:CD001544.

Johnson BE, Porter J: Preoperative evaluation of the gynecologic patient. Obstet Gynecol 2008;111:1183–1194.

Johnson N, Barlow D, Lethaby A, et al: Surgical approach to hysterectomy for benign gynecological disease. Cochrane Database Syst Rev 2006;Issue 2:CD003677.

Keshavarz H, Hillis SD, Kieke BA, Marchbanks PA: Hysterectomy surveillance—United States, 1994–1999 MMWR Surveill Summ 2002;51(SSO5):1–8.

Kovac SR: Decision-directed hysterectomy: A possible approach to improve medical and economic outcomes. Intl J Obstet Gynecol 2000;71:159–169.

Kovac SR, Barhan S, Lister M, et al: Guidelines for the selection of the route of hysterectomy: Application in a resident clinic population. Am J Obstet Gynecol 2002;187:1521–1527.

Kovac SR: Clinical opinion: Guidelines for hysterectomy. Am J Obstet Gynecol 2004;191:635–640.

Le Tohic A, Dhainaut C, Yazbeck C, et al: Hysterectomy for benign uterine pathology among women without previous vaginal delivery. Obstet Gynecol 2008;111: 829–837.

Mahid SS, Polk HC Jr, Lewis JN, Turina M: Opportunities for improved performance in surgical specialty practice. Ann Surg 2008;247:380–388.

Nationwide Inpatient Sample (NIS) of the Healthcare Cost and Utilization Project (HCUP). Available at: www.hcupnet.ahrq.gov. Retrieved December 28, 2007.

Schulpher M, Manca A, Abbott J, et al: Cost effectiveness analysis of laparoscopic hysterectomy compared with standard hysterectomy: Results from a randomised trial. BMJ 2004;328:134.

Stovall TG, Ling FW, Crawford DA: Hysterectomy for chronic pelvic pain of presumed uterine etiology. Obstet Gynecol 1990;75:676–679.

Wilson W, Taubert KA, Gewitz M, et al: Prevention of infective endocarditis: Guidelines from the American Heart Association, A guideline from the American Heart Association Rheumatic Fever, Endocarditis, and Kawasaki Disease Committee, Council on Cardiovascular Disease in the Young, and the Council on Clinical Cardiology, Council on Cardiovascular Surgery and Anesthesia, and the Quality of Care and Outcomes Research Interdisciplinary Working Group [published erratum appears in Circulation 2007;116:e376–377. Circulation 2007;116:1736–1754.

Wu JM, Wechter ME, Geller EJ, et al: Hysterectomy rates in the United States, 2003. Obstet Gynecol 2007;110:1091–1095.

Outcomes of Hysterectomy

Matthew D. Barber M.D., M.H.S.
Mark D. Walters M.D.

5

Hysterectomy is a highly effective treatment for many gynecologic disorders. Patient satisfaction is generally very high after hysterectomy and tends to be related to the initial indication for surgery and patient expectation. The Maine Women's Health Study evaluated the effect of hysterectomy for nonmalignant disorders on quality of life (Carlson et al, 1994a). The indications for surgery were similar to those reported from national statistics (www.hcupnet.ahrq.gov, 2007; Keshavarz, 2002). They documented a marked improvement abnormal uterine bleeding, pelvic pain, urinary symptoms, fatigue, and psychological and sexual symptoms at 1 year in the majority of patients. In the Maryland Women's Health Study patients were followed for up to 2 years after hysterectomy for nonmalignant conditions (Kjerulff et al, 2000). Symptoms related to the underlying indication for surgery, as well as associated symptoms of depression and anxiety and quality of life, improved after hysterectomy (Table 5-1). However, each study reported that about 8% of patients had new symptoms, such as depression and lack of interest in sex, or lack of improvement in quality of life (Table 5-2). Although women with pelvic pain and depression did not show the same level of improvement as other groups, there was significant improvement over baseline (Hartmann et al, 2004). Low socioeconomic status and concurrent bilateral oophorectomy also have been shown to lower the likelihood of satisfactory outcome in some studies (Kjerulff et al, 2000). Farquhar and associates (2008) found significant reductions in pelvic pain, abdominal pain, urinary frequency, and depression 5 years after hysterectomy in a prospective cohort of premenopausal women. Women 5 years after hysterectomy had similar bladder, bowel, and sexual function to a parallel cohort of women with normal menses who had not undergone a hysterectomy.

This chapter will discuss in detail the symptom- and indication-based long-term outcomes of hysterectomy, reviewing both the positive and negative effects of this surgery on women. It will also compare the outcomes of subtotal (supracervical) hysterectomy to total hysterectomy and summarize the outcomes of hysterectomy relative to several nonhysterectomy alternatives for treatments of heavy menstrual bleeding and uterine fibroids (Table 5-3). A more detailed discussion of short-term outcomes including perioperative complications and the relative risks and benefits of different routes of hysterectomy can be found elsewhere in this text (Chapters 4 and 11).

Bleeding

Hysterectomy always provides a definitive cure of irregular or excessive menstrual bleeding. The exception is subtotal (supracervical) hysterectomy, after which cyclic bleeding can be seen in 3% to 24% of patients postoperatively.

Table 5-1 Frequency of Signs and Symptoms and Disturbances in Quality of Life before and after Hysterectomy*

Indicator	Before Hysterectomy	After Hysterectomy			
		6 mo (*n* = 1225)	12 mo (*n* = 1188	18 mo (*n* = 1174)	24 mo (*n* = 1162)
Clinical sign/Symptom					
Vaginal bleeding	59.2	0.5	0.5	0.3	0.3
Pelvic pain	63.1	11.4	8.5	7.8	7.8
Back pain	43.1	17.5	16.4	17.7	17.4
Activity limitation	57.5	5.9	4.1	3.2	2.4
Sleep disturbance	40.9	22.7	21.8	22.3	20.6
Fatigue	70.0	27.4	26.7	27.2	24.7
Abdominal bloating	47.8	15.0	13.5	13.0	12.1
Urinary incontinence	19.5	6.3	8.5	7.0	8.3
Psychological function					
Depression	28.0	11.6	11.9	10.7	12.4
Anxiety	65.4	29.9	30.6	28.1	25.1
Quality of life					
Limited physical function	47.7	28.1	23.6	24.4	23.3
Limited social function	23.1	6.8	5.1	5.9	4.9
Poor health perception	78.6	31.8	32.0	34.5	31.9

*In the Maryland Women's Health Study (*n* = 1299). Values are percentages. All before-after comparisons demonstrate significant improvement at *p* < .001.
Data from Kjerulff KH, Langenberg PW, Rhodes JC, et al: Effectiveness of hysterectomy. Obstet Gynecol 2000;95:319–326.

Table 5-2 Frequency of Positive or Negative Outcomes at 24 Months after Hysterectomy*

Indicator	Outcome†	
	Problem Relieved	Problem Acquired
Clinical sign/symptom		
Vaginal bleeding	99.7	0.2
Pelvic pain	89.4	2.8
Back pain	71.0	7.9
Activity limitation	99.6	1.2
Sleep disturbance	64.4	10.9
Fatigue	68.7	8.4
Abdominal bloating	81.1	5.7
Urinary incontinence	75.7	4.5
Psychological function		
Depression	73.0	7.3
Anxiety	67.6	11.6
Quality of life		
Limited physical function	63.4	12.9
Limited social function	88.6	3.6
Poor health perception	60.8	7.7

*In the Maryland Women's Health Study (*n* = 1299). Values are percentages.
†*Problem relieved*: problem no longer experienced at the "problematic-severe" level among women who did report having the problem at this level before hysterectomy. *Problem acquired*: problem reported at the "problematic-severe" level among women who did not have the problem at this level before hysterectomy.
Data from Kjerulff KH, Langenberg PW, Rhodes JC, et al: Effectiveness of hysterectomy. Obstet Gynecol 2000;95:319–326.

Table 5-3 Summary of Randomized Controlled Trial Evidence Comparing Hysterectomy versus Alternative Treatments for Dysfunctional Uterine Bleeding or Fibroids

Alternative Treatment (Population)	No. of Trials (n)	Bleeding	Quality of Life	Pain	Sexual Health	Bulk Symptoms	Satisfaction	Additional Tx	Adverse Events	Quality of Evidence
Endometrial ablation (DUB)	7 (1167)	Favors hyst	ND*	Favors hyst	ND	ND	ND	Favors hyst	Favors ablation	Low to moderate
Medications (DUB)	1 (57)	NA	ND	ND	ND	NA	ND	NA	Favors meds	Low
Uterine artery embolization (fibroids)	3 (391)	Favors hyst	ND	ND	ND	ND	ND	Favors hyst	ND	Moderate
LNG-IUS (mixed DUB and fibroids)	1 (236)	Favors hyst	ND	NA	Favors hyst	NA	NA	Favors hyst	Favors LNG-IUS	Moderate

DUB, dysfunctional uterine bleeding; Favors hyst, studies favor hysterectomy; LNG-IUS, levonorgesterel intrauterine system; meds, medications, N, total number of study participants; NA, not applicable (no trials evaluated outcome); ND, no difference; Tx, treatments.

*Improvements in quality of life are similar overall for hysterectomy and for endometrial ablation; however, hysterectomy is favored for some domains (social functioning, energy, pain, and general health).

Adapted from the Society of Gynecologic Surgeons (SGS) Systematic Review Group Guidelines on hysterectomy versus alternative treatments for heavy menstrual bleeding, presented at the 2010 Annual meeting of the Society of Gynecologic Surgeons, Tucson, AZ.

Hysterectomy should be considered a second-line therapy in most cases of abnormal menstrual bleeding because it results in permanent loss of fertility and has greater risk, higher cost, and longer recovery than most alternative treatments. Hormonal therapies (such as oral contraceptive pills and oral or intramuscular medroxyprogesterone acetate), nonsteroidal anti-inflammatory medications (particularly mefenamic acid and naproxen sodium), and medicated intrauterine devices (IUDs) effectively treat abnormal menstrual bleeding in many patients. However, a significant proportion of patients eventually require further treatment, including hysterectomy. The Maine Women's Health Study prospectively evaluated a cohort of women with abnormal uterine bleeding treated medically over a 1-year period (Carlson et al, 1994b). Overall, they had a significant improvement in symptoms of pain and bleeding and in quality of life. However, 23% still underwent a hysterectomy in the 12-month follow-up period.

Few randomized clinical trials comparing medical therapy to hysterectomy for treatment of abnormal menstrual bleeding exist. One study by Kuppermann and associates (2004) randomized 63 premenopausal women who had failed previous treatment with medroxyprogesterone acetate for excessive menstrual bleeding to receive either hysterectomy or expanded medical therapy, typically oral contraceptive pills with or without nonsteroidal anti-inflammatory drugs (NSAIDs). At 6 months, women in the hysterectomy group had greater improvement in scores of mental health, and greater improvement in symptom resolution, interference with sex, sexual desire, health distress, sleep problems, and satisfaction with health. During the 2 years of follow-up, 53% of those who had received expanded medical treatment eventually requested and received hysterectomy, with resulting improvements in quality of life.

A large randomized trial of 236 women age 35 to 49 with excessive menstrual bleeding compared hysterectomy to a levonorgestrel-releasing intrauterine system (LNG-IUS) (Hurskainen et al, 2004). After 5 years of follow-up, both groups reported high (>90%) satisfaction with treatment. In those who received the LNG-IUS, 75% reported amenorrhea or minimal spotting; however, 42% of subjects eventually underwent a hysterectomy during the follow-up period.

Endometrial ablation is an effective alternative to hysterectomy for treatment of excessive menstrual bleeding. To date, there have been seven randomized trials with a total of 1192 participants comparing either abdominal or vaginal hysterectomy to endometrial ablation in women with abnormal uterine bleeding (Lethaby et al, 2009). Compared to hysterectomy, endometrial ablation is associated with a shorter operative time, shorter recovery period, and lower postoperative complication rate. However, although hysterectomy eliminates menstrual bleeding, endometrial ablation results in amenorrhea in only 45% of patients and recurrent excessive bleeding is seen in 15% to 25% of cases. Approximately 9% to 34% of patients who receive endometrial ablation subsequently undergo hysterectomy. A systematic review performed by the Cochrane Collaboration found that hysterectomy had a significant advantage over endometrial ablation for the improvement in anemia as well as overall satisfaction and general health for up to 4 years after surgery (Lethaby et al, 2009). Although many quality-of-life scales reported no differences between surgical groups, there was some evidence of a greater improvement in some health domains (social functioning, energy, pain, and general health) for hysterectomy patients. Most adverse events were significantly more likely to occur after hysterectomy and before discharge from hospital. However, after discharge from hospital, the only difference was a lower rate of infection among those receiving endometrial ablation (odds ratio [OR] = 0.2, confidence interval

[CI] 0.1–0.5). The overall cost of endometrial ablation was lower than that of hysterectomy, but the cost differences narrow over time because of the need for eventual hysterectomy in a proportion of those who receive ablation, or re-treatment with other alternatives to hysterectomy including uterine fibroid embolization and myomectomy. The relative advantages and disadvantages of these therapies are discussed in Chapter 12.

Uterine fibroid embolization (UFE) offers an alternative to hysterectomy in women with symptomatic uterine fibroids, particularly those with uterine fibroids and heavy menstrual bleeding. Women with symptomatic uterine fibroids who are of reproductive age but who are not interested in childbearing are candidates for UFE. Three randomized clinical trials including a total of 391 women have compared UFE to hysterectomy for the treatment of heavy menstrual bleeding in women with uterine fibroids. Overall, hysterectomy offers better control of bleeding than UFE and requires fewer additional treatments but demonstrates no differences in quality of life, sexual health, or frequency of adverse events. The EMMY trial randomized 177 patients with uterine fibroids and menorrhagia to UFE (n = 88) or hysterectomy (n = 89) (Volkers et al, 2007). Of those who received UFE, 62% reported resolution of menorrhagia at 24 months and 4% described their menorrhagia as being unchanged. In both groups hemoglobin levels increased significantly compared to baseline (at 24 months: UFE, +1.37 g/dL; hysterectomy, +2.03 g/dL; $p <$ .001 for each) with the increase in hemoglobin being significantly greater for hysterectomy patients (p = .037). Two years after treatment, 23.5% of UFE patients had undergone a hysterectomy for inadequate symptom control. This finding is similar to the REST trial, in which 20% of patients receiving UFE required invasive procedure (hysterectomy or repeat UFE) within 2 years after the procedure for continued or recurrent symptoms compared with none in those who received a hysterectomy (The REST Investigators, 2007).

For simple dysfunctional uterine bleeding, a short trial of oral contraceptives followed by second-generation ablation is the most cost-effective strategy. Hysterectomy is more cost-effective for achieving amenorrhea, which likely improves with more follow-up time. Patient preferences of treatment also play an important role (Wade et al, 2006).

Pelvic Pain/Endometriosis

Hysterectomy is an effective therapy for carefully selected patients with chronic pelvic pain. However, unlike abnormal menstrual bleeding, symptom relief is not guaranteed, with as many as 22% of patients having persistent pelvic pain after surgery. Medical management of chronic pelvic pain, including oral contraceptive pills, anti-inflammatory drugs, and analgesics result in a significant improvement in pain and quality of life. However, after 1 year of therapy approximately half will still report significant pelvic pain and almost one quarter will undergo a hysterectomy. Hysterectomy provides an effective therapy for many women with pelvic pain who fail nonsurgical management. In the Maine Women's Health Study, 65% of subjects reported some degree of pelvic pain prior to hysterectomy. Twelve months after surgery only 5% of these women had persistent pelvic pain. Back pain, dyspareunia, and abdominal bloating also improved significantly after hysterectomy. Three percent of patients in this study developed new pelvic pain during the 1-year follow-up period. Similarly, the Maryland Women's Health Study found that 88.5% and 89.4% of women with pelvic pain who underwent hysterectomy were relieved

Figure 5-1 Reoperation-free survival estimates for women with pelvic pain due to endometriosis undergoing hysterectomy with and without ovarian preservation and laparoscopic excision with ovarian preservation. (From Shakiba K, Bena JF, McGill KM, et al: Surgical treatment of endometriosis: A 7-year follow-up on the requirement for further surgery. Obstet Gynecol 2008;111:1285–1292; reprinted with permission.)

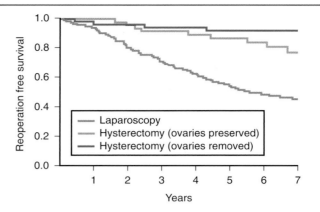

of pain at 1 and 2 years after surgery, respectively. Less than 4% of patients acquired new pelvic pain during the 2-year study period. In this study, women with pelvic pain fared less well after hysterectomy than those who had hysterectomy for other reasons, particularly if they also had depression. However, substantial improvements in symptoms and quality of life were still seen in this patient group. Two randomized trials comparing total abdominal hysterectomy to subtotal abdominal hysterectomy also demonstrated a substantial improvement in pelvic pain postoperatively, with no difference between groups. In contrast, the trial by Thakar and associates (2004) had very few patients with pelvic pain at baseline, but found a significant increase in general pain scores in both groups 1 year after surgery.

Hysterectomy is often considered in patients with pelvic pain from endometriosis if fertility is no longer desired and medical or conservative surgical therapy has proved inadequate. LGN-IUS has recently been shown to be an effective nonsurgical approach for reducing pelvic pain, dyspareunia, and dysmenorrhea in patients with endometriosis. It is likely with the increasing use of the LGN-IUS in this population, that rate of hysterectomy for endometriosis and pelvic pain will decline. Nonetheless, hysterectomy with or without oophorectomy is a successful approach for treating pelvic pain associated with endometriosis for many women who have failed medical treatment and less invasive surgical approaches. It is important to note that some women with endometriosis will not have persistent relief of pain and that residual endometriosis can be seen even after hysterectomy. Shakiba and associates (2008) investigated the rates of requiring additional surgery after various surgical treatments for endometriosis (Fig. 5-1). In women who underwent hysterectomy with ovarian preservation, the 2-, 5-, and 7-year reoperation-free percentages were 95.7%, 86.6%, and 77.0%, respectively. In women who underwent hysterectomy without ovarian preservation, the percentages were 96.0%, 91.7%, and 91.7%, respectively. However, in women between 30 and 39 years of age, removal of the ovaries did not significantly improve the surgery-free time. Hysterectomy with or without ovarian preservation compared favorably to those women who underwent laparoscopic excision with uterine and ovarian preservation, whose the surgery-free percentages were 79.4%, 53.3%, and 44.6%, respectively, at 2, 5, and 7 years. Use of hormone replacement after total abdominal hysterectomy with bilateral oophorectomy for pelvic pain and endometriosis is associated with a very low risk of recurrent pelvic pain (0.9% per year).

Clinical trials suggest that hysterectomy is more likely to result in improvement of pelvic pain than is endometrial ablation (Lethaby et al, 2009). In women with symptomatic uterine fibroids, UFE appears to result in similar reduction in pelvic and abdominal pain as hysterectomy (Volkers et al, 2007).

Sexual Function

Although there has been considerable debate about the effect of hysterectomy on sexual function, current evidence suggests that hysterectomy results in *improved* or *unchanged* sexual function in the majority of women in the first 1 to 5 years after surgery. Only a small proportion of women will have a decline in sexual function after hysterectomy during this period. Available research provides information about the short-term effect of hysterectomy on dyspareunia, frequency of intercourse, orgasm, libido/sexual interest, vaginal dryness, and overall sexual function. The long-term effect of hysterectomy on sexual function, particularly any effect beyond 5 years, is largely unknown.

Studies that address the effect of hysterectomy on dyspareunia demonstrate either no change or an improvement in this symptom in the majority of women. The Maryland Women's Health Study demonstrated a significant decline in the number of woman who reported dyspareunia 12 and 24 months after hysterectomy when compared to the preoperative period (Hartmann et al, 2004). Eighty-one percent of the women in this study who experienced frequent dyspareunia preoperatively had an improvement in this symptom at 24 months after hysterectomy, but only 1.9% of women without preoperative dyspareunia developed it by 24 months after surgery. In the Maine Women's Health Study, 39% of women complained of dyspareunia preoperatively and only 8% had this complaint 12 months after hysterectomy. By comparison, women in this study who were managed nonsurgically showed no decline in the mean frequency of dyspareunia.

Hysterectomy appears to have little impact on the frequency of intercourse. In the Maryland Women's Health Study, the mean number of sexual relations per month increased from 2.3 per month preoperatively to 2.9 per month 24 months after hysterectomy. Another study found that 56% of the subjects in their study reported an increase in sexual frequency 18 months after hysterectomy, while 27% reported no change and 17% had a decrease in frequency. Similarly, most well-designed studies that have evaluated libido or sexual interest have demonstrated either no change or an improvement after hysterectomy. In the Maryland Women's Health Study, 70.8% of women with low libido preoperatively were improved 12 months after hysterectomy, while only 4.3% of women who had normal libido preoperatively developed low libido at 12 months after surgery. In the Maine Women's Health Study, 36% of women had decreased sexual interest preoperatively while 8% had this problem 12 months after hysterectomy. The proportion of women who developed decreased sexual interest as a new symptom postoperatively was not significantly different from the proportion of women with this complaint in a group who was managed nonsurgically. Farquhar and associates (2008) found no difference in sexual frequency in premenopausal women 5 years after a hysterectomy compared to a parallel cohort of women with normal menses who did not undergo hysterectomy.

There is disagreement in the literature on the effect hysterectomy has on postoperative orgasmic function. The Maryland Women's Health Study demonstrated a significant increase in the proportion of women who experienced orgasms after hysterectomy, from 62.8% prior to surgery to 71.5% 24 months after hysterectomy. However, four smaller prospective cohort studies demonstrated no change in orgasmic function after hysterectomy. Farquhar and associates (2008) found similar orgasmic function and overall quality of sex life 5 years after hysterectomy compared to women with normal menses who had not received a hysterectomy. Lowenstein and associates (2005) evaluated vaginal and clitoral sensation before and 3 months after hysterectomy in 27 women. They demonstrated a quantifiable sensory loss in the vagina after hysterectomy, with preservation of clitoral sensation. Only a minority of patients reported a decline in their sexual function, however, which the authors attributed to the relative importance of clitoral as compared to vaginal sensation in sexual function. One prospective study of 109 women undergoing abdominal or vaginal hysterectomy noted that in more than 75%, sexual arousal, intensity of orgasms, and the effect of nipple stimulation were the same or increased after uterus and cervix were removed (Goetsch, 2005). However, 25% of subjects noted decreased ease of arousal after hysterectomy and 16% noted decreased intensity of orgasms after surgery.

Vaginal dryness appears to improve in a small proportion of women after hysterectomy, but most women with preoperative vaginal dryness continue to have this symptom postoperatively. Development of vaginal dryness after hysterectomy when it does not exist preoperatively largely depends upon postoperative hormonal status.

The "eVALuate" study (Garry et al, 2004) involved two parallel randomized trials, one comparing laparoscopic with abdominal hysterectomy and the other comparing laparoscopic with vaginal hysterectomy. Body image and sexual function were improved in all groups 4 months and 1 year after surgery, with no differences between the three routes of hysterectomy. Randomized controlled studies comparing hysterectomy and uterus-sparing treatment options are few, but no negative impact on sexual functioning has been reported. Hysterectomy results in greater improvements in sexual desire and a greater decrease in pelvic problems that interfere with sexual intercourse than does expanded medical therapy (oral contraceptive pills with or without NSAIDs) in women with menorrhagia who previously failed medroxyprogesterone acetate treatment (Kuppermann et al, 2004). In one large trial comparing hysterectomy to LNG-IUS, sexual satisfaction improved significantly and sexual problems decreased after hysterectomy, but no changes in sexual satisfaction or sexual problems were noted 6 or 12 months after LNG-IUS (Halmesmaki et al, 2007). In the EMMY Trial, no differences in sexuality and body image were observed between the UFE and the hysterectomy at 24 months after procedure (Hehenkamp et al, 2007). On average, both after UFE and hysterectomy, sexual functioning and body image scores improved, but this figure reached statistical significance only in the UFE group. Trials comparing hysterectomy to endometrial ablation have generally shown no differences in postprocedure sexual function between these treatments.

Ovarian Function

The effect of hysterectomy on ovarian function is contradictory but is most likely dependent on the age of the patient at the time of surgery. In a prospective cohort study, serum follicle-stimulating hormone was measured in women after hysterectomy and a control group for 5 years (Farquhar et al, 2005). It was estimated that women after hysterectomy with retention of both ovaries reached menopause 3.7 years (95% confidence interval [CI] 1.5–6.0 years) earlier than women who did not have a hysterectomy. Women with a unilateral oophorectomy at the time of hysterectomy reached menopause 4.4 years (95% CI 0.6–7.9 years) earlier than women who had both ovaries left in at the time of hysterectomy.

Bladder Function

Many studies have demonstrated an adverse effect on bladder function after radical hysterectomy for cervical cancer. The effect of simple hysterectomy on lower urinary tract function is less clear, however. A systematic review of the literature published in 2000 (Brown et al, 2000), relying heavily on observational studies, concluded that hysterectomy increased the odds of urinary incontinence by 60% in women over the age of 60. No increased risk was found in younger women.

In contrast, the majority of prospective cohort studies that subjectively evaluate lower urinary tract symptoms before and after hysterectomy demonstrate either a significant improvement or no change in bladder symptoms 3 months to 5 years after surgery. A study of identical twins suggested that hysterectomy does not predispose women to stress urinary incontinence (Miller et al, 2008). Data from the Maryland Health Study suggest that most women with urinary incontinence preoperatively will have a significant reduction in urinary incontinence after surgery; however, approximately 10% of women can be expected to develop new or worsening urinary incontinence in the first 2 years after surgery (Kjerulff et al, 2002). The Maine Women's Health Study demonstrated a significant *reduction* in urinary incontinence, urinary urgency and urinary frequency 12 months after hysterectomy (Carlson et al, 1994a). No significant change in urinary symptoms was seen in the nonsurgically managed population of this cohort. Similarly, Farquhar and associates (2008) demonstrated a significant reduction of urinary frequency and nocturia 5 years after hysterectomy in premenopausal women, with no change in rates of stress or urge urinary incontinence. A randomized trial comparing hysterectomy to endometrial ablation found no difference in bladder function 2 years after the procedure.

It does not appear that there is a difference in long-term urinary symptoms among the different types of routes of hysterectomy for benign disease. One randomized trial of total abdominal hysterectomy versus subtotal hysterectomy found urinary symptoms and incontinence were reduced by 44% to 88% from baseline 2 years after surgery, with no differences between groups; another study demonstrated a significant reduction in urinary incontinence in the total abdominal hysterectomy group but no reduction in those who received a subtotal hysterectomy. Thakar and associates (2002) found that significantly fewer women had stress incontinence, urinary urgency, frequency, nocturia, interrupted stream, and incomplete bladder emptying 1 year after both total and subtotal abdominal hysterectomy, with no difference between groups. A recent meta-analysis concluded that 1 year after surgery, there is no statistical difference in the risk for developing urinary incontinence after a supracervical versus total hysterectomy (Robert et al, 2008).

Bowel Function

The effect of hysterectomy on postoperative bowel dysfunction is controversial. In a population-based cross-sectional study of 1058 women, self-reported constipation was significantly more common in subjects with a prior hysterectomy than in women without prior hysterectomy (22% versus 9%, respectively), as was straining at defecation and a feeling of incomplete emptying. Similarly, a case-control study found that women who had a hysterectomy 2 to 8 years prior were significantly more likely to have decreased bowel frequency than control subjects. In contrast, several prospective cohort studies that evaluated women before and 3 months to 5 years after hysterectomy found either no change or an improvement in bowel function postoperatively. Only two studies have prospectively examined this issue and included a control group of women who did not get a hysterectomy. The Maine Women's Health Study found that 9% of women who received a hysterectomy developed new-onset constipation by 12 months after surgery compared to 1% of women who received nonsurgical management. Farquhar and associates (2008) found a significant improvement in constipation symptoms 5 years after a hysterectomy with no differences in constipation rates compared to a cohort of women with normal menses who did not receive a hysterectomy. Randomized comparisons of total and subtotal hysterectomy demonstrate no change in constipation after surgery and no differences between groups.

Pelvic Organ Prolapse

Hysterectomy appears to increase the risk of subsequent pelvic organ prolapse; however, the development of symptomatic prolapse typically occurs many years after the hysterectomy. Also, it is unknown whether the patients who had had hysterectomy also had mild pelvic floor relaxation (thus, the future prolapse represents a progression of disease) and whether various techniques of vaginal cuff closure affect future hysterectomy rates. In a consecutive series of 693 patients who presented to the Mayo Clinic (Webb et al, 1998) for surgical management of post-hysterectomy vaginal vault prolapse, the median time from hysterectomy to prolapse repair was 15.8 years. A retrospective cohort study of 149,554 women (Olsen et al, 1997) age 20 and older found that in women who developed pelvic organ prolapse or urinary incontinence, the mean interval between hysterectomy and surgery for prolapse was 19.3 years. The Oxford Family Planning Association Study (Mant et al, 1997) followed 17,032 women aged 25 to 39 for an average of 17 years. The annual incidence of surgery for pelvic organ prolapse was 0.16% per year. In women who had undergone hysterectomy for reasons other than prolapse, surgical incidence rate increased to 0.29% per year. The cumulative risk of prolapse surgery rose from 1% at 3 years after hysterectomy to 5% 15 years after hysterectomy.

Similarly, Dallenbach and colleagues (2007) found that the risk of prolapse repair was 4.7 times higher in women whose initial hysterectomy was indicated by prolapse and 8.0 times higher if preoperative prolapse grade 2 or more was present. Other risk factors for requiring subsequent prolapse repair after hysterectomy that were identified in this study included history of vaginal delivery (adjusted OR 5.0, 95% CI 1.3–19.7), and sexual activity (adjusted OR 6.2, 95% CI 2.7–14.5). Vaginal hysterectomy was not a risk factor when preoperative prolapse was taken into account. Surgical technique at the time of hysterectomy, including the performance of prophylactic culdoplasty at vaginal hysterectomy, can decrease development of subsequent pelvic organ prolapse as demonstrated in the trial by Cruikshank and Kovac (1999).

Quality of Life and Psychosocial Function

Hysterectomy results in an increased health-related quality of life (HRQOL), improved general health perception, and improved psychological outcomes in a majority of women. A small proportion of women will have decline in quality of life or a worsening of psychological symptoms after undergoing hysterectomy. Both the Maine and Maryland Women's Health studies demonstrated significant improvement in all aspects of HRQOL as well as decreased anxiety and depression 12 to 24 months after hysterectomy. In the Maryland study, nearly three quarters of patients with preoperative depression and two thirds of women with preoperative anxiety no longer had the psychological condition 12 months after their hysterectomy. However, 3% to 12% of patients in the Maine study developed new-onset depression, anxiety, or negative feelings about themselves as a woman after the hysterectomy. The presence of depression prior to the hysterectomy appears to be the most important predictor of postoperative depression after surgery. Women younger than age 40, less educated women, those with a conflict about childbearing, and those undergoing oophorectomy may also be at higher risk of depression after hysterectomy.

The available data indicate that the laparoscopic and vaginal approaches to hysterectomy lead to equal or greater quality of life compared to abdominal hysterectomy in the first few weeks after the procedure (Nieboer et al, 2009). There are scant data evaluating the impact of different routes of hysterectomy on quality of life over the long term, however. One randomized trial found that general psychological well-being is equal after laparoscopic and abdominal hysterectomy 6 months after surgery. Trials comparing total and subtotal hysterectomy demonstrate improved HRQOL in both groups. The trial by Thakar and associates (2004) also found improvements in anxiety, depression, and social dysfunction 6 and 12 months after surgery, with no difference between those who had their cervix removed and those whose cervix was left in situ. Similarly, vaginal, abdominal, and laparoscopic hysterectomy each appears to result in similar improvements in HRQOL, as recently demonstrated in the "eVALuate" study.

Overall, hysterectomy appears to provide similar or greater improvements in quality of life compared to nonhysterectomy alternatives. Compared with medical treatments, hysterectomy offers better short-term improvement in HRQOL measured at 6 months. This superior effect appears to diminish over time, however (Kuppermann et al, 2004). Hysterectomy results in similar improvements in HRQOL and greater perception of overall general health 5 years after surgery than in women receiving LNG-IUS over the same time period (Hurskainen et al, 2004). Similarly, hysterectomy appears to result in similar improvements in HRQOL as endometrial ablation, although there was some evidence of a greater improvement in some health domains (social functioning, energy, pain, and general health) for hysterectomy patients (Lethaby et al, 2009). The EMMY trial found that both UFE and hysterectomy improved HRQOL. No differences were observed between groups regarding HRQOL at 24-month follow-up, although patients who received hysterectomy were more satisfied than those who received UFE ($p < .02$) (Hehenkamp et al, 2008). Similarly, the REST trial found no significant differences between those who received a hysterectomy and those who received a UFE at 1 year in any of the eight domains assessed by the SF-36, a generic HRQOL measure (REST investigators, 2007).

Subtotal versus Total Hysterectomy

Until recently, information about the relative risks and benefits of preservation of the cervix at the time of hysterectomy (subtotal hysterectomy) has been based on retrospective studies and nonrandomized comparisons. In the last several years, however, several well-designed prospective randomized trails comparing total abdominal hysterectomy to subtotal abdominal hysterectomy have been reported. The Cochrane Review on this topic identified three randomized trials including a total of 733 women (Lethaby et al, 2006). Length of surgery and amount of blood lost during surgery are significantly reduced during subtotal hysterectomy when compared with total hysterectomy, but there was no evidence of a difference in the risk of transfusion. Febrile morbidity was less likely (OR = 0.43, CI 0.25–0.75) and ongoing cyclic vaginal bleeding 1 year after surgery was more likely (OR = 11.3, CI 4.1–31.2) after subtotal when compared with total hysterectomy. There is no evidence of a difference in the rates of other complications, recovery from surgery, or readmission rates.

As mentioned earlier, randomized trials comparing total abdominal hysterectomy with subtotal hysterectomy have found no advantage of cervical preservation at the time of hysterectomy with regard to sexual function. Similarly, a prospective cohort of 413 women undergoing either vaginal hysterectomy, subtotal abdominal hysterectomy, or total abdominal hysterectomy found significant improvements in sexual pleasure 6 months after surgery in all groups. The persistence and development of bothersome problems during sexual activity were similar for all three techniques.

Thakar and colleagues (2002) performed a multicenter randomized double-blind clinical trial of total and subtotal abdominal hysterectomy in 279 women. They demonstrated an improvement in urinary frequency, nocturia, and stress urinary incontinence in both groups, with no difference between the two groups 12 months after surgery. Sexual function and bowel function did not change significantly in either group. Of women who received a subtotal abdominal hysterectomy, 7% had persistent cyclic bleeding and 2% developed cervical prolapse beyond the introitus. Hysterectomy by either technique led to significant reductions in most symptoms, including pelvic pain, back pain, urinary incontinence, and voiding dysfunction. In contrast, a Danish trial of 319 patients found that women who received a total abdominal hysterectomy were less likely to have urinary incontinence than those who underwent subtotal abdominal hysterectomy 1 year after surgery (9% vs. 18%). Additionally, 20% of those who received a subtotal hysterectomy had persistent vaginal bleeding postoperatively. As previously noted, a recent meta-analysis concluded that 1 year after surgery there is no statistical difference in the risk for developing urinary incontinence after a subtotal versus total hysterectomy (Robert et al, 2008).

There are no randomized trials comparing laparoscopic hysterectomy to laparoscopic subtotal hysterectomy. One retrospective study of 240 women who received a laparoscopic subtotal hysterectomy reported that over 90% were satisfied with their surgery (Lieng et al, 2008). However, 24% reported experiencing vaginal bleeding up to 3 years following their hysterectomy, although this was rated as minimal in 90% of cases. Similarly, 38% continued to experience menstrual pain 3 years after surgery, although this was significantly less intense than preoperatively.

Suggested Readings

Brown JS, Sawaya G, Thom DH, Grady D: Hysterectomy and urinary incontinence: A systematic review. Lancet 2000;356:535–539.

Carlson KJ, Nichols DH, Schiff I: Current concepts: Indications for hysterectomy. N Engl J Med 1993;328:856–860.

Carlson KJ, Miller BA, Fowler FJ: The Maine Women's Heath Study: I. Outcomes of hysterectomy. Obstet Gynecol 1994a;83:556–565.

Carlson KJ, Miller BA, Fowler FJ: The Maine Women's Health Study: II. Outcomes of nonsurgical management of leiomyomas, abnormal bleeding and chronic pelvic pain. Obstet Gynecol 1994b;83:566–572.

Cruikshank SH, Kovac S: Randomized comparison of three surgical methods used at the time of vaginal hysterectomy to prevent posterior enterocele. Am J Obstet Gynecol 1999;180:859–865.

Dallenbach P, Kaelin-Gambirasio I, Dubuisson JB, Boulvain M: Risk factors for pelvic organ prolapse repair after hysterectomy. Obstet Gynecol 2007;110:625–632.

Farquhar CM, Sadler L, Harvey SA, Stewart AW: The association of hysterectomy and menopause: A prospective cohort study. Br J Obstet Gynaecol 2005;112:956–962.

Farquhar CM, Sadler L, Stewart AW: A prospective study of outcomes five years after hysterectomy in premenopausal women. Aust NZ J Obstet Gynecol 2008;48:510–516.

Garry R, Fountain J, Mason S, et al: The eVALuate study: Two parallel randomized trails, one comparing laparoscopic with abdominal hysterectomy, the other comparing laparoscopic with vaginal hysterectomy. BMJ 2004;328:129–133.

Goetsch M: The effect of total hysterectomy on specific sexual sensations. Am J Obstet Gynecol 2005;192:1922–1927.

Halmesmaki K, Hurskainen R, Teperi J, et al: The effect of hysterectomy or levonorgestrel-releasing intrauterine system on sexual functioning among women with menorrhagia: A 5-year randomized controlled trial. Br J Obstet Gynaecol 2007;114:563–568.

Hartmann KE, Ma C, Lamvu GM, et al: Quality-of-life and sexual function after hysterectomy in women with preoperative pain and depression. Obstet Gynecol 2004;104:701–709.

Hehenkamp WJK, Volkers NA, Bartholomeus W, et al: Sexuality and body image after uterine artery embolization and hysterectomy in the treatment of uterine fibroids: A randomized comparison. Cardiovasc Intervent Radiol 2007;30:866–875.

Hehenkamp WJK, Volkers NA, Birnie E, et al: Symptomatic uterine fibroids: Treatment with uterine artery embolization or hysterectomy—results from the Randomized Clinical Embolisation versus Hysterectomy (EMMY) trial. Radiology 2008;246:823–832.

Hurskainen R, Teperi J, Rissanen P, et al: Clinical outcomes and costs with the levonorgestrel-releasing intrauterine system or hysterectomy for treatment of menorrhagia: Randomized trial 5-year follow-up. JAMA 2004;291:1456–1463.

Keshavare H, Hillis SD, Kieke BA, Marchbanks PA: Hysterectomy surveillance-United States, 1994–1999. MMWR Surveill Summ 2002;51(SS05):1–8.

Kjerulff KH, Langenberg PW, Rhodes JC, et al: Effectiveness of hysterectomy. Obstet Gynecol 2000;95:319–326.

Kjerulff KH, Langenberg PW, Greenaway L, et al: Urinary incontinence and hysterectomy in a large prospective cohort study in American women. J Urol 2002;167:2088–2092.

Kuppermann M, Varner RE, Summitt RL, et al: Effect of hysterectomy vs. medical treatment on health-related quality of life and sexual functioning: The Medicine or Surgery (MS) Randomized Trial. JAMA 2004;291:1447–1455.

Lethaby A, Shepperd S, Farquhar C, Cooke I: Endometrial resection and ablation versus hysterectomy for heavy menstrual bleeding. Cochrane Database of Syst Rev 1999;Issue 2:CD000329. Last updated May 2009.

Lethaby A, Ivanova V, Johnson N: Total versus subtotal hysterectomy for benign gynaecological conditions. Cochrane Database of Syst Rev 2006;Issue 2:CD004993.

Lieng M, Qvigstad E, Istre O, et al: Long-term outcomes following laparoscopic supracervical hysterectomy. Br J Obstet Gynaecol 2008;115:1605–1610.

Lowenstein L, Yarnitsky D, Gruenwald I, et al: Does hysterectomy affect genital sensation? Eur J Obstet Gynecol 2005;119:242–245.

Mant J, Painter R, Vessey M: Epidemiology of genital prolapse: Observations from the Oxford Family Planning Association Study. Br J Obstet Gynaecol 1997;104:579–585.

Martin DC: Hysterectomy for treatment of pain associated with endometriosis. J Minim Invasive Gynecology 2006;13:566–572.

Miller JJR, Botros SM, Beaumont JL, et al: Impact of hysterectomy on stress urinary incontinence: An identical twin study. Am J Obstet Gynecol 2008;198:565.

Nationwide Inpatient Sample (NIS) of the Healthcare Cost and Utilization Project (HCUP). Available at: www.hcupnet.ahrq.gov. Retrieved December 28, 2007.

Nieboer TE, Johnson N, Lethaby A, et al: Surgical approach to hysterectomy for benign gynaecological disease. Cochrane Database of Syst Rev 2009;Issue 3:CD003677.

Olsen AL, Smith VJ, Bergstrom JO, et al: Epidemiology of surgically managed pelvic organ prolapse and urinary incontinence. Obstet Gynecol 1997;89:501–506.

The REST Investigators: Uterine-artery embolization versus surgery for symptomatic uterine fibroids. N Engl J Med 2007;256:360–370.

Rhodes JC, Kjerulff KH, Langenberg PW, Guzinski GM: Hysterectomy and sexual function. JAMA 1999;282:1934–1941.

Robert M, Soraisham A, Sauve R: Postoperative urinary incontinence after total abdominal hysterectomy or supracervical hysterectomy: A meta-analysis. Am J Obstet Gynecol 2008;198:264.

Shakiba K, Bena JF, McGill KM, et al: Surgical treatment of endometriosis: A 7-year follow-up on the requirement for further surgery. Obstet Gynecol 2008;111:1285–1292.

Spies JB, Cooper JM, Worthington-Kirsch R, et al: Outcomes of uterine embolization and hysterectomy for leiomyomas: Results of a multicenter study. Am J Obstet Gynecol 2004;191:22–31.

Stovall TG, Ling FW, Crawford DA: Hysterectomy for chronic pelvic pain of presumed uterine etiology. Obstet Gynecol 1990;75:676–679.

Thakar R, Ayers S, Clarkson P, et al: Outcomes after total versus subtotal abdominal hysterectomy. N Engl J Med 2002;347:1318–1325.

Thakar R, Ayers S, Georgakapolou A, et al: Hysterectomy improves quality of life and decreases psychiatric symptoms: A prospective and randomized comparison of total versus subtotal hysterectomy. Br J Obstet Gynaecol 2004;111:1115–1120.

Volkers NA, Hehenkamp WJK, Birnie E, et al: Uterine artery embolization versus hysterectomy in the treatment of symptomatic uterine fibroids: 2 years' outcome from the randomized EMMY trial. Am J Obstet Gynecol 2007;196:519.e1–519.e11.

Wade SW, Magee G, Metz L, Broder MS: Cost-effectiveness of treatments for dysfunctional uterine bleeding. J Reprod Med 2006;51:553–562.

Webb MJ, Aronson MP, Ferguson LK, et al: Post-hysterectomy vaginal vault prolapse; primary repair in 693 patients. Obstet Gynecol 1998;92:281–285.

Weber AM, Walters MD, Schover LR, et al: Functional outcomes and satisfaction after abdominal hysterectomy. Am J Obstet Gynecol 1999;181:530–535.

Abdominal Hysterectomy

6

Beri M. Ridgeway M.D.

 Video Clips on DVD

6-1 Total Abdominal Hysterectomy, Basic Techniques

6-2 Total Abdominal Hysterectomy, Endometriosis

6-3 Total Abdominal Hysterectomy, Fibroid Uterus

Over 500,000 hysterectomies were performed in the United States in 2003 for benign disease, of which two thirds were performed via the abdominal route (Wu et al, 2007). Despite advancements in laparoscopy and data supporting vaginal hysterectomy outcomes, the abdominal route is still more popular than the vaginal and laparoscopic routes combined. Furthermore, despite advances in medical management and less invasive techniques for the treatment of benign gynecologic conditions such as menorrhagia, the rate of hysterectomy does not seem to be decreasing.

Once the decision to perform a hysterectomy has been made, the type and route of hysterectomy must be decided. Chapter 4 contains a detailed discussion on choosing the route of hysterectomy. Factors that lead to the choice of the abdominal route include vaginal shape and access to the uterus, uterine size and shape, extent of extrauterine disease, need for concurrent procedures, surgeon experience and preference, and patient preference. Generally speaking, abdominal hysterectomy for benign disease is indicated for the following: large fibroid uterus (especially when the uterus is broad), suspected presence of disease outside the uterus (adnexal disease, severe adhesive disease, endometriosis, bowel disease), and insufficient access to the vagina. Though many skilled laparoscopists would argue that laparoscopy should be used for the preceding indications, the abdominal approach is completely acceptable and may be safer in the general gynecologist's hands (Garry et al, 2004; McPherson et al, 2004).

The preoperative and perioperative considerations for abdominal hysterectomy are described in Chapter 4. This chapter will review the basic techniques of abdominal hysterectomy as well as techniques for difficult abdominal hysterectomies.

Case 1: Uterovaginal Prolapse

CM is a 34-year-old gravida 2, para 2 woman who presents with the complaint of symptomatic uterovaginal prolapse. She reports the feeling of a bulge in her vagina since her last delivery. She denies urinary or bowel complaints and is sexually active and denies any dysfunction. She has two healthy children and states that she definitely does not desire any additional children. Her medical and surgical histories are unremarkable and she has never had an abnormal Papanicolaou (Pap) smear or abnormal bleeding. Physical examination reveals a small, anteflexed uterus with stage III uterovaginal prolapse with predominant anterior vaginal wall prolapse. Her laboratory studies are unremarkable and a recent Pap smear and human papillomavirus (HPV) DNA assay are negative. Urodynamics reveal normal voiding function and no evidence of detrusor overactivity or stress urinary incontinence. The treatment options including conservative and surgical management are discussed at length with the patient, including uterine-sparing procedures, and she desires hysterectomy. Given the patient's young age and significant pelvic organ prolapse, a total abdominal hysterectomy, sacral colpopexy, and Burch colposuspension are planned.

Discussion of Case

As quality of life issues become more important and the stigma of pelvic floor disorders decreases, women are seeking treatment for pelvic organ prolapse with increasing frequency. Treatment options include observation, pelvic muscle exercises, pessary placement, and surgical management. Although surgical treatment options include uterine-sparing procedures, the outcomes data for these operations are newer and less studied compared to the procedures that include hysterectomy. Uterovaginal prolapse often facilitates vaginal hysterectomy, which can be combined with vaginal apex suspension. Vaginal procedures to treat prolapse are associated with good anatomic outcomes. However, according to the Cochrane review, the abdominal sacral colpopexy is better than vaginal sacrospinous colpopexy, in terms of a lower rate of recurrent apical prolapse and less dyspareunia, but is associated with higher cost and a slower return to activities of daily living (Maher et al, 2008). Given this patient's young age and stage III uterovaginal prolapse, it is reasonable to offer the most aggressive therapy that has the strongest data supporting long-term anatomic success.

The patient elected abdominal sacral colpopexy with total abdominal hysterectomy. Alternatively, a supracervical hysterectomy could be considered, especially if cervical elongation was not present. Patients without cervical dysplasia, uterine hyperplasia, premalignancy, known or suspected malignancy, or cervical fibroids may have the choice between total and subtotal hysterectomy. Subtotal hysterectomy is defined as the removal of the uterine corpus at or below the level of the internal os with attempted ablation of the endocervical canal after removal of the corpus. Historically, the supracervical or subtotal hysterectomy was abandoned in favor of total hysterectomy because of problems related to the retained cervix. However, subtotal hysterectomy has gained a renewed interest as one technique to reduce the effects of hysterectomy on urinary and sexual function. Unfortunately, to date, the possible benefits of supracervical hysterectomy with regard to perioperative morbidity and postoperative sexual and urinary function are not supported by research. In three randomized controlled trials using laparotomy for access, there were no differences in complications including infection; blood loss requiring transfusion; or urinary tract, bowel, or vascular injury (Learman et al, 2003; Thakar et al, 2002; Gimbel et al, 2003). Reported rates of postoperative cyclical vaginal bleeding in women randomized to subtotal hysterectomy were 5% to 20%. Approximately 1.5% of participants had a second operation within 3 months to remove the cervix. Additionally, choosing to preserve the cervix to conserve sexual and urinary function has not been supported by prospective randomized trials (Lethaby et al, 2006). There were no differences in postoperative stress or urge urinary incontinence, urinary frequency, or incomplete bladder emptying in most studies. One European study did find a higher incidence of urinary incontinence after subtotal hysterectomy (Gimbel et al, 2003). In regard to sexual function, there was no difference in any outcome in any of the prospective studies. Despite the lack of data supporting superior outcomes for subtotal hysterectomy, the decision between total and subtotal hysterectomy is often highly personal. Many patients have strong preexisting ideas about retaining the cervix and this should be discussed with the patient preoperatively in detail. Also, future studies using laparoscopic or robotic techniques may show different results.

Candidates interested in subtotal hysterectomy must have normal results from a recent cytologic cervical examination and a normal gross appearance of the cervix documented before surgery. Clinicians should also consider testing for high-risk human papillomavirus strains. In general, unless the patient is at high risk for ovarian cancer or the ovaries appear abnormal intraoperatively, we do not advocate prophylactic oophorectomy in a premenopausal woman undergoing hysterectomy by any route. Please see Chapter 9 for further discussion of prophylactic oophorectomy.

Surgical Technique

See DVD Video 6-1 for video demonstration of simple abdominal hysterectomy.

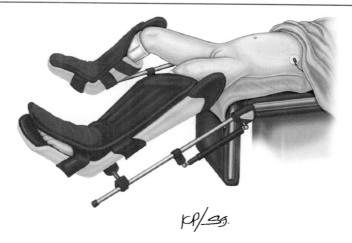

Figure 6-1 The low dorsal lithotomy position allows for vaginal and rectal access.

Surgical Technique

There are many variations in the technique of abdominal hysterectomy. Given that there are no randomized controlled trials comparing various surgical techniques, slight variation in technique likely results in minimal or no change in outcome.

After general anesthesia is induced and the patient is intubated, the abdominal hysterectomy begins with proper positioning of the patient. Abdominal hysterectomy can be performed in the dorsal supine or dorsal lithotomy position (Fig. 6-1). If vaginal access is necessary for other procedures or if a difficult abdominal hysterectomy is anticipated, the dorsal lithotomy position may be advantageous because an additional surgical assistant can stand between the legs in close proximity to the surgical field. When placing the patient in the dorsal lithotomy position, she should be positioned in the low lithotomy position using adjustable cushioned stirrups, such as Allen or Yellofin stirrups. Care must be taken to not overflex or extend the joints. Additionally, the weight of the patient's leg should rest on the heel as opposed to the calf or lateral leg. The arms can be tucked and cushioned to help prevent nerve injury or secured to arm boards. If tucked, arm sleds may be necessary in patients who are obese. If the arms are secured to arm boards, they should not extend beyond 90 degrees and all operative personnel must take care not to rest or place any weight against the arms. The pubic hair is clipped to the level of the pubic symphysis. An examination under anesthesia is performed. Careful attention should be paid to uterine size, contour, and width; uterine mobility; cervical size and location; ovarian size; and evidence of masses or signs of endometriosis. This information will help guide the decision of what type of skin incision to make. A single dose intravenous antibiotic and antiembolic prophylaxis are routinely given. The patient's abdomen, vagina, and upper thighs are prepared with povidone-iodine or hibiclens and the patient is draped. A Foley catheter attached to a continuous drainage system is inserted into the bladder.

Based on the planned procedures, patient body habitus, presence of prior surgical scar, and uterine or other disease, a laparotomy incision is made. The anatomic considerations for the different incision types are covered in Chapter 2. In the case of abdominal hysterectomy, this includes several incision types: Pfannenstiel incision, vertical midline incision, Maylard incision, and Cherney incision. The Pfannenstiel incision is the least invasive, preserving the rectus muscles and is ideal in normal-weight patients who have normal-sized uteri and don't require additional procedures.

The Pfannenstiel incision is performed by making a horizontal incision 2 cm above the pubic symphysis with a scalpel. The width of the incision depends on the planned procedure. Once the skin is open, the subcutaneous tissue is divided sharply or with electrocautery. Upon identification of the fascia, it is incised and the fascial incision is extended laterally to the border of the skin incision. Kocher clamps are applied to the superior edge of the fascial incision and the rectus muscles are dissected bluntly or with electrocautery from the fascia. Perforating vessels are cauterized as this dissection takes place. Similarly, the rectus muscles are dissected from the inferior aspect of the fascial incision. The rectus muscles are then separated in the midline. Starting near the superior aspect of the fascia, the preperitoneal fat is separated until the peritoneum is identified. Once identified, it is grasped with two clamps and elevated. After palpating for underlying structures such as bowel, the peritoneum is opened bluntly or sharply with Metzenbaum scissors. After the defect is created and proper cavity entry is assured, one finger is used to explore the underside of the peritoneum for adhesions. The peritoneum is then opened vertically to the superior extent of the fascial incision and inferiorly toward the bladder. As one gets close to the bladder, the peritoneum should be taken down in layers to avoid cystotomy. If necessary, the peritoneal incision can be extended laterally to create more space and avoid the bladder. Ultimately, the incision should be taken down to the pubic symphysis which requires division of the pyramidalis muscles.

For cases of an enlarged uterus (typically ≥ 16 weeks), pelvic mass, or cancer, or when procedures above the umbilicus are anticipated, a vertical incision may be appropriate. In these cases, a vertical skin incision is made with a scalpel from the pubic symphysis to the umbilicus. If necessary, the incision can be carried through the umbilicus or to the left of the umbilicus to the xiphoid process. The subcutaneous tissue is divided sharply or with electrocautery. The fascia is identified and opened sharply, then extended vertically for the length of the incision. Kocher clamps are applied to one side of the fascia and elevated. The rectus muscles are dissected from the fascia with the goal of identifying where the rectus muscles meet in the midline. Once this area is identified, the rectus muscles are separated, the preperitoneal fat is cleared, and the peritoneum is grasped with two sets of pick-ups and opened sharply or bluntly. The peritoneum is incised superiorly and inferiorly with good visualization of the bladder.

For cases when lateral access is required, a Maylard incision may be useful. A horizontal skin incision is made 2 cm above the pubic symphysis with the scalpel. The subcutaneous tissue is divided and the fascia is identified and opened sharply. The fascial incision is opened in a horizontal fashion to the border of the skin incision. The rectus muscles are identified and the lateral aspect of the rectus muscle is moved medial, exposing the inferior epigastric vessels. A right-angle clamp is passed under the vessels and used to bring two ties of No. 0 polyglactin 910 under the vessels. The vessels are then suture-ligated and divided. Once this has been performed bilaterally, the rectus muscles are divided with electrocautery. The peritoneum is identified and opened as described above.

The Cherney incision is useful when a transverse skin incision is desired and more operative space is required. The initial steps are similar to those of the Pfannenstiel skin incision. However, once the anterior rectus sheath is opened, the rectus muscles are identified, and the tendons of the rectus abdominis and pyramidalis muscles are transected 1 to 2 cm above their insertion into the pubic symphysis. The muscles can then be moved cephalad to provide better access to the pelvis. This incision should be kept in mind when one is struggling during a difficult hysterectomy, as a Pfannenstiel incision can be converted to a Cherney when visualization is suboptimal.

Once the laparotomy is accomplished, an examination of the upper abdomen via palpation is performed. A variety of self-retaining retractors are available to assist with visualization, including the Bookwalter, Balfour, Turner-Warwick, and O'Connor-O'Sullivan. The bowel is gently packed cephalad with moistened laparotomy sponges and the retractor is applied. Great care must be taken to choose retractor blades of the appropriate length to avoid iatrogenic nerve injury. This is of most concern when using lateral blades because retractors that are too long will place pressure on the psoas muscle and femoral nerve. Thin patients are especially at risk for this nerve injury.

The pelvic anatomy is examined (Fig. 6-2). Restoration of normal anatomy is achieved with adhesiolysis, if necessary. The uterus is grasped at each cornu with a long clamp such as a Kelly or Kocher clamp and elevated toward the incision (Fig. 6-3). This clamp should incorporate the cornu, round ligament, and fallopian tube. Traction and countertraction is a key principle for the successful completion of any hysterectomy. The uterus is deviated to the patient's left side, placing tension on the right round ligament. The round ligament is grasped with forceps and a suture is placed directly below the round ligament through the mesosalpinx approximately 3 to 4 cm from the cornu (Fig. 6-4). The same suture is then placed through the round ligament at this same location and tied. Electrocautery is used to desiccate and transect the

Figure 6-2 Pertinent pelvic anatomy is examined prior to starting the hysterectomy.

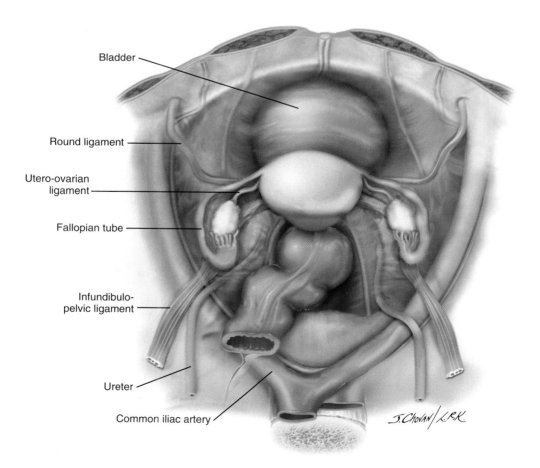

Bladder

Round ligament

Utero-ovarian ligament

Fallopian tube

Infundibulo-pelvic ligament

Ureter

Common iliac artery

Figure 6-3 The uterus is grasped at each cornu with a long clamp such as a Kelly or Kocher clamp and elevated toward the incision. Each clamp should incorporate the cornu, round ligament, and fallopian tube.

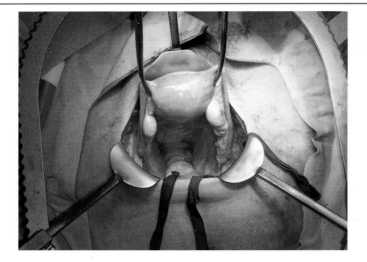

Figure 6-4 The round ligament is grasped with forceps and a suture is placed directly below it through the mesosalpinx approximately 3 to 4 cm from the cornu. The same suture is then placed through the round ligament at this same location, tied, and held if desired.

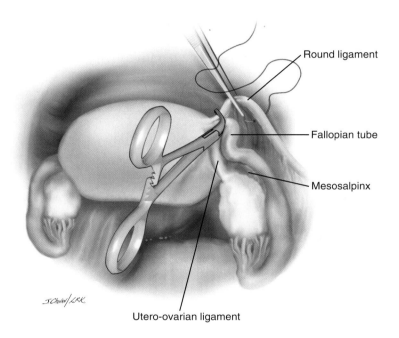

Round ligament

Fallopian tube

Mesosalpinx

Utero-ovarian ligament

round ligament medial to the suture. The suture is tagged and placed laterally over the retractor, thereby holding the peritoneum open laterally.

The anterior leaf of the broad ligament is opened inferiorly to the level of the uterine vessel and then medially along the vesicouterine peritoneal fold separating the bladder peritoneum from the lower uterine segment in preparation for bladder flap development. The surgical assistant can place an opened tonsil clamp below the peritoneum and guide the surgeon's dissection. This dissection is carried to the midportion of the vesicouterine peritoneum. An identical procedure is performed on the contralateral side. When anatomy is not distorted, the area to incise is easily identified by grasping the peritoneum with atraumatic forceps and identifying where it becomes pliable and loose. The posterior leaf of the broad ligament can be dissected sharply or with electrocautery lateral to the infundibulopelvic ligament to open up this space further. With the anterior and posterior leaves of the broad ligament open, the ureter is identified in the retroperitoneum (Fig. 6-5). This vital step should be

Figure 6-5 With the anterior and posterior leaves of the broad ligament open, the ureter is identified in the retroperitoneum. Note the uterine vessels are skeletonized.

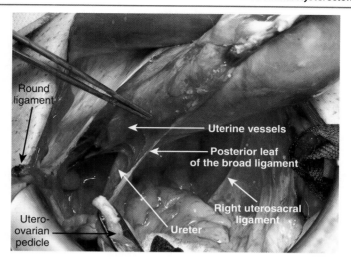

performed during every hysterectomy to help prevent ureteral injury. With the leaves of the broad ligament separated, the areolar tissue is gently separated with a blunt instrument such as rounded forceps or the suction tip. Placing these instruments at an angle toward the medial leaf of the broad ligament and moving them in a craniocaudad fashion, the ureter is identified. If the ureter cannot be identified, the gentle blunt dissection can be carried toward the bifurcation of the common iliac artery where the ureter crosses this structure at the pelvic brim. The use of ureteral catheters is advocated by some surgeons; however, in our experience, prophylactic ureteral catheterization is not helpful and can be associated with ureteral injury (Kuno et al, 1998). Others advocate ureteral identification through palpation; however, the internal iliac artery, ovarian vessels, and vessels of the broad ligament are easily confused with the ureter.

Once the ureter is identified, either the infundibulopelvic ligament or the utero-ovarian ligament is clamped and transected, depending on whether a salpingo-ophorectomy is planned or not. In cases in which an oophorectomy is planned, a defect is created in the posterior broad ligament inferior to the ovary with the ureter in sight. This defect is extended toward the infundibulo-pelvic ligament. Typically, three clamps are passed from lateral to medial through this defect lateral to the ovary, making certain that the entire ovary is included in the surgical specimen (Fig. 6-6A). The ligament is then transected and suture ligated. We use a free tie of No. 0 polyglactin 910 behind the most proximal clamp, followed by suture ligation with the same suture type using the fore-aft technique behind the most distal clamp. Tying the pedicle before suturing it prevents formation of an expanding hematoma through inadvertent puncture of the ovarian vessels. The clamp on the specimen side is then removed after suture ligation. The free ends of the suture can be used to tie the adnexa to the clamp on the cornu to improve visualization.

If an ovary-sparing procedure is planned, a defect is created in the posterior broad ligament lateral to the uterus and inferior to the utero-ovarian ligament (see Fig. 6-6B). Two clamps are placed through this defect and the cornual clamp is advanced to prevent back-bleeding. The utero-ovarian ligament is then suture-ligated as described earlier. These procedures are performed bilaterally.

The uterus is elevated cephalad and the bladder dissection is performed. The vesicouterine peritoneum is elevated and sharp dissection is performed with

Figure 6-6 A, If oophorectomy is being done, a defect is created in the posterior broad ligament inferior to the ovary, with the ureter in sight. Three clamps are passed through this defect lateral to the ovary, making certain that the entire ovary is included in the surgical specimen. **B,** In an ovary-sparing procedure, a defect is created in the posterior broad ligament lateral to the uterus and inferior to the utero-ovarian ligament. Two clamps are placed through this defect and the cornual clamp is advanced to prevent back-bleeding.

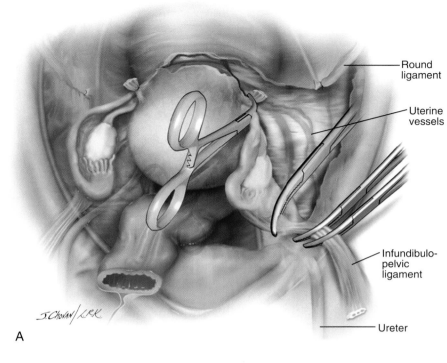

A

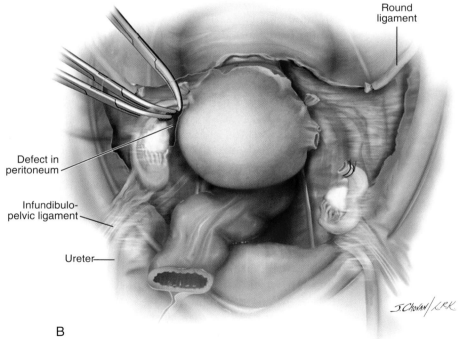

B

the tips of the scissors pointing toward the uterus. An avascular plane exists between the lower uterine segment and bladder, which allows for its mobilization. With caution, the bladder is taken down past the cervix. We perform this portion solely with sharp dissection, as blunt dissection and electrocautery have been associated with cystotomy and vesicovaginal fistula formation. If the dissection is difficult, as after a previous cesarean section, an intrafascial technique can be used. Above the bladder, the serosa and endopelvic fascia cover-

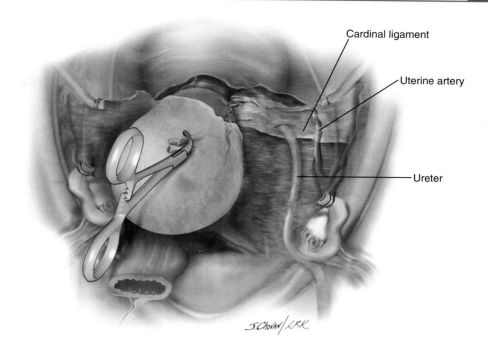

Figure 6-7 The posterior leaf of the broad ligament is incised down to the level of the uterosacral ligament, and the ureter and blood vessels are more thoroughly visualized.

Cardinal ligament

Uterine artery

Ureter

ing the cervix are opened in a transverse fashion with electrocautery. This step allows the fascia to be pushed down which also ultimately moves the bladder as well. The posterior leaf of the broad ligament is then incised to the level of the uterosacral ligament, further opening the retroperitoneum to better identify the ureter (Fig. 6-7). This incision can be performed sharply or with electrocautery.

The uterine vessels are then skeletonized, removing excess tissue so that the ureter drops even further and so that the pedicle contains only vascular structures. The excess connective tissue is picked up with forceps and separated from the vascular structures using sharp dissection or electrocautery. Great care must be taken to avoid opening the uterine vessels. With the uterine vessels exposed, a large curved clamp is placed perpendicular to the vessels at the junction of the cervix and lower uterine segment (Fig. 6-8). For this step, we typically use a curved Heaney clamp. The clamp is placed with the tips on the uterus and a slow clamping motion is used so that the clamp slides off the uterus, assuring that the entire pedicle is included. A second clamp is placed to prevent back-bleeding. Either a scalpel or scissors are used to transect the pedicle, which is then suture ligated using No. 0 polyglactin 910. When placing these stitches, it is important to place the needle at the inferior corner of the clamp tip in order to secure the entire pedicle. Either the suture can be tied directly behind the clamp or the needle can be passed through the lateral aspect of the pedicle for extra security prior to tying. This step is performed bilaterally.

Additional clamps are placed on each side, with each clamp placed medial to the previous pedicle, close to the cervix, further avoiding the ureter (Fig. 6-9). These bites incorporate the cardinal ligaments and uterosacral ligaments, and a series of pedicles may be required depending on uterine size. As one nears the cervix, one may choose to use a straight Heaney or Kocher clamp; with each bite, care must be taken to slide off the uterine corpus and cervix. As one progresses, always double-check to make sure the bladder has been dissected sufficiently and the rectum is not close. If there is any doubt, addi-

Figure 6-8 A large curved clamp is placed perpendicular to the uterine vessels at the junction of the cervix and lower uterine segment.

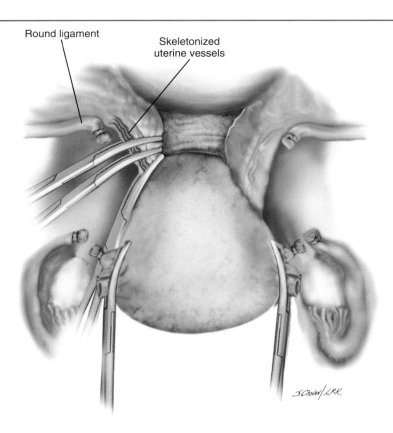

Round ligament

Skeletonized uterine vessels

Figure 6-9 Additional clamps are placed on each side, with each clamp placed medial to the previous pedicle, close to the cervix, further avoiding the ureter. These bites incorporate the cardinal and uterosacral ligaments and a series of pedicles may be required depending on uterine size and cervical length.

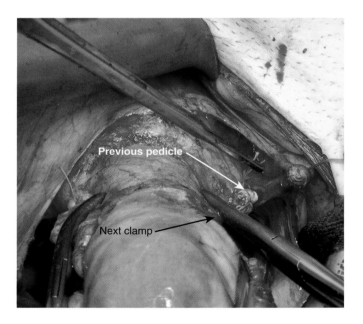

Previous pedicle

Next clamp

tional bladder dissection can be performed or the rectovaginal septum may be dissected to avoid injury. Once the location of the external cervical os is confirmed via palpation, a large curved clamp may be placed below the cervix bilaterally in preparation for amputation (Fig. 6-10). In a hysterectomy for benign indications, place this clamp as close to the cervix as possible to prevent vaginal shortening. The cervix and uterus are amputated with a scalpel or

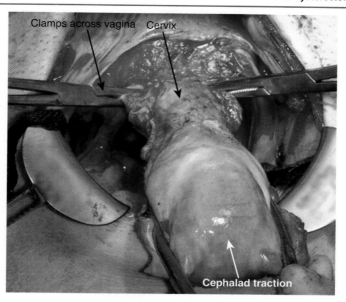

curved scissors (Fig. 6-11A, B). Check the specimen to assure that the entire cervix has been removed. The specimen and the scissors are passed off the table and considered contaminated.

Admittedly, there are many ways to close the vaginal cuff. Typically, we place a figure-of-eight stitch of No. 0 polyglactin 910 in the midportion of the vaginal cuff approximating the anterior and posterior cuff and marking the midline. Figure-of-eight stitches are placed on each side of the midline making sure that there are no spaces between bites. All sutures are tagged and not tied at this point. Once one approximates the corner, a transfixing stitch is placed and the clamp is removed. The remaining sutures are tied. Tagging the corner stitches allows one to identify the borders of the vaginal cuff if additional sutures are required (Fig. 6-12). Alternatively, the cuff angle stitches can be placed and the intervening cuff can be closed using a running, locking suture. We do not advocate closing the cuff with only two angle stitches, as this can narrow and distort the upper vagina. The cuff is inspected for hemostasis and additional sutures are placed if necessary. Some surgeons prefer leaving the cuff open to heal by secondary intention. There appears to be no increase in postoperative febrile morbidity when the cuff is not closed (Neuman et al, 1993).

Emerging data support the use of an angle stitch, often called a Richardson stitch, in order to prevent apical prolapse (Rahn et al, 2008; also see Chapter 1 for the original description). To do this, the cardinal and uterosacral ligaments are incorporated into the cuff angles bilaterally.

The abdomen is irrigated with warm saline or water and all operative pedicles are observed. Once hemostasis is assured, additional procedures are performed if planned, the retractor and laparotomy sponges are removed, and the incision is closed.

Cystoscopy is not routinely performed after abdominal hysterectomy; however, it should be considered. Recently published data describe a lower urinary tract (bladder and ureteral) injury rate of 1.7% after total abdominal hysterectomy (Ibeanu et al, 2009). As routine cystoscopy becomes cost-effective when the ureteral injury rate exceeds 1.5%, the addition of this

Figure 6-11 A, The cervix and uterus are amputated with a scalpel or curved scissors. **B,** The vaginal cuff is ready to be closed.

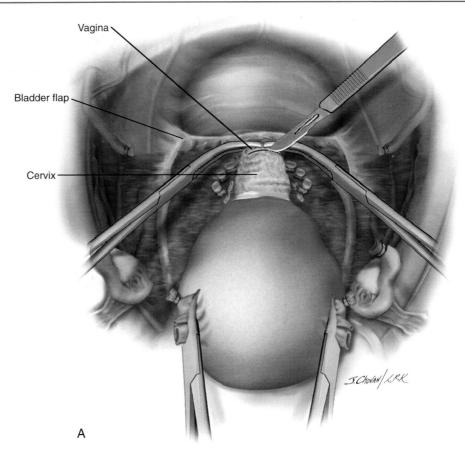

Vagina

Bladder flap

Cervix

A

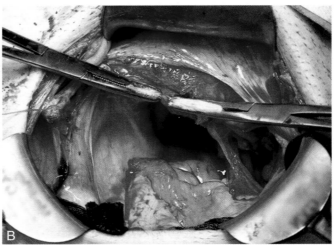

B

procedure after total abdominal hysterectomy merits some consideration, especially in difficult cases (Visco et al, 2001).

The placement of an intraperitoneal drain is not recommended after routine hysterectomy. However, it can be considered in cases of intra-abdominal infection. If a drain is to be used, a closed suction drain such as the Jackson-Pratt drain should be placed through a separate stab incision in the lower abdominal wall and should not exit through the incision itself.

Figure 6-12 The vaginal cuff is closed. The lateral sutures mark the cuff border.

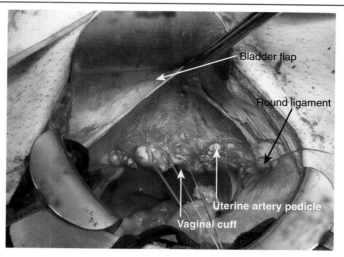

Case 2: Chronic Pelvic Pain

RJ is a 42-year-old gravida 3, para 2, aborta 1 with a 15-year history of chronic pelvic pain. The patient was diagnosed with stage IV endometriosis in her 20s and underwent laparoscopic excision of endometriosis prior to becoming pregnant. Since her last pregnancy 6 years ago, the patient's pain has been increasing in frequency and severity. The pain is worst immediately before and during the patient's menses. She also complains of severe dyspareunia on deep penetration. She denies urinary or bowel complaints. She has tried the following medications with limited success: continuous oral contraceptives, progestins, and depo lupron. She is becoming frustrated with her chronic pelvic pain and dysmenorrhea that requires her to miss work several days a month. Her past medical history is significant for depression and surgical history is significant for laparoscopic excision of endometriosis and a dilation and curettage. She has never had an abnormal Pap smear or abnormal bleeding. Physical examination reveals an immobile, small, anteflexed uterus. No masses are palpable, though the entire pelvis feels fixed. Nodularity is present on rectovaginal examination. Her laboratory studies are unremarkable and a recent Pap smear and HPV DNA assay are negative. Given that she has completed childbearing and has failed medical management, a total abdominal hysterectomy and excision of endometriosis are planned.

Discussion of Case

Endometriosis is a debilitating condition that can lead to chronic pain, dyspareunia, and infertility. Although the exact prevalence is unknown, studies demonstrate that it is relatively common, affecting 1% of women undergoing major surgery for all gynecologic indications and 12% to 32% of women of reproductive age undergoing laparoscopy to determine the cause of pelvic pain. Pain is the most common symptom associated with endometriosis, and approximately three quarters of symptomatic patients experience pelvic pain or dysmenorrhea (Sinaii et al, 2008). Other symptoms include dysmenorrhea, subfertility, deep dyspareunia, cyclical bowel or bladder symptoms, abnormal menstrual bleeding, and chronic fatigue (Kennedy et al, 2005).

Because this patient has documented stage IV endometriosis, debilitating chronic pelvic pain, and has tried and failed multiple medical therapies, definitive surgical therapy is appropriate. Given the patient's age, preoperative discussion and consent should be made with the patient as to whether her ovaries should be conserved or removed, after carefully reviewing the pros and cons of each option.

Surgical Technique

See DVD Video 6-2 for video demonstration of total abdominal hysterectomy in a patient with a frozen pelvis secondary to stage IV endometriosis.

Despite extensive research, the optimal treatment of endometriosis is unclear. Treatment of endometriosis must be individualized and depends on severity of symptoms, the extent and location of disease, whether there is a desire for pregnancy, the age of the patient, medication side effects, surgical complication rates, and cost. Medical treatment options include expectant management, analgesia, hormonal medical therapy (oral contraceptive pills, gonadotropin-releasing hormone [GnRH] agonists, progestins, danazol, and aromatase inhibitors). Surgical intervention includes conservative (spare uterus and ovaries) and definitive (hysterectomy and possible bilateral salpingo-oophorectomy) choices. Indications for surgical management of endometriosis include severe, incapacitating, or acute symptoms; symptoms that have failed to resolve with medical therapy; and the presence of advanced disease. Definitive, rather than conservative, surgery for treatment of endometriosis should be considered when incapacitating symptoms persist following conservative surgery, moderate to severe disease is present and future pregnancy is not desired, or hysterectomy is indicated for coexisting pelvic disease. The decision to perform a definitive procedure is primarily dependent upon the patient's interest in maintaining childbearing potential. The ovaries may be conserved in younger women (before age 45) to avoid premature development of menopausal symptoms and decisions regarding estrogen replacement. However, removal of both ovaries is appropriate when the ovaries are extensively damaged by endometriosis or when the woman is approaching menopause.

There are many variations to anatomy of the patient condition that may make the abdominal hysterectomy difficult. When a difficult hysterectomy is anticipated, preoperative planning is essential. We recommend the use of the low lithotomy position for these cases, as it provides access to the vagina, bladder, and rectum. The benefit of a skilled assistant cannot be underestimated. Furthermore, additional operative time should be booked. Depending on the preoperative hemoglobin level, patient co-morbidities, and anticipated findings, one may consider having cross-matched blood products available. The use of mechanical bowel preparations remains controversial. It has been reported that some general surgeons will not perform a primary reanastomosis after bowel injury if the patient has not undergone a mechanical bowel preparation. However, new evidence suggests that aggressive mechanic bowel preparations may do more harm than good, leading to increased spillage of bowel contents and an increase in anastomotic leaks (Mahajna et al, 2005; Wille-Jorgensen et al, 2005).

Once the difficult hysterectomy is started, exposure of pertinent anatomy is necessary. For these cases, a vertical skin incision should be considered and the use of a Bookwalter retractor may assist in achieving maximal exposure. One of the most important intraoperative skills necessary to perform a difficult abdominal hysterectomy is the ability to identify and reestablish normal anatomy. In almost all gynecologic conditions, the retroperitoneal spaces remain free of distortion and are therefore a good starting place to establish normal anatomy.

Typically, we do not advocate the use of routine ureteral catheterization in complicated cases; however, in this case of documented, extensive endometriosis, ureteral catheterization can be helpful. Deep infiltrating endometriosis and previous surgical excision of endometriosis can lead to significant scarring and anatomic distortion, making it very difficult to identify the ureter. After a laparotomy is performed, retractors are placed and the pertinent anatomy is identified. The bladder dome is opened with electrocautery and ureteral catheters are placed. If one has experience placing ureteral catheters, they may be placed cystoscopically before starting the case or intraoperatively. Alternatively, a urologic consultant may be called.

The key retroperitoneal spaces in the pelvis are identified, including rectovaginal and vesicovaginal septa in the center of the pelvis and the pararectal and paravesical spaces in the lateral pelvis. See Chapter 2 for a detailed description of the pertinent anatomy. To open the pararectal and paravesical spaces, the lateral pelvic peritoneum is incised over the psoas muscle. Dividing the peritoneum lateral to the external iliac artery and opening the retroperitoneal space is safely accomplished, as there are no vital structures at this level of the pelvis. The dissection proceeds medially, reflecting the medial peritoneum off the retroperitoneal space, revealing the external iliac artery and vein. Once these structures are identified, the dissection is carried cephalad to the bifurcation of the common iliac, where the ureter is identified. The ureter is retracted medially and the hypogastric artery laterally and the pararectal space is developed.

The paravesical space is opened by identifying the external iliac artery and vein and retracting the areolar and adipose tissue medially. On the medial aspect of the paravesical space is the superior vesical artery. The tissue located between the pararectal and paravesical spaces is the parametrium or cardinal ligament and it contains the uterine vessels. To specifically identify the origin of the uterine artery, the dissection is carried along the anterior surface of the hypogastric artery until the first main medial branch (uterine artery) is identified. As the ureter has been identified on the medial aspect of the pelvic peritoneum, the ureter is mobilized from the peritoneum to protect it from injury. With the ureter identified, it is dissected from the paracervical tunnel in the course of more distal mobilization, which may be required to manage an expanded lower uterine segment or cervix.

It is common to also find an obliterated posterior cul-de-sac or bladder flap that is severely scarred in cases in which the preceding dissections are necessary. Techniques to safely open these spaces are described later in this chapter.

Once these spaces and all pertinent anatomy are identified, it is safe to proceed with the hysterectomy as described.

Case 3: Menorrhagia and Fibroids

A 39-year-old gravida 5, para 5 woman has a long history of menorrhagia. The patient notes that her bleeding has increased during the last year. Currently, she bleeds every 26 days for a total of 7 days, noting clots during the first 2 days. She was diagnosed with iron deficiency anemia 3 years ago and required a blood transfusion 8 months ago after an episode of severe menorrhagia. She has been treated unsuccessfully with nonsteroidal anti-inflammatory drugs (NSAIDs), oral contraceptive pills, and GnRH agonists. Her past medical and surgical histories are otherwise unremarkable and a recent Pap smear is normal. Physical examination reveals a 16-week-size uterus with an irregular contour consistent with multiple fibroids. An endometrial biopsy is performed demonstrating secretory endometrium, and an ultrasound demonstrates an enlarged uterus measuring 16 × 9 × 9 cm with a large posterior fundal fibroid and normal-appearing ovaries. The patient has completed childbearing and is interested in definitive therapy. After a discussion of her options, she elects hysterectomy.

Discussion of Case

Uterine myomas are very common with the estimated cumulative incidence by age 50 of greater than 80% in black women and almost 70% in white women (Day Baird et al, 2003). African-American race, nulliparity, early menarche, and family predisposition have all been associated with the development of fibroids. Fibroids can lead to bulk symptoms such as pelvic pain and pressure, heavy or irregular bleeding, urinary symptoms, and reproductive dysfunction. These symptoms are related to the number, size, and location of the tumors.

Relief of symptoms is the major goal in management of women with significant symptoms. The type and timing of any intervention should be individualized, based upon factors such as size and location of the myomas, severity of symptoms, patient age, reproductive plans, and obstetric history. Treatment options include medical and surgical management. Medical management includes NSAIDs and hormonal therapy (oral contraceptive pills, progestins, GnRH agonists, levonorgestrel intrauterine device [IUD], aromatase inhibitors). Other treatment options include endometrial ablation and uterine artery embolization. Surgical treatment includes myomectomy (hysteroscopic, laparoscopic, or open) and hysterectomy, with hysterectomy being definitive therapy.

Leiomyomas are the most common indication for hysterectomy, accounting for 30% of hysterectomies in white and over 50% of hysterectomies in black women. The main advantage of hysterectomy over other invasive interventions is that it eliminates both current symptoms and the chance of recurrent problems from leiomyomas. For many women, such as our patient, who have completed childbearing, this freedom from future problems makes hysterectomy an attractive option.

Surgical Technique

See DVD Video 6-3 for video demonstration of total abdominal hysterectomy in a patient with large uterine fibroids.

The technique for abdominal hysterectomy in a patient with fibroids is dependent on the size and location of the tumors. A careful examination in the office and imaging (ultrasound or magnetic resonance imaging [MRI]) may assist in preoperative planning. The patient should be consented for a vertical and horizontal skin incision. The examination under anesthesia performed in the operating room is critical to decide on incision type.

Once the incision has been made, restoration of anatomy, including adhesiolysis, is performed. A retractor is set up and the bowel is packed away with moistened laparotomy sponges. Attempt to mobilize the uterus through the incision by manually maneuvering it through the defect or elevating it with Kelly or Kocher clamps that have been placed on the cornua. Carefully identify all pertinent structures, as large fibroids can significantly distort the anatomy.

If there is one predominant fibroid distorting the anatomy or making visualization difficult, a myomectomy can be performed. In these cases, the area is infiltrated with dilute vasopressin (20 U vasopressin in 100 mL normal saline), the serosa covering the fibroid is opened sharply or with electrocautery and the myoma is shelled out. Depending on the amount of bleeding, the defect can be left open or closed.

The steps of hysterectomy are similar to those described previously and may require a combination of techniques described in Cases 1 and 2. Dissection of the retroperitoneum and identification of the ureter is critical in cases with fibroids as the distal course of the ureter can be significantly distorted. Aggressive elevation and retraction of the uterine corpus to the contralateral side will help open the pelvic sidewall for dissection. If the ureter cannot be identified, dissection can be performed more cephalad where the ureter crosses the bifurcation of the common iliac vessels at the pelvic brim. As one progresses toward the cervix with pedicle bites, visualization may become difficult secondary to the large size of the uterus. In these cases, once the uterine vessels are occluded, the uterine corpus is amputated, similar to the technique used in supracervical hysterectomy. At this point, Kocher clamps are applied to the cervix and a trachelectomy is performed, followed by vaginal cuff closure as described earlier.

The Difficult Abdominal Hysterectomy and Special Cases

Supracervical Hysterectomy

Although there are no data supporting improved sexual function and urinary outcomes after supracervical hysterectomy compared to total abdominal hysterectomy, the decision to retain the cervix is often highly personal and the patient should be consulted. There are, of course, times when performing a supracervical hysterectomy can reduce morbidity and prevent potential complications. This is especially true in patients who have significant scarring between the cervix and bladder or rectum in cases of endometriosis, pelvic adhesive disease, or pelvic inflammatory disease. Furthermore, when a patient is hemodynamically unstable, complete removal of the cervix may not be prudent as the goal should be to complete the operation as fast as possible.

Performing a supracervical hysterectomy starts with the same steps as the total abdominal hysterectomy described earlier. Once the cardinal and broad ligaments are clamped at the level of the internal os, the uterus is amputated. Amputation can be performed sharply or with electrocautery. To avoid cyclic bleeding from retained lower uterine segment endometrium, the endocervix

Figure 6-13 In subtotal or supracervical hysterectomy the uterus is amputated from the cervix at the level of the internal os.

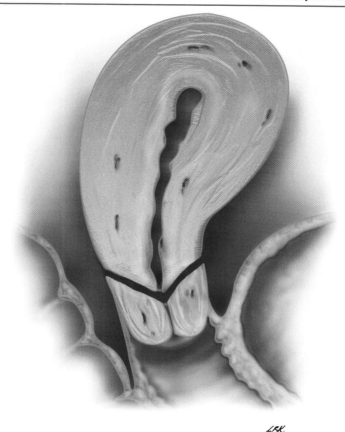

is carefully resected or cauterized. We prefer to perform a reverse cone (Fig. 6-13) and cauterize the remainder of the endocervix. The cervical stump is then closed with No. 0 polyglactin 910 in a running or interrupted fashion.

Obliterated Rectovaginal Septum

To protect the rectum, one must have the ability to open the rectovaginal septum. Usually this can be accomplished by making an incision along the junction between the cervix and vagina and dissecting the avascular plane. However, if this area is scarred the initial incision must be made higher on the cervix or posterior uterus to create a plane between the cervical serosa and stroma. Once this plane has been developed sharply, the avascular plane will be encountered and blunt dissection can be applied. In the case of significant endometriosis, a majority of the septum can be scarred. In such cases, a probe or end-to-end anastomosis sizer may be placed in the vagina and rectum to identify the lumina. With these in place, the septum can be opened with a combination of sharp and blunt dissection. This will often lead to some bleeding, which can be controlled with pressure, suture ligation, and hemostatic aids. Bipolar electrocautery can be used judiciously; however, this may increase the risk of bowel injury. Alternatively, if one is able to gain access to the anterior vagina after bladder flap development and ligation of the uterine vessels, the anterior vagina may be entered sharply. Kocher clamps are applied to the anterior vagina, which is then retracted caudad. The cervix is grasped with a single-tooth tenaculum and retracted cephalad, inverting the uterus. The posterior vagina is then incised and dissected from the rectum. With any technique, rigid proctoscopy can be performed at the end of the case to rule out proctotomy.

Scarring of the Vesicouterine Septum

This variation is most commonly seen after cesarean section or rarely with endometriotic implants. There are several options for addressing this anatomic distortion. If normal bladder peritoneum can be identified at the dome or even laterally, the dissection can be started in this area. The peritoneum is dissected off the underlying bladder toward the cervix, thereby establishing a plane between the bladder and peritoneum. As one nears the diseased area, the dissection will be directly over the bladder muscularis and one may encounter bleeding. This can easily be controlled with electrocautery. Remaining in this plane will eventually develop the bladder flap. Alternatively, the incision can be made higher on the uterus. To accomplish this, the bladder and uterine serosa are dissected above the vesicouterine peritoneum with scissors or electrocautery dissection. One essentially creates a plane, leaving the uterine serosa and some myometrium and stroma on the bladder. If neither of the foregoing techniques work, the dome of the bladder can be opened, thereby allowing one to palpate the cervix through the bladder. With palpation, one can see where the bladder is attached to the cervix and use this as a starting point for dissection. At the end of the surgery, the bladder should be closed in layers and drained continuously. If these options are not viable or the surgeon does not feel comfortable performing this type of dissection, the surgeon can always perform a supracervical hysterectomy. If the patient does not have uterine or cervical malignancy, this option may help avoid complications such as cystotomy and proctotomy. Additionally, amputating the uterine corpus improves visualization and may aid in identifying the rectovaginal and vesicouterine planes.

Unsuspected Malignancy

In cases in which unsuspecting malignancy is discovered at the time of surgery, management depends on the type of malignancy and experience of the surgeon. In an ideal situation, a consultant surgeon such as a gynecologic oncologist should be called. Staging procedures performed by a specialist appear to lead to better patient outcomes (Vernooij et al, 2007). If a gynecologic oncologist is not available, one can consider calling a urologist; however, it is completely acceptable to close the incision and arrange for prompt consultation with an appropriate specialist for a second procedure.

Obesity

Obesity is a chronic disease that is increasing in prevalence in all age groups. Patients who are obese often have multiple weight-related co-morbidities that increase their surgical risk further. Morbidly obese patients benefit from vaginal or laparoscopic surgeries, if feasible, to avoid abdominal wall morbidities. When performing an abdominal hysterectomy on an obese patient, preoperative planning is essential. The patient should be evaluated by an anesthesiologist or internal medicine specialist for preoperative clearance. Ideally, the patient's health status can be optimized prior to surgery. An examination under anesthesia or preoperative imaging may assist in deciding the type of incision.

We will often place these patients in Allen stirrups so that a second surgical assistant can stand between the legs. Although obese patients are at increased risk for postoperative wound infections and separations, inadequate surgical exposure can lead to increased intraoperative morbidity. Avoid making the skin incision in the pannus fold as this area often remains moist and is a nidus for infection. We choose a larger self-retaining retractor, such as the Bookwalter, due to the stability and versatility it provides. We also use longer instruments. Once the operation is complete, a mass closure can be performed. The use of a subcutaneous drain is controversial.

Cesarean Hysterectomy

A hysterectomy following a cesarean section occurs in 0.05% to 0.1% of deliveries (Glaze et al, 2008). In the majority of cases, this procedure is performed emergently for severe uterine hemorrhage that cannot be controlled by conservative measures. Such hemorrhage may be due to an abnormally implanted placenta, uterine atony, uterine rupture, coagulopathy, or laceration of a pelvic vessel. However, it may also be performed in nonemergent cases including cervical cancer and known abnormal placentation. Generally speaking, it is best to perform a cesarean hysterectomy only as a last resort because it is associated with increased morbidity due to the highly vascular pelvic organs. When one is confronted with uncontrollable hemorrhage, conservative measures must be instituted rapidly. If these prove ineffective, the decision to proceed with hysterectomy should be made quickly, as indecisiveness places the patient at even higher risk for morbidity secondary to hypovolemia and coagulopathy. When bleeding of this magnitude is encountered, first notify those responsible for anesthesia and nursing so that they can begin aggressive resuscitation with fluids and blood products.

Peripartum hysterectomy differs from nongravid hysterectomy in several important respects. The uterus is significantly larger and blood vessels throughout the pelvis are greatly dilated, including varices in the mesosalpinx. Additionally, the tissues are friable, and if the cervix has undergone significant dilation and effacement, it will be soft and may be difficult to identify. All of these factors can lead to massive hemorrhage that may obscure the operative field.

The steps of the hysterectomy are identical to those described for case 1. Fortunately, in the postpartum uterus, surgical planes are usually easy to identify and develop. Every attempt should be made to identify the ureter and avoid ligating it. However, control of hemostasis is the primary concern; repair of lower urinary tract injury can be done, if needed, after hemostasis has been achieved and coagulopathy and hypovolemia have been corrected. Supracervical hysterectomy may be safer than total hysterectomy and should be considered unless there is specific indication for removal of the cervix.

Suggested Reading

Baggish MS: Abdominal hysterectomy. In Baggish MS, Karram MM: Atlas of Pelvic Anatomy and Gynecologic Surgery, 2nd ed. Philadelphia, WB Saunders, 2006.

Day Baird D, Dunson DB, Hill MC, et al: High cumulative incidence of uterine leiomyoma in black and white women: Ultrasound evidence. Am J Obstet Gynecol 2003;188:100–107.

Garry R, Fountain J, Mason S, et al: The eVALuate study: two parallel randomised trials, one comparing laparoscopic with abdominal hysterectomy, the other comparing laparoscopic with vaginal hysterectomy. BMJ 2004;328(7432):129. Erratum in BMJ 2004;328(7438):494.

Gimbel H, Zobbe V, Andersen BM, et al: Randomised controlled trial of total compared with subtotal hysterectomy with one-year follow up results. Br J Obstet Gynaecol 2003;110:1088–1098.

Glaze S, Ekwalanga P, Roberts G, et al: Peripartum hysterectomy: 1999 to 2006. Obstet Gynecol 2008;111:732–738.

Ibeanu OA, Chesson RR, Echols KT, et al: Urinary tract injury during hysterectomy based on universal cystoscopy. Obstet Gynecol 2009;113(1):6–10.

Johnson N, Barlow D, Lethaby A, et al: Methods of hysterectomy: Systematic review and meta-analysis of randomized controlled trials. BMJ 2005;330:1478.

Johnson N, Barlow D, Lethaby, A, et al: Surgical approach to hysterectomy for benign gynaecological disease. Cochrane Database Syst Rev 2006;(2):CD003677.

Kennedy S, Bergqvist A, Chapron C, et al: ESHRE guideline for the diagnosis and treatment of endometriosis. Hum Reprod 2005;20:2698–2704.

Kuno K, Menzin A, Kauder HH, et al: Prophylactic ureteral catheterization in gynecologic surgery. Urology 1998;52(6):1004–1008.

Learman LA, Summitt RL Jr, Varner RE, et al: A randomized comparison of total or supracervical hysterectomy: Surgical complications and clinical outcomes. Total or Supracervical Hysterectomy (TOSH) Research Group. Obstet Gynecol 2003;102:453–462.

Lethaby A, Ivanova V, Johnson NP: Total versus subtotal hysterectomy for benign gynaecological conditions. Cochrane Database Syst Rev 2006;(2):CD004993.

Mahajna A, Krausz M, Rosin D, et al: Bowel preparation is associated with spillage of bowel contents in colorectal surgery. Dis Colon Rectum 2005;48:1626–1631.

Maher C, Baesler K, Glazener CMA, et al. Surgical management of pelvic organ prolapse in women. Cochrane Incontinence Group. Cochrane Database Syst Rev 2007;(3):CD004014.

Management of Uterine Fibroids. Summary, Evidence Report/Technology Assessment: Number 34. AHRQ Publication No. 01-E051, Jan 2001. Agency for Healthcare Research and Quality, Rockville, MD, Available at: www.ahrq.gov/clinic/epcsums/utersumm.htm. Retrieved March 7, 2005.

McPherson K, Metcalfe MA, Herbert A, et al: Severe complications of hysterectomy: The VALUE study. Br J Obstet Gynaecol 2004;111(7):688–694.

Neuman M, Beller U, Ben Chetrit A, et al: Prophylactic effect of the open vaginal vault method in reducing febrile morbidity in abdominal hysterectomy. Surg Gynecol Obstet 1993;176(6):591–593.

Nichols DH, Clarke-Pearson DL: Gynecologic, Obstetric and Related Surgery, 2nd ed. Philadelphia, Mosby, 2000.

Olive DL, Schwartz LB: Endometriosis. N Engl J Med 1993;328:1759.

Rahn DD, Stone RJ, Vu AK, et al: Abdominal hysterectomy with or without angle stitch: Correlation with subsequent vaginal vault prolapse. Am J Obstet Gynecol 2008;199(6):669.e1–4.

Sangi-Haghpeykar H, Poindexter AN: Epidemiology of endometriosis among parous women. Obstet Gynecol 1995;85:983–992.

Sinaii N, Plumb K, Cotton L, et al: Differences in characteristics among 1,000 women with endometriosis based on extent of disease. Fertil Steril 2008;89:538.

Thakar R, Ayers S, Clarkson P, et al: Outcomes after total versus subtotal abdominal hysterectomy. N Engl J Med 2002;347:1318–1325.

Vernooij F, Heintz P, Witteveen E, van der Graaf Y: The outcomes of ovarian cancer treatment are better when provided by gynecologic oncologists and in specialized hospitals: A systematic review. Gynecol Oncol 2007;105(3):801–812.

Visco AG, Taber KH, Weidner AC, et al: Cost-effectiveness of universal cystoscopy to identify ureteral injury at hysterectomy. Obstet Gynecol 2001;97(5 Pt 1):685–692.

Wille-Jorgensen P, Guenaga KF, Matos D, Castro AA: Pre-operative mechanical bowel cleansing or not? An updated meta-analysis. Colorectal Dis 2005;7:304–310.

Wu JM, Wechter ME, Geller EJ, et al: Hysterectomy rates in the United States, 2003. Obstet Gynecol 2007;110(5):1091–1095.

Vaginal Hysterectomy and Trachelectomy: Basic Surgical Techniques

7

Mark D. Walters M.D.

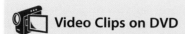

Video Clips on DVD

7-1 Vaginal Hysterectomy
7-2 Anterior Cul-de-sac Entry

7-3 Electrosurgical Device-Assisted
      Vaginal Hysterectomy
7-4 Vaginal Trachelectomy

Once the decision to perform a hysterectomy has been made, the type and route of hysterectomy must be chosen, and efforts are made to accomplish the surgery as safely as possible. Chapter 4 discusses the pre- and perioperative considerations and informed consent procedure when planning a hysterectomy. The choice of the route of hysterectomy should be individualized to the patient and the indication for surgery. Vaginal hysterectomy has well-documented advantages and relatively lower complication rates in comparison to other types of hysterectomy and should be the route of choice, if possible. For women with benign uterine disease requiring a hysterectomy, there are few absolute contraindications to the vaginal route, and these contraindications tend to be somewhat operator-dependent. In general, if the uterus is too large, or the vagina too narrow for the uterus to be removed safely through the vagina, then a laparoscopic or abdominal alternative must be undertaken. If there is extrauterine disease, such as an adnexal mass, or obliteration of tissue planes adjacent to the uterus, as with severe endometriosis or pelvic adhesive disease, then a vaginal hysterectomy may not be possible. However, in most other cases, assuming that the gynecologic surgeon is skilled and experienced in vaginal surgery, a vaginal hysterectomy can usually be accomplished.

This chapter will review the basic techniques of vaginal hysterectomy and trachelectomy for benign uterine disease. Techniques for more difficult vaginal hysterectomy as with large uterine fibroids, obliterated cul-de-sac, or total prolapse are discussed in detail in Chapter 8.

Case 1: Menorrhagia

GW is a 46-year-old gravida 3, para 2, aborta 1 woman who presents complaining of worsening menorrhagia with menses lasting 8 to 9 days per month. She states that during the first several days she changes a pad every 1 to 2 hours. Her menses are associated with significant cramping and some low back pain especially during the first 3 days. She has tried medical management with continuous oral contraceptive pills without success. Her physical examination reveals a 6-week-size mobile uterus without adnexal disease or significant pelvic organ prolapse. Her laboratory studies are unremarkable aside from a hematocrit of 31.5%. A Papanicolaou (Pap) smear showed no malignant cells. Office hysteroscopy was benign-appearing without polyps or fibroids, and an office endometrial biopsy was benign. The options of further medical management, levonorgestrel-releasing intrauterine device, endometrial ablation, or hysterectomy were discussed and she prefers a vaginal hysterectomy if possible. She states that she definitely does not desire any further children. She works full-time in a demanding field and prefers the more definitive resolution of her problem.

Discussion of Case

Abnormal bleeding, specifically frequent, heavy menses, can occur within a histologically normal uterus or may be associated with adenomyosis, uterine fibroids, or neoplasia. The spectrum of menorrhagia can range greatly with some women even to the point of iron therapy and blood transfusions. Given that she has continued symptoms in spite of medical management, resulting in anemia and decreased quality of life, it is reasonable to consider hysterectomy as part of her treatment plan. Although treatments such as medicated intrauterine devices or endometrial ablation are effective in many women, hysterectomy has been shown to have a very high satisfaction rate in women with these symptoms and essentially a 100% cure rate of bleeding, cramping, and dysmenorrhea. After a careful informed consent with review of the risks, benefits, and alternatives, and documentation that no further child-bearing is desired, a hysterectomy is chosen.

The gynecologist must assess this patient with pelvic examination to determine whether a vaginal hysterectomy is feasible and do that if possible. Alternatives such as total laparoscopic hysterectomy or laparoscopic supracervical hysterectomy would be reasonable for this patient, if desired by her and her surgeon. In general, unless she is at high risk for ovarian cancer or has a strong desire for ovarian removal, we do not favor prophylactic removal of ovaries in a premenopausal woman having a hysterectomy by whatever route. See Chapter 9 for further discussion of prophylactic oophorectomy.

Surgical Technique

See DVD Video 7-1 for video demonstration of the techniques for vaginal hysterectomy.

Before surgery appropriate perioperative intravenous antibiotics and antiembolic prophylaxis are routinely given. Vaginal hysterectomy begins with appropriate positioning of the patient. Vaginal hysterectomy is performed with the patient in the dorsal lithotomy position with her feet in "candy-cane" (Fig. 7-1) or Allen stirrups. The patient's buttocks should extend slightly over the edge of the table so that the posterior retractor can easily be placed. The thighs are somewhat abducted and the hips flexed. Excessive flexion and abduction of the thigh should be avoided, as this can lead to position-induced injuries. "Candy-cane" stirrups are preferable for deep vaginal surgery and when two vaginal surgical assistants are needed. An examination under anesthesia is performed to confirm the uterine size, degree of uterine mobility, the width of the vaginal canal, and the presence or absence of pelvic (especially adnexal) disease. The freedom of the cul-de-sac should be noted and a rectovaginal bimanual examination done. Elongation of the cervix is noted to help identify the point at which the incision through the vagina should begin. The vaginal, perineal, and lower abdominal areas are prepped in the normal fashion and the patient is sterilely draped. The urinary bladder is then emptied with a catheter. This catheter can be left in for intermittent emptying of the bladder or continuous drainage, or it can be removed and the bladder periodically catheterized.

A weighted speculum is placed in the vagina to depress the posterior vaginal wall, and the anterior vaginal wall is lifted with a Heaney retractor. The cervix is grasped with two single-toothed or a double-toothed tenacula, and downward traction is placed on the cervix. Vasoconstrictors such as vasopressin or a pre-

Figure 7-1 The patient is placed in candy-cane stirrups with her hips flexed and buttocks extending slightly over the edge of the table.

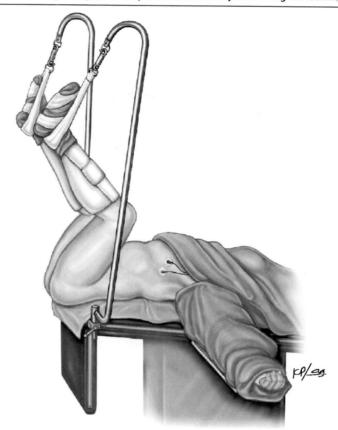

pared solution of 0.5% lidocaine with 1:200,000 epinephrine are used routinely if no contraindications exist. Vasopressin injected in the cervix or pericervical tissue just before incision has been shown in randomized trials to decrease operative blood loss, without an increase in morbidity (Kammerer-Doak et al, 2001), but does not improve postoperative pain control (Ascher-Walsh et al, 2009). A paracervical block also can be given before vaginal hysterectomy if desired; this has been shown to decrease postoperative pain and narcotic requirements after surgery (O'Neal et al, 2003; Long et al, 2009). The surgeon should remember that the maximum amount of lidocaine with epinephrine used should not exceed 7 mg/kg or 500 mg total in the healthy adult, and the dose of bupivacaine with epinephrine, if used, should generally not exceed 225 mg. Should a medical contraindication to the use of vasopressors or epinephrine be present, injectable saline provides the benefits of hydrodistention but without the benefit of vasoconstriction or any increase in cardiovascular risks.

Either a knife or electrosurgical instrument is used to make the initial incision through the vaginal mucosa at the cervicovaginal junction (Fig. 7-2). The position and depth of this incision are important because they determine access to the appropriate planes that will lead to the anterior and posterior cul-de-sacs. The appropriate location of the incision is at the site of the bladder reflection, which is indicated by the crease formed in the vaginal mucosa when the cervix is pushed slightly upward. If this location cannot be identified, one should make the incision low rather than high to avoid any potential bladder injury. The circumferential incision is accomplished and continued down to the cervical stroma. Downward traction of the tenacula and gentle countertraction by the retractors help to determine the appropriate depth of the incision. Once the

Figure 7-2 A scalpel is used to make the initial incision through the vaginal mucosa at the cervicovaginal junction.

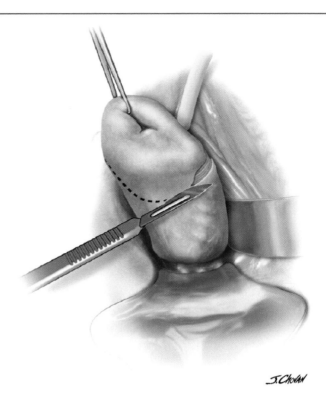

appropriate depth of the incision is reached the vaginal tissue will fall away from the underlying cervical tissue because there is a direct plane between these two tissues.

The vagina is mobilized both anteriorly and posteriorly using sharp dissection. Careful palpation of the subvaginal tissues posteriorly will usually help identify the location of the cul-de-sac before entry. The posterior cul-de-sac is sharply entered with Mayo scissors (Fig. 7-3) and then explored digitally for any adhesive disease, masses, or bowel (Fig. 7-4). At times, bleeding may be encountered from the posterior vaginal cuff, and this is controlled with a running interlocking suture or perhaps cauterization. A long-weighted Steiner-Auvard vaginal speculum is then placed in the posterior cul-de-sac.

The uterus is pulled outward and somewhat to the opposite side. One half of an opened Heaney clamp is introduced into the posterior cul-de-sac, rotated nearly to the horizontal, and the uterosacral ligament is clamped (Fig. 7-5). The pedicle is cut with either Mayo scissors or a scalpel. The author prefers to ligate the pedicle with an absorbable suture, usually No. 0 Vicryl on the CT-1 needle. Pop-off sutures are convenient for the flow of the surgery. The cut pedicle is suture-ligated with a transfixing-type suture in which the needle enters the upper part of the ligament pedicle just behind the tip of the Heaney clamp; it is withdrawn, and then reintroduced into the pedicle at its midpoint. The uterosacral ligament sutures are usually tagged for later identification. It is convenient to alternate clamping of the pedicles on opposite sides instead of clamping up one side of the uterus and then the other. This helps to gradually improve uterine mobility and exposure, and decreases back-bleeding that can occur from the uterine vessels.

Sharp dissection with Mayo or Metzenbaum scissors is used to mobilize the bladder anteriorly off the cervix (Fig. 7-6A). There is never a benefit in rushing to enter the anterior cul-de-sac, as this will likely lead to accidental cystotomies. Also, forceful blunt dissection of the bladder off the cervix (with a finger or

Figure 7-3 After the vagina is dissected from the cervix the posterior cul-de-sac is sharply entered with Mayo scissors.

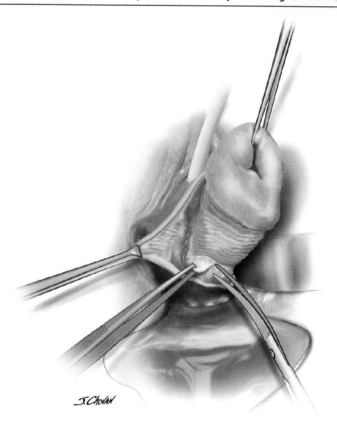

Figure 7-4 After sharp entry into the posterior cul-de-sac the peritoneal cavity is digitally explored for any adhesive disease, masses, or bowel, and to verify that damage to the rectum has not occurred.

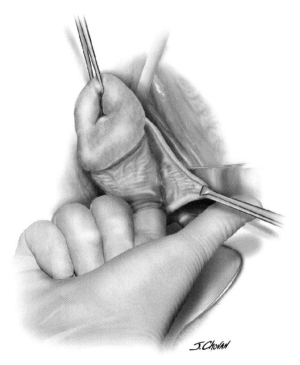

retractor) is discouraged as lacerations into the bladder can occur. No blind attempt should be made to enter the anterior cul-de-sac until the vesicouterine space has been developed and the peritoneum visualized (see Fig. 7-6B; see DVD Video 7-2 for video demonstration of entry into anterior cul-de-sac 📹). Once the bladder has been adequately mobilized with or without peritoneal

Figure 7-5 The Heaney clamp is introduced into the posterior cul-de-sac and rotated toward the horizontal, and the uterosacral ligament is clamped.

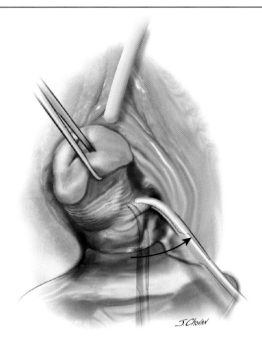

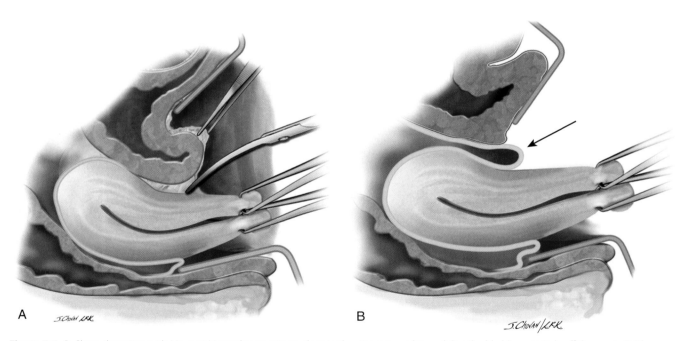

Figure 7-6 A, Sharp dissection with Mayo or Metzenbaum scissors close to the uterus is used to mobilize the bladder anteriorly off the cervix. **B,** The bladder is dissected off the uterus until the lower edge of the peritoneum is seen (*arrow*).

entry, the cardinal ligaments can be clamped on each side. These pedicles, which should include peritoneal tissue posteriorly, are sutured in a similar fashion as the uterosacral ligaments. Sequential clamps on each side should be made adjacent to each other to avoid any dead space between pedicles which may increase bleeding during the surgery.

After the cardinal ligaments have been incised bilaterally, the uterus usually begins to descend somewhat, making visualization of the anterior cul-de-sac easier. A retractor is gently placed in the vesicouterine space to elevate the

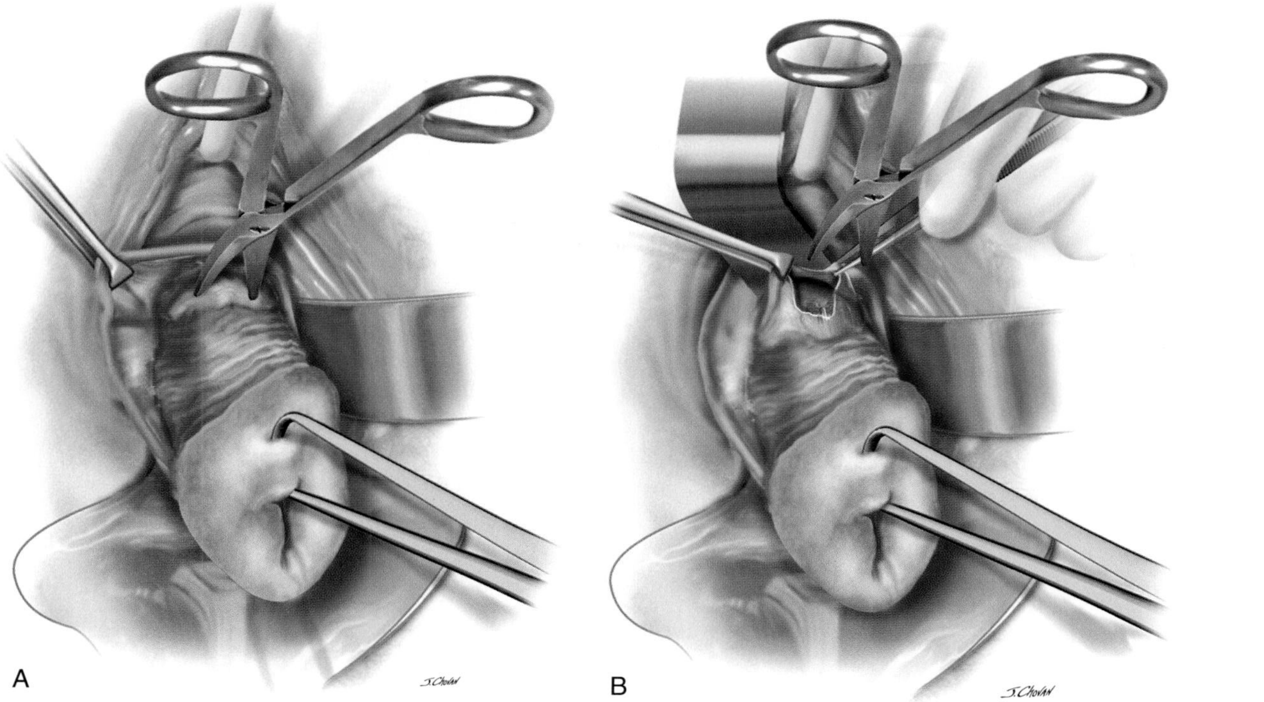

Figure 7-7 A, The anterior peritoneum is carefully inspected and palpated to differentiate it from the bladder. **B,** The anterior peritoneum is incised with scissors.

bladder off the uterus and attempts are made to directly visualize the lower edge of the anterior cul-de-sac peritoneum (see DVD Video 7-2 for video demonstration 🎥). Movement of the surgeon's finger over this tissue should provide a sliding feel to identify the peritoneum. Entering into the cul-de-sac should be done at this time if possible with a scissor (Fig. 7-7A, B) and a finger placed into the peritoneum to verify that the bladder has not been entered. A Heaney retractor is then placed anteriorly using a finger to protect the bladder. The next clamp, which will probably include the uterine vessels, should incorporate the anterior and posterior peritoneal reflections if the anterior cul-de-sac has been entered. The placement of these clamps should be perpendicular to the longitudinal access of the cervix, nearly horizontal (Fig. 7-8A, B; also see Fig. 13-2A), and the tips of the clamps should slide off the cervix and uterus to ensure that all of the perimetrial and vascular tissues have been included. This placement will help avoid excessive bleeding and, by staying close to the cervix, will help avoid ureteral injury. The uterine vessels are then suture-ligated with a fixation stitch (see Fig. 7-8B); some surgeons prefer double-ligation of the uterine vessels.

Depending on the size of the uterus, several more clamps may be needed on each side, perhaps including the round ligaments. If morcellation of the uterine fundus is necessary, it is generally done at this point (see Chapter 8 and videos). When the adnexal pedicles are palpated and felt to be small enough to be ligated, then the uterus can be delivered posteriorly into the vagina. The fundus is grasped with a tenaculum and pulled gently downward to expose the utero-ovarian ligament. With an index finger as guide, a Heaney or long Kelly clamp is placed close to the uterus at a right angle to the pedicle (Fig. 7-9). The last pedicle usually includes the fallopian tube, ovarian ligaments, and perhaps the round ligament. We prefer placing two clamps completely across the

Figure 7-8 A, The uterine vessels are clamped with a Heaney clamp, incorporating posterior and anterior peritoneum if possible. Note that the handle of the clamp is rotated to near horizontal to facilitate suture placement. **B,** The uterine vessels are cut and sutured.

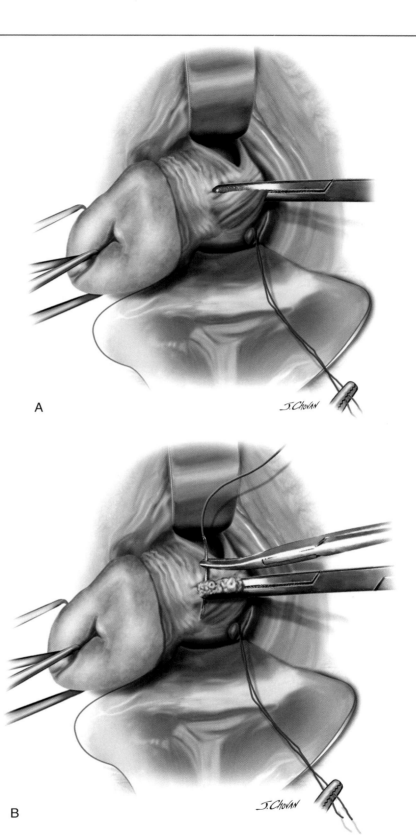

A

B

Figure 7-9 The uterus is delivered through the posterior cul-de-sac and the fallopian tube and the round and ovarian ligaments are clamped close to the uterus before cutting. Note that a finger is behind the pedicle to prevent accidental cutting of bowel or other structures.

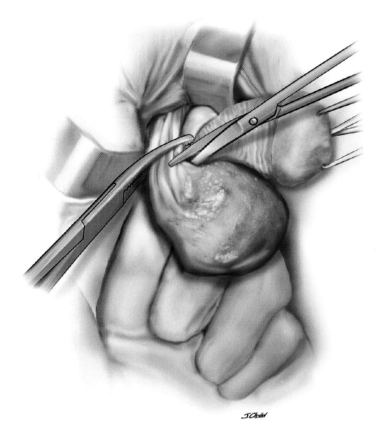

pedicle and double-ligating the pedicle, first with a free suture, followed by a suture-ligature. Other surgeons singly clamp the pedicle or may double-clamp the pedicle with clamps from above and below that meet in the center. After the pedicle is clamped, it is incised close to the uterus. This is usually repeated on the other side and the uterus and cervix removed, then handed off and sent for pathologic examination. We then gently retract the clamps and palpate the ovaries and tubes to make sure that they are normal and there is no unsuspected pelvic disease. During the operative dictation the surgeon should always make a note of the condition of the tubes and ovaries if they are left in place. The ovarian suture ligatures are then held without tension so that the pedicles and the spaces between the ovarian pedicle and uterosacral ligaments can be carefully examined for bleeding. Additional sutures or electrocautery may be used to achieve excellent hemostasis of all pedicles.

If the adnexa are to be removed as per the preference of the patient, or if an abnormality or lesion is found in the ovaries and the patient previously gave consent, then the ovaries or tubes can be removed at this time. This step is discussed in detail in Chapter 9.

Instead of the traditional methods of clamping, cutting, and suture-ligating the uterine pedicles, some surgeons prefer to use electrosurgical bipolar vessel-sealing devices to seal or fuse the tissues and blood vessels. The tissue fusion instrument consists of a disposable device with a pistol-grip, Heaney-type clamp, and retractable scalpel to cut tissue after fusion. The clamp jaws are used in the same fashion as Heaney clamps used in a standard hysterectomy. Pedicles are clamped, sealed or fused, and then cut before the clamp is released. The device is then advanced to the next pedicle and the process is repeated (see DVD Video 7-3 for video demonstration of electrosurgical device-assisted vaginal hysterectomy 📹). This technology is popular and has been shown in several small studies to decrease operating and anesthesia times, and blood loss, without an increase in morbidity. It is perhaps useful in some hysterectomies but no randomized trials compared to traditional surgery have been done to verify clinical benefit, nor have proper cost analyses been done.

A McCall culdoplasty or uterosacral ligament vaginal suspension is usually done after a vaginal hysterectomy to help resupport the vaginal apex and to help minimize the risk of future vaginal vault prolapse or enterocele. Adding this maneuver was shown in a randomized surgical trial compared to simple vaginal closure to lower the risk of future vaginal prolapse (Cruikshank and Kovac, 1999). The vagina is then closed with No. 2-0 Vicryl suture. Because the rate of ureteral obstruction is very low with simple vaginal hysterectomy, we do not routinely perform a cystoscopy. However, if the surgery is complex, or if culdoplasty or uterosacral ligament suspension is done, then cystoscopy after intravenous injection of indigo carmine is advised. A vaginal pack and Foley catheter may be placed overnight, if desired.

Case 2: Cervical Bleeding after a Prior Supracervical Hysterectomy

SL is a 48-year-old gravida 2, para 2 woman who underwent a laparoscopic supracervical hysterectomy with morcellation 2 years earlier because of symptomatic uterine fibroids. Her surgery was accomplished without complication and she had good relief of heavy menses and pelvic pressure and discomfort from the fibroids. Unfortunately, approximately 1 year after surgery, she developed vaginal spotting 5 or 6 days per month that occurred somewhat unpredictably and occasionally after intercourse. She had no pain or dyspareunia related to this. She is sexually active and generally prefers to retain her cervix; however, she finds the bleeding particularly annoying and would like resolution of this difficulty. Physical examination reveals a normal-appearing cervix that descends within 4 cm of the hymen with gentle traction. There are no masses on bimanual and rectovaginal examinations and her cervix appears to move freely within the pelvis. A Pap smear and endocervical curettage were both benign. She is scheduled for trachelectomy procedure.

Discussion of Case

Supracervical hysterectomy is a popular procedure in the United States, especially among laparoscopic surgeons. Potential benefits of laparoscopic supracervical hysterectomy include a more rapid surgery, fewer lower urinary tract and vascular complications, and quicker recovery. Randomized trials have only compared open total abdominal hysterectomy versus open supracervical hysterectomy, so the benefits of this procedure at laparoscopy remain to be verified in randomized controlled trials. Some also believe that sexuality is less affected after a supracervical hysterectomy, compared to when the cervix is removed, but this claim remains unproved.

The long-term complications of supracervical hysterectomy include cyclic vaginal bleeding in 11% to 17% of cases and the need for trachelectomy because of symptoms in up to 23% of cases, at a mean of 14 months after the time of hysterectomy (Okaro et al, 2001; Ghomi et al, 2005). An additional risk of supracervical hysterectomy relates to the lifetime development of benign or neoplastic conditions that require further removal of the cervical stump. Complications of trachelectomy reported in the largest published series included 9% incidence of infection and perioperative bleeding, and a 2% incidence of intraoperative bowel or bladder injury (Hilger et al, 2005). Future studies are required to delineate the relative risks and advantages of supracervical hysterectomy compared to other types of hysterectomy.

In our patient with cyclic bleeding from her cervix, few options are available to her, short of trachelectomy, if she wants complete relief from her bleeding. Although trachelectomy can be done abdominally and laparoscopically, the vaginal approach is the most direct and probably the safest, assuming the cervix is technically accessible through the vagina. Since she has mild prolapse of her cervix, a McCall culdoplasty or uterosacral ligament colpopexy should be done to support the vaginal cuff and help prevent future apical prolapse.

Surgical Technique

See DVD Video 7-4 for video demonstration of vaginal trachelectomy. 📹

Figure 7-10 Vaginal trachelectomy. Two Heaney clamps are used to clamp proximal to the cervix before removal. The bladder, ureters, and rectum were previously pushed superiorly to avoid damage. (From Baggish MS, Karram MM: Atlas of Pelvic Anatomy and Gynecologic Surgery, 2nd ed. Philadelphia, Elsevier, 2006.)

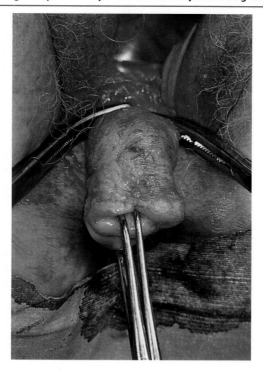

The trachelectomy is accomplished using patient positioning and techniques that start a vaginal hysterectomy. After examination under anesthesia and vaginal prep and sterile draping, the bladder is emptied with a catheter and a weighted speculum is placed in the vagina. The cervix is grasped with a single-tooth tenaculum and downward traction placed on the cervix. Vasoconstrictors can be used at the cervicovaginal junction. With either a knife or electrosurgical instrument the initial incision is made through the vaginal mucosa at the cervicovaginal junction. Curved Mayo scissors are used to dissect the vagina and bladder off the cervix anteriorly and posteriorly until the entire cervical stump is palpated. Careful palpation of the posterior cul-de-sac is made and, if it is felt to be free of adhesions and bowel and no vaginal suspension is needed, then Heaney clamps can be placed extraperitoneally just above the cervical stump bilaterally (Fig. 7-10). The cervix is excised with scalpel or scissors, and the tissue is ligated with No. 0 Vicryl suture. If culdoplasty or uterosacral colpopexy is to be done, then Mayo scissors are used to enter the posterior cul-de-sac sharply. A finger is inserted into the posterior cul-de-sac and peritoneal cavity to examine for bowel adhesions that may have adhered to the cervical stump or cul-de-sac. A finger can reach around the top of the cervix and also palpate whether it is adhered to the bladder anteriorly. If adhesions are present, they should be carefully dissected off the cervix through the posterior colpotomy incision. After the top of the cervix is free of bowel and adhesions, the finger can be placed around the cervix to help delineate the anterior vesicocervical space. When the anterior peritoneum is identified it is entered sharply and examined carefully to determine that no cystotomy has been made. A Heaney retractor is placed anteriorly and a long-weighted speculum is placed posteriorly.

As with a vaginal hysterectomy a Heaney clamp is used to clamp, cut, and ligate both uterosacral ligaments and they are held for later identification (see Fig. 7-10). A second clamp of both cardinal ligaments is made and they are also ligated with No. 0 Vicryl suture. Any additional tissue connected laterally to the cervix can be clamped close to the cervix, incised with scissors, and suture-ligated. The cervix is then sent for pathologic examination. As with a vaginal hysterectomy, if an electrosurgical bipolar sealing device is chosen by the surgeon, it can be used to occlude the blood vessels in the uterosacral and cardinal ligaments before removal of the cervix.

As after a vaginal hysterectomy, a McCall culdoplasty or uterosacral ligament vaginal suspension is done to help resupport the vaginal cuff and to minimize the risk of future vaginal apex prolapse. The vagina is then closed and a vaginal pack and Foley catheter are placed, if desired. Because of a small rate of cystotomy and ureteral obstruction after trachelectomy, the surgeon may wish to perform cystoscopy after intravenous injection of indigo carmine to exclude bladder damage and to verify patency of both ureters.

Suggested Readings

Ascher-Walsh CJ, Capes T, Smith J, et al: Cervical vasopressin compared with no premedication and blood loss during vaginal hysterectomy. Obstet Gynecol 2009;113:313–318.

Cruikshank SH, Kovac SR: Randomized comparison of three surgical methods used at the time of vaginal hysterectomy to prevent posterior enterocele. Am J Obstet Gynecol 1999;180:859–865.

Ghomi A, Hantes J, Lotze EC: Incidence of cyclical bleeding after laparoscopic supracervical hysterectomy. J Minim Invasive Gynecol 2005;12:201–205.

Gimbel H, Zobbe V, Andersen BM, et al: Randomised controlled trial of total compared with subtotal hysterectomy with one-year follow-up results. Br J Obstet Gynaecol 2003;110:1088–1098.

Hilger WS, Pizarro AR, Magrina JR: Removal of the retained cervical stump. Am J Obstet Gynecol 2005;193:2117–2121.

Hoffman CP, Kennedy J, Borschel L, et al: Laparoscopic hysterectomy: The Kaiser Permanente San Diego experience. J Minim Invasive Gynecol 2005;12:16–24.

Ibeanu OA, Chesson RR, Echols KT, et al: Urinary tract injury during hysterectomy based on universal cystoscopy. Obstet Gynecol 2009;113:6010.

Kammerer-Doak DN, Rogers RG, Maybach JJ, Mickelson MT: Vasopressin as an etiologic factor for infection in gynecologic surgery: A randomized double-blind placebo-controlled trial. Am J Obstet Gynecol 2001;185:1344–1348.

Karram MM: Vaginal hysterectomy. In Baggish MS, Karram MM: Atlas of Pelvic Anatomy and Gynecologic Surgery, 2nd ed. Philadelphia, WB Saunders, 2006.

Kuppermann M, Summitt RL Jr, Varner RE, et al: Sexual functioning after total compared with supracervical hysterectomy: A randomized trial. Total or Supracervical Hysterectomy (TOSH) Research Group. Obstet Gynecol 2005;105:1309–1318.

Learman LA, Summitt RL Jr, Varner RE, et al: A randomized comparison of total or supracervical hysterectomy: Surgical complications and clinical outcomes. Total or Supracervical Hysterectomy (TOSH) Research Group. Obstet Gynecol 2003;102:453–462.

Lethaby A, Ivanova V, Johnson NP: Total versus subtotal hysterectomy for benign gynecological conditions. Cochrane Database of Systematic Reviews 2006;Issue 2:CD004993.

Levy B, Emery L: Randomized trial of suture versus electrosurgical bipolar vessel sealing in vaginal hysterectomy. Obstet Gynecol 2003;102:147–151.

Long JB, Eiland RJ, Hentz JG, et al: Randomized trial of preemptive local analgesia in vaginal surgery. Int Urogynecol J 2009;20:5–10.

Nichols DH, Randall CL: Vaginal Surgery, 2nd ed. Baltimore, Williams & Wilkins, 1983.

Okaro EO, Jones KD, Sutton C: Long-term outcome following laparoscopic supracervical hysterectomy. Br J Obstet Gynaecol 2001;108:1017–1020.

O'Neal MG, Beste T, Shackelford DP: Utility of preemptive local analgesia in vaginal hysterectomy. J Obstet Gynecol 2003;189:1539–1542.

Thakar R, Ayers S, Clarkson P, et al: Outcomes after total versus subtotal abdominal hysterectomy. N Engl J Med 2002;347:1318–1325.

Difficult Vaginal Hysterectomy

8

Matthew D. Barber M.D., M.H.S.

 Video Clips on DVD

8-1 Uterine Morcellation Techniques   **8-3** Difficult Posterior Entry
8-2 Difficult Anterior Entry   **8-4** Uterovaginal Prolapse

Previous chapters have discussed the advantages of vaginal hysterectomy over other approaches and described its basic technique. There are few absolute contraindications to the vaginal approach for hysterectomy; however, there are a few factors that generally preclude this approach, including (1) the suspicion of malignancy; (2) the presence of known extrauterine disease or adnexal disease; (3) a narrow pubic arch (<90 degrees); (4) a narrow vagina (narrower than 2 fingerbreadths, especially at the apex); and (5) a fixed, immobile uterus. In the absence of all of these factors, vaginal hysterectomy should be the approach of choice whenever feasible given its well-documented advantages.

Some conditions and patient characteristics can make vaginal hysterectomy technically challenging. Many of these are easily identified preoperatively and can be anticipated. These conditions include the enlarged uterus, uterine prolapse, and the undescended uterus. This chapter discusses the surgical approaches to these difficult cases and describes techniques to facilitate their safe and successful completion. It also discusses techniques to manage surgical challenges that may not be anticipated and may be encountered even in cases initially thought to be simple and straightforward, such as difficult anterior or posterior entry into the peritoneal cavity and pelvic adhesive disease. By mastering the techniques described in this chapter, the gynecologic surgeon can increase the proportion of hysterectomies that can be successfully performed vaginally to the ultimate benefit of their patients.

Patient Selection and Preparation

Considerations for the selection of route of hysterectomy and a discussion of routine pre- and perioperative patient preparation can be found in Chapter 4. Once it is determined that the patient is an appropriate candidate for hysterectomy, the choice of route of surgery is largely dependent upon the patient's medical history, the findings during pelvic examination, and the surgeon's

Figure 8-1 Vulvar slant as an indication of type of pelvis. **A,** With a narrow android or anthropoid pelvis, the soft tissue slant of the vulva is perpendicular to the long axis of the body. **B,** A vulvar slant of approximately 45 degrees is associated with a gynecoid pelvis, which is more favorable for vaginal surgery. **C,** The axis of the platypelloid pelvis. (Reproduced with permission from Nichols DH, Randall CL [eds]: Vaginal Surgery, 4th ed. Philadelphia, Lippincott Williams & Wilkins, 1996.)

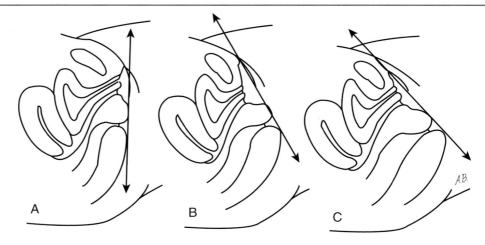

experience and skill. The gynecologic surgeon must use his or her judgment to select the best approach for the individual patient. Suspected malignancy or the presence of an adnexal mass are contraindications to vaginal hysterectomy. However premalignant conditions such as cervical intraepithelial neoplasia (CIN) III or complex endometrial hyperplasia are often best performed via the vaginal route. Factors in the patient's medical history that suggest the possibility of a difficult or technically challenging vaginal hysterectomy include uterine enlargement; a history of endometriosis, pelvic adhesive disease, or pelvic inflammatory disease; and a history of previous pelvic surgery. However, in appropriately selected patients the skilled vaginal surgeon can often successfully perform a hysterectomy via the vaginal approach in patients with these conditions. In patients with a history of endometriosis or previous pelvic surgery it is often useful to review the operative notes from previous surgeries to help determine the degree of pelvic adhesive disease when making the assessment of whether vaginal hysterectomy is appropriate. Additionally, patients with a history of or suspicion for extrauterine disease may benefit from preoperative imaging such as transvaginal ultrasonography or pelvic magnetic resonance imaging (MRI) in order to help determine the appropriateness of the vaginal approach. Nulliparity or history of cesarean section may increase the degree of difficulty of a vaginal hysterectomy, but should not be considered contraindications. Specific patient selection criteria for each of these conditions will be discussed in greater detail later in the chapter.

On preoperative physical examination, the surgeon should make careful note of the following factors in order to assess the degree of difficulty of performing a vaginal hysterectomy: (1) size and shape of the bony pelvis with particular note of the angle of the pubic arch; (2) the vaginal caliber, particularly at the apex; (3) the mobility of the uterus in all dimensions; and (4) the size and shape of the uterus. A pubic arch angle of less than 90 degrees generally precludes vaginal hysterectomy, and a wide pubic arch angle will facilitate the vaginal approach. In addition to the pubic arch angle, Nichols and Randall (1996) advocate assessing the slant the vulva makes with the body axis (vulvar slant) as a way of assessing the adequacy of the bony pelvis for vaginal surgery (Fig. 8-1). They noted that the gynecoid pelvis, which has the most room for vaginal surgery, has a vulvar slant of about 45 degrees with the horizontal, but the android and anthropoid pelvis is often contracted and associated with a vulvar slant that is about 90 degrees or perpendicular with the horizontal. The platypelloid pelvis, which may also be constricted, has a vulvar slant of approximately 30 degrees. During bimanual examination, the surgeon should carefully assess the uterine mobility in all directions. Adequate mobility in the lateral and anteroposterior (AP) directions is a prerequisite for vaginal hysterectomy. Although lack of uterine descent is often discussed as a contraindication to vaginal hysterectomy, the descent of the cervix and uterus noted on preoperative examination is less important than mobility in the lateral and AP directions for predicting successful vaginal hysterectomy. As will be discussed later in the chapter, vaginal hysterectomy can often be successfully completed in women without uterine descent noted on preoperative examination, presuming adequate vaginal caliber and uterine mobility in the other planes. Moreover, uterine descent often improves significantly after the patient is placed under anesthesia and the pelvic floor muscles are relaxed. Some surgeons advocate assessing uterine descent preoperatively by performing a "traction test" whereby the cervix is grasped with a single-tooth tenaculum and traction is applied on the uterus. We generally do not advocate the use of the traction test as it can be painful to the patient and is not necessarily predictive of the degree of descent that will be present when the patient is under anesthesia or the likelihood of success of vaginal hysterectomy. The surgeon should also assess the vaginal caliber during preoperative examination, paying particular attention to the caliber of the upper vagina. If the width of the vagina at the apex is less than 2 fingerbreadths, then it is unlikely that a vaginal hysterectomy can be accomplished safely and the laparoscopic or abdominal approach is more appropriate. Conversely, a wide vaginal caliber will increase the likelihood of successful vaginal hysterectomy and is particularly desirable in the face of other factors that might make the vaginal hysterectomy more challenging, such as an enlarged uterus and poor uterine descent. During preoperative physical examination, the surgeon should also assess the uterine size and shape. With the skilled use of morcellation and other uterine size reducing techniques there is no upper limit of uterine size that necessarily precludes the vaginal approach; however, we generally do not advocate vaginal hysterectomy for uterus greater than 16 weeks in size. Details of the appropriate selection of vaginal hysterectomy for patients with the enlarged uterus are discussed in detail later in the chapter.

While all patients undergoing vaginal hysterectomy should be counseled that a laparotomy or laparoscopy may be necessary to complete the hysterectomy if vaginal removal is not possible, this is particularly true for the patient whose hysterectomy is expected to be difficult. In these patients, it is often useful to inform the operating room staff to have the equipment for a laparoscopy or laparotomy readily available in case conversion is necessary. As with all hysterectomies, the standard perioperative intravenous antibiotics and antiembolic prophylaxis are routinely given prior to surgery. Factors that will increase the likelihood of successful and safe completion of a vaginal hysterectomy that is anticipated to be difficult include proper patient positioning, a careful examination under anesthesia, adequate lighting and instrumentation, and good surgical assistance. Although vaginal hysterectomy can be performed using either Allen or candy-cane stirrups, the candy-cane stirrups are particularly helpful in cases that are expected to be difficult. Compared with Allen stirrups and other similar boot stirrups, the candy-cane stirrups provide increased exposure to the deep pelvis and adequate room for two operative assistants. (See Chapter 7 for a discussion of appropriate patient positioning using candy-cane stirrups.) After proper patient positioning, an examination under anesthesia (EUA) should be performed to confirm the preoperative assessment and more carefully evaluate the uterine size, degree of uterine mobility, the width of the

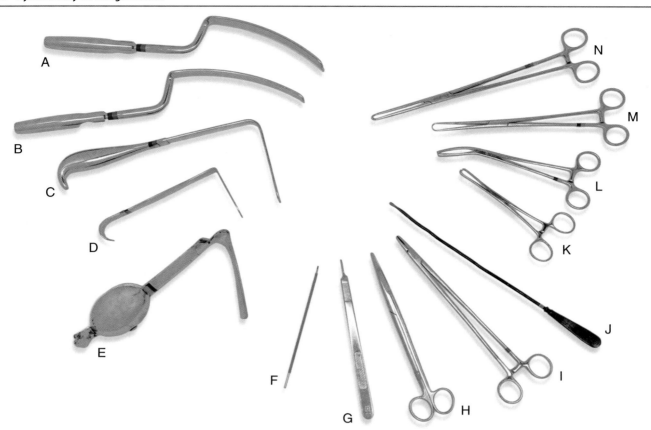

Figure 8-2 Instruments useful for difficult vaginal hysterectomy: Briesky-Navratil vaginal retractors (a, b); long Heaney retractor (c); short Heaney retractor (d); Steiner-Auvard speculum (e); Bovie extender (f); long scalpel handle (g); long heavy Mayo scissors (h); long needle driver (i); flexible uterine sound (j); Leahy tenaculum (k); Jacobson double-tooth tenaculum (l); single tooth tenaculum (m); and long Allis clamp (n).

vaginal canal, and the presence or absence of pelvic disease. A rectovaginal examination should be performed to assess the freedom of the posterior cul-de-sac. The EUA provides the surgeon with the best assessment of whether or not the hysterectomy can be performed successfully and safely via the vaginal route and it is at this point that the final decision about whether or not to proceed with the vaginal approach should be made.

Good visualization is important for any surgery but especially for the difficult vaginal hysterectomy. To maximize visualization, it is valuable to have two surgical assistants, ideally with at least one of them also a skilled vaginal surgeon. Good operative lighting is essential. In some instances, the use of a headlamp or lighted retractor or suction device can be valuable. A number of instruments can be useful for difficult vaginal surgery beyond those found in the typical vaginal hysterectomy set including a long needle drivers; long heavy Mayo scissors; a weighted speculum with an extra-long blade (Steiner-Auvard speculum); long Allis clamps; a number of different tenacula including the single-tooth, Jacobson, and Leahy varieties; Briesky-Navratil vaginal retractors; long and short right-angle retractors (Heaney retractors); a flexible uterine sound; a Bovie extender; and a scalpel with a long handle (Fig. 8-2). A cystoscope should also be available to evaluate the integrity of the bladder and ureters during or at the end of surgery. In cases in which blood loss may be increased such as the large fibroid uterus, the use of a surgical blood salvage/autotransfusion system (CellSaver®, Haemonetics Corp., Braintree, MA) can be considered.

Case 1: Menometrorrhagia, Dysmenorrhea, and Uterine Fibroids

L.D. is a 42-year-old gravida 2, para 2 female who presents with painful, irregular, heavy menses. She reports a 3-year history of painful menses that are partially relieved with nonsteroidal anti-inflammatory drugs (NSAIDs). She states that her menses occur every 2 to 4 weeks and last 8 to 9 days with a heavy flow that includes blood clots. She uses approximately 10 to 12 pads per day to manage this bleeding. Previous treatments have included oral contraceptives and depot-medroxyprogesterone acetate, which did not relieve her symptoms. Her past surgical history is significant only for a previous postpartum tubal ligation. Bimanual examination reveals an irregularly shaped 12-week-size uterus that is freely mobile in all directions. Several fibroids appear to be located in the uterine fundus but the lower uterine segment and cervix are normal size. Her pubic arch angle is approximately 120 degrees and her vaginal caliber is approximately 3 fingerbreadths in width. Office hysteroscopy reveals a distorted uterine cavity but no intramural fibroids or polyps. An endometrial biopsy performed 2 months previously reveals proliferative endometrium. Her laboratory values reveal a hematocrit of 30.0%. The options of further medical management, uterine fibroid embolization, myomectomy, and hysterectomy were discussed and she prefers a vaginal hysterectomy if possible.

Discussion of Case

Uterine fibroids are a common cause of excessive and irregular menstrual bleeding and dysmenorrhea. Other symptoms that can be attributable to uterine fibroids include pelvic pain and bulk symptoms such as urinary frequency and urgency, rectal pressure, pelvic pressure, and increasing abdominal girth. Hysterectomy can be considered in a woman with symptomatic uterine fibroids who no longer desires fertility, particularly if the severity of symptoms is such that they interfere with her daily life. Given the severity of this patient's symptoms, the lack of response to medical management, and resulting anemia, it is reasonable to consider hysterectomy in this case. Myomectomy by either laparoscopy or laparotomy and uterine fibroid embolization are also options, but hysterectomy remains the most effective and definitive method

for relieving this patient's symptoms. As was noted in Chapter 3, uterine fibroids and menstrual irregularities are the most common indications for hysterectomy in reproductive age women. Uterine fibroids are the most common reason for uterine enlargement, but adenomyosis and malignancy are other potential sources that should be considered. When the uterus is enlarged, bimanual examination is usually adequate to make a diagnosis of uterine fibroids, particularly when intramural and subserosal fibroids are present, because they often result in a characteristic irregularity of the uterine contour as in this patient. Although the vaginal, laparoscopic, or abdominal approach to hysterectomy might be reasonable in this patient, the vaginal approach offers several distinct advantages. When vaginal access is adequate and the uterus is enlarged, vaginal hysterectomy can often be accomplished safely using uterine size reduction techniques such as wedge morcellation, uterine bisection, and intramyometrial coring. A randomized trial comparing the vaginal to the abdominal route for women with enlarged uteri (200 to 1300 g) demonstrated decreased operating time, febrile morbidity, postoperative narcotic use, and hospital stay for those who received vaginal hysterectomy (with or without morcellation) compared to total abdominal hysterectomy (Benassi et al, 2002). Similarly, several clinical trials have demonstrated advantages of vaginal hysterectomy over laparoscopically assisted vaginal hysterectomy (LAVH) in women with enlarged uteri including decreased hospital stay, less operating room time, quicker discharge, and less blood loss (Sesti et al, 2008a; 2008b; Hwang et al, 2002). One trial suggested that vaginal hysterectomy also had a lower complication rate than LAVH in women with enlarged fibroid uteri (Darai et al, 2001). There are currently no randomized comparisons of total laparoscopic hysterectomy and vaginal hysterectomy performed exclusively for enlarged uteri, but generally the laparoscopic approach is associated with greater operating time and cost (Johnson et al, 2006). This patient has a number of characteristics that make her ideal for the vaginal approach including adequate vaginal caliber and pubic arch angle, a mobile uterus with a surgically accessible lower uterine segment, and fibroids confined to the uterine fundus.

Vaginal Hysterectomy for the Enlarged Uterus

Patient Selection

As noted earlier, during the preoperative bimanual examination a careful assessment of uterine shape is essential, as it is often more important than actual size for identifying the appropriate patient for vaginal hysterectomy in the face of uterine fibroids. Before beginning any uterine size reduction or morcellation procedure, the uterine vessels must be ligated bilaterally and the peritoneal cavity should be entered both anteriorly and posteriorly. If the cervix or lower uterine segment is enlarged or contains fibroids that prevent uterine artery ligation or entry into the peritoneal cavity then the procedure should not be performed vaginally, regardless of size. In contrast, if the lower uterine segment is accessible surgically and the uterine fundus is mobile, then even very large uteri (up to 20-week size) can be removed transvaginally by an appropriately skilled surgeon. The presence of lateral or anterior fibroids tend to make transvaginal removal more difficult. In contrast, posterior fundal myomas are often easily removed transvaginally.

With increasing skill the gynecologic surgeon can become adept at removing large uteri transvaginally. For most gynecologic surgeons, it is probably reasonable to attempt transvaginal hysterectomy in patients with up to 12- to 14-week-size uteri (or 300 cm^2). Although the upper limit of uterine size for which a vaginal hysterectomy should be done has not been established, many skilled vaginal surgeons would consider 16- to 18-week size as a reasonable and practical upper limit. In our experience, removing uteri larger than this, although often technically feasible, can be a significant struggle associated with long operating times and increased blood loss.

In women with uterine fibroids and anemia, gonadotropin-releasing hormone (GnRH) agonists preoperatively should be considered. A common regimen is leuprolide acetate 3.75 mg given intramuscularly at monthly intervals for 3 months preoperatively. A meta-analysis of 26 randomized trials comparing preoperative GnRH agonists to no treatment or placebo found that those who received preoperative GnRH agonists increased their hematocrit an average of 3%, decreased their uterine volume an average of two gestational sizes (i.e., from 14 weeks to 12 weeks), and decreased intraoperative blood loss an average of 58 mL (Lethaby et al, 2001). Additionally, because of the decrease in uterine volume, women who received preoperative GnRH agonists were more likely to receive a vaginal hysterectomy than those who did not.

Surgical Techniques (Video 8-1)

Transvaginal removal of an enlarged uterus begins similar to that of a routine vaginal hysterectomy. A careful EUA should be performed to confirm the size, shape, and mobility of the uterus as well as the adequacy of vaginal access. The hysterectomy proceeds in the standard fashion until the uterine arteries are ligated bilaterally. After entry into the anterior and posterior cul-de-sacs, it is helpful to digitally palpate the uterus to confirm the location and size of the uterine fibroids. When the uterus is enlarged from uterine fibroids or adenomyosis, uterine debulking techniques such as uterine bivalving, intramyometrial coring, wedge morcellation, and myomectomy are often necessary to successfully complete the hysterectomy vaginally. The employment of uterine debulking techniques becomes necessary when all accessible pedicles have been cut and ligated and no further uterine descent is possible for the delivery of the fundus through the anterior or posterior cul-de-sac. Each of these uterine debulking techniques may be used alone but often are used in combination with each other, so the surgeon should be familiar with each technique. Hoffman and Spellacy (1995) noted that the versatility in the application of the various morcellation techniques is a key factor to successful transvaginal removal of the enlarged uterus.

Prior to proceeding with uterine morcellation the following criteria should be met regardless of technique planned:

1. The uterine arteries should be ligated bilaterally. If an additional pedicle on the broad ligament beyond the uterine artery can be ligated prior to beginning morcellation, this is desirable.

2. The anterior and posterior cul-de-sacs should be entered. There are circumstances where the surgeon may consider proceeding with morcellation without having entered the anterior or posterior cul-de-sacs but these are uncommon and should be approached with caution. (See section on difficult anterior and posterior entry later in the chapter.)

3. Long retractors should be placed anteriorly and posteriorly to protect the bladder and rectum respectively. We prefer to use a long weighted speculum such as the Steiner-Auvard speculum posteriorly and a long right-angle Heaney retractor anteriorly.

4. The bladder should drained either continuously or at frequent intervals throughout the case.

Because the uterine vessels have been ligated and steady traction is applied to the uterus throughout the procedure compressing collateral vessels, the amount of bleeding from any of the uterine debulking techniques is limited. Prior to beginning any of the uterine debulking procedures, it is useful to place Heaney clamps or single-tooth tenacula bilaterally on the uterine fundus just above the highest ligated pedicle. This ensures that the pedicles will not be lost, maintains uterine orientation, and provides useful lateral landmarks for morcellation. Careful observation for nearby intestines or intestinal adhesions should be made throughout in order to prevent accidental bowel injury. It may be desirable to use the Trendelenburg position and pack the bowel out of the pelvis using long laparotomy sponges.

Bivalving or Hemisection (See Fig. 8-3 and Video 8-1)

Uterine bivalving or hemisection is performed by splitting the uterus in the midline into halves before removal. This allows one half of the uterus to be temporarily displaced into the pelvis, providing greater mobility and visualization for surgical removal of the other half of the uterus. Bivalving is best performed on mildly enlarged uteri that are symmetrical. Bivalving is begun by grasping the uterine cervix at 3 o'clock and 9 o'clock with tenacula. Using a scalpel or heavy scissors the uterus is divided longitudinally in the midline (Fig. 8-3B). Continuous traction should be placed on both tenacula throughout the procedure. Once the uterine fundus is accessible, a finger or vaginal retractor is placed behind the uterus to protect the pelvic viscera and the fundus is completely divided. If the uterine fundus is not accessible, then morcellation or myomectomies should be performed, as needed (Fig. 8-3C), until delivery of the fundus occurs and the upper pedicles can be ligated.

Intramyometrial Coring (See Fig. 8-4 and Video 8-1)

Intramyometrial coring was first introduced by Lash in 1941. This technique facilitates removal of the enlarged uterus through decreasing the uterine width by increasing its length. Coring is most easily performed on moderately sized symmetrically enlarged uteri without multiple fibroids. It is a particularly useful technique when the vaginal canal and pubic arch are somewhat narrow. While applying firm traction to the cervix, the myometrium is incised circumferentially using a scalpel or heavy scissors parallel to the long axis of the uterine cavity at the level of the uterocervical junction below (Fig. 8-4C). The incision is continued circumferentially parallel to the uterine serosa maintaining a thin shell of myometrium superficially to avoid perforation into the serosa. Care should be taken to avoid creating multiple planes. As the cervix is pulled, the myometrium is "cored out" so that the endometrial cavity and a layer of myometrium are pulled toward the surgeon, collapsing the bulky

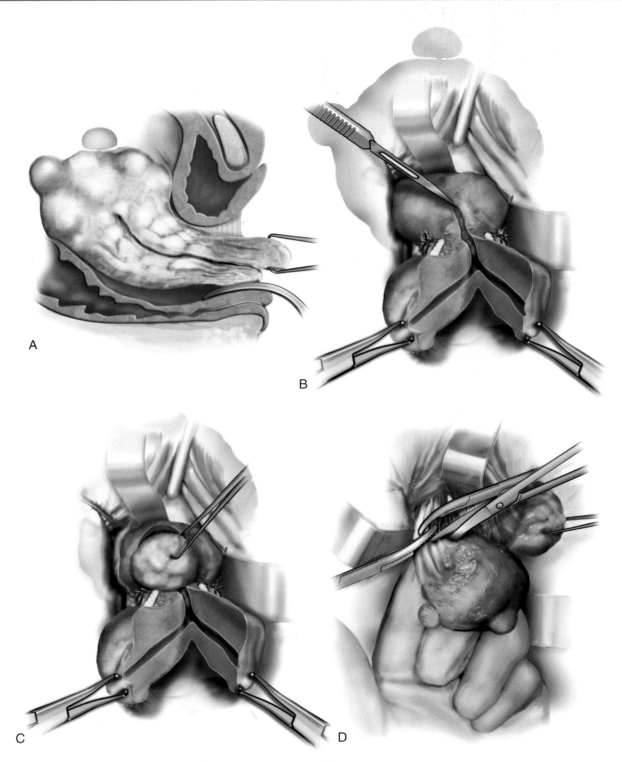

Figure 8-3 Technique of bivalving or hemisection of the uterus. **A,** Sagital view of the uterus with multiple leiomyomas. **B,** The scalpel incises up the midportion of the uterus longitudinally. **C,** Vaginal myomectomy. **D,** Delivery of the uterus after its size has been reduced and clamping of the adnexal pedicle.

Figure 8-4 Technique of intramyometrial coring. **A,** While applying firm traction to the cervix, the myometrium is incised circumferentially using a scalpel parallel to the long axis of the uterine cavity at the level of the uterocervical junction. **B** and **C,** The incision is continued circumferentially parallel to the uterine serosa maintaining a thin shell of myometrium superficially to avoid perforation into the serosa. **D,** As the cervix is pulled, the myometrium is "cored out," collapsing the bulky uterus and allowing access to the upper pedicles.

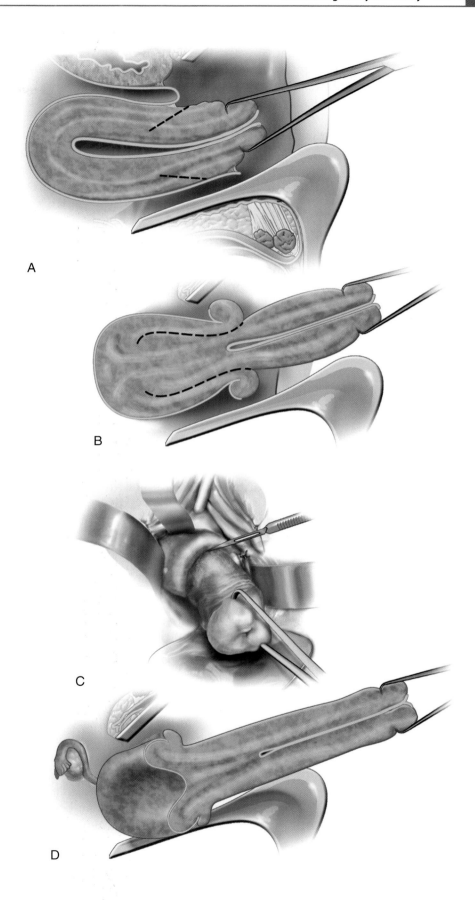

A

B

C

D

uterus and allowing access to the upper pedicles (see Fig. 8-4D). As the uterine fundus enlarges, the plane of dissection should stay close to the uterine serosa in order to ensure that the removed core is large enough to reduce uterine volume sufficiently to allow delivery of the fundus. Because the coring technique is intraserosal, it is a particularly useful technique when uterine adhesions are present, as will be discussed later in the chapter.

Wedge Morcellation (See Fig. 8-5 and Video 8-1 🎥)

Wedge morcellation is the most versatile uterine debulking technique and is the procedure of choice when other techniques fail. Wedge morcellation begins by amputating the cervix with a wedge-shaped incision into the uterine corpus. Alternatively, the surgeon can begin wedge morcellation after bivalving the cervix. The surgeon maintains orientation of the uterus and continuous traction by placing Heaney clamps or single-tooth tenacula bilaterally on the uterine fundus just distal to the highest ligated pedicle. It is generally recommended that these clamps not be moved or removed until the uterine fundus has been debulked enough to be delivered. V-shaped pieces of tissue are removed piecemeal from the anterior and posterior uterine walls in order to centrally debulk the uterus. (See Fig. 8-5 and Video 8-1 for two variations in the technique. 🎥) A tenaculum is applied to the tissue that is to be excised and traction applied. Excision is performed with a long-handled scalpel or heavy Mayo scissors. Several different kinds of uterine tenacula including single-tooth, double-tooth (Jacobson), and Leahey tenacula should be available to assist with the morcellation process. Uterine myomas are removed as encountered. Morcellation is continued until the round ligament, utero-ovarian ligament, and fallopian tube are accessible and can be clamped, cut, and ligated.

Although the process of morcellation will vary for each patient based on the size and location of the fibroids, there are a few technical points worth noting. Enucleation of fibroids is simpler and quicker than morcellation of the uterine body. After excision of the cervix, intramural fibroids involving lower uterine segment will be accessible and easily removed. The endometrial cavity is often accessible to digital palpation at this point, allowing direct access for enucleation of submucosal fibroids. Repetitive enucleation of the largest accessible central fibroid should be performed until there are no fibroids readily accessible. Morcellation of the uterine myometrium can then begin. Whenever possible, morcellation should occur inside the serosal surfaces of the uterus. This will minimize the risk of injury to pelvic viscera. Any excision that includes the serosal surface should be performed entirely under direct vision with care to avoid surrounding structures. The posterior aspect of the uterus is typically more accessible and more easily seen than the anterior aspect and it is often useful to debulk as much of the posterior uterus as possible before proceeding anteriorly, particularly when a posterior fibroid is present. The surgeon should digitally palpate the anterior and posterior uterine surfaces regularly throughout the surgery in order to remain oriented and evaluate the progress of the uterine debulking. Morcellation should continue until the uterine fundus can be delivered or the upper pedicles become accessible for ligation. Once the top of the uterine fundus is readily accessible both anteriorly and posteriorly, hemisection of the remaining uterus can be a useful technique to achieve final delivery of the fundus to allow completion of the case.

Myomectomy (See Video 8-1 🎥)

Myomectomy is often necessary during other uterine debulking techniques but can, on occasion, be useful in isolation. This is particularly true for isolated

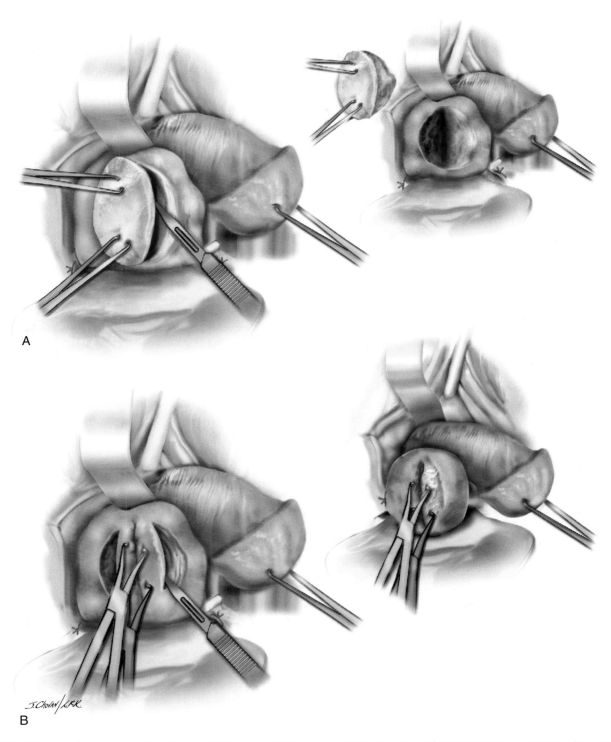

A

B

J.Chovan/ERK

Figure 8-5 Technique of posterior uterine wedge morcellation. **A,** An elliptical wedge of tissue is removed from posterior uterus. **B,** Edges of the initial incision are brought together with two tenacula and another wedge of tissue is removed. The procedure is continued until the uterus can be completely delivered.

anterior or posterior fibroids. If accessible, the fibroid can be grasped through either the anterior or posterior peritoneal incisions and pulled to the operative field. The serosa is incised and the myoma can be enucleated. In the case of a large isolated fibroid, this is often enough to debulk the uterus to allow completion of the hysterectomy. If the uterine arteries cannot be ligated because of an anterior or posterior lower uterine segment fibroid, myomectomy can be considered. In this situation, it is often useful to inject a hemostatic agent over the myoma such as dilute vasopressin (20 units/100 mL saline).

Case 2: Menorrhagia and Dysmenorrhea in a Nulliparous, Obese Patient

B.G. is a 41-year-old obese female gravida 0 with a body mass index of 34 kg/m^2 who presents with a 4-year history of worsening menorrhagia and dysmenorrhea. She reports regular menses that last 6 to 8 days with heavy flow and associated blood clots requiring 10 to 12 pads per day. Her menses have become increasingly painful, causing her to miss work 1 or 2 days per month in spite of taking ibuprofen 600 mg every 6 hours. In addition to NSAIDs, she has tried oral contraceptive pills and the levonorgestrol intrauterine device without relief. Her gynecologic history is notable for a history of infertility, ultimately resulting in the adoption of two children, aged 6 and 9. On physical examination, she is noted to have a globular 6- to 8-week-size uterus that is freely mobile in the lateral and AP dimensions but has only minimal uterine descent. Saline-infusion sonography reveals a uterus measuring 8 × 5 × 4 cm without evidence of uterine fibroids or intracavitary lesions. The ovaries are normal bilaterally. An endometrial biopsy demonstrates proliferative endometrium and a Papanicolaou (Pap) smear performed 8 months ago is normal. Given the impact her symptoms are having upon her life, she decides to proceed with hysterectomy and wonders if she is a candidate for the vaginal route.

Discussion of Case

Menorrhagia and dysmenorrhea associated with a slightly enlarged globular uterus without evidence of fibroids or other intracavitary lesions suggests a diagnosis of adenomyosis. Symptomatic adenomyosis is most commonly seen in women aged 35 to 50, which is consistent with this patient. Given the failure of medical management to relieve her symptoms, the significant impact the symptoms are having on her quality of her life, and the fact that future childbearing is not an issue for this patient, in spite of her nulliparity, hysterectomy is appropriate for this patient. Uterine-sparing options often used for menorrhagia, such as endometrial ablation and uterine artery embolization, often provide inadequate symptom relief when adenomyosis is the cause.

Two factors in this case that warrant further discussion when considering route of hysterectomy include the patient's nulliparity with relative lack of uterine descent and her obesity. In spite of its frequent mention, nulliparity is not a contraindication to the vaginal route. Many nulliparous women and women who have not delivered vaginally have adequate vaginal caliber to allow successful completion of a vaginal hysterectomy. In one series of 300 hysterectomies in women without previous vaginal delivery, the authors planned the vaginal route in 75% and, among these, successfully completed the hysterectomy vaginally in 92%. (Le Tohic et al, 2008). Similarly, in a series of 492 consecutive hysterectomies in nulliparas, Sheth was able to successfully perform a vaginal hysterectomy in 75% (Sheth, 1999). Even in the case of minimal uterine descent, if the upper vagina allows adequate access for transection of the uterosacral and cardinal ligaments, uterine mobility will improve, making the remainder of the vaginal hysterectomy easier to accomplish. Moreover, as was previously discussed, the amount of uterine descent noted on preoperative examination often underestimates the degree of descent found after the patient is placed under anesthesia. This patient has a uterus that is only slightly enlarged and, despite lacking significant uterine descent, otherwise has good uterine mobility. Assuming that the size of her bony pelvis is adequate, vaginal hysterectomy would be a reasonable approach. On the other hand, if the uterus is not mobile, the bony pelvis or vaginal caliber is small, or there is a contraindication to morcellation, then the laparoscopic (or abdominal) approach are more appropriate.

Obesity increases the difficulty of any hysterectomy, whether performed abdominally, laparoscopically, or vaginally. However, the obese patient will benefit considerably if an abdominal incision can be avoided. Compared with vaginal and laparoscopic hysterectomy, abdominal hysterectomy in obese women is associated with increased risk of infection, wound separation, and other morbidity as well as prolonged hospital stay and convalescence. Raffi and associates (2005) compared the morbidity of vaginal hysterectomy in obese and nonobese women and found no difference in morbidity, operative time, or length of stay suggesting that the general benefits of the vaginal route extend to the obese patient. Given this, vaginal hysterectomy is a reasonable choice for this patient even if this means struggling somewhat in the face of minimal uterine descent. Another reasonable option in this patient would be either a total or supracervical laparoscopic, robotic, or single port hysterectomy. The surgeon's skill and the patient's preference should ultimately determine whether to proceed vaginally or laparoscopically when performing the hysterectomy for this patient.

Surgical Technique: Lack of Uterine Descent

As in the case of the enlarged uterus, when planning a vaginal hysterectomy in the patient with minimal uterine descent, a careful EUA should be performed to confirm good uterine mobility in the lateral and AP planes and adequate vaginal caliber. The surgeon should confirm that there is enough room at the vaginal apex that the uterosacral ligaments will be successfully ligated. Uterine descent often improves considerably after the patient is placed under anesthesia. This is particularly true if using general anesthesia with muscle relaxants. Even if descent does not improve substantially with anesthesia, with appropriate uterine mobility and adequate space at the apex, it is safe to proceed using the vaginal route. As with all challenging hysterectomies, the surgeon should pay careful attention to patient positioning, lighting, and surgical assistance to optimize the chance of success. In the case of poor uterine descent, it is particularly important to have good surgical assistants experienced with vaginal surgery. A number of the instruments mentioned previously can be of particular value during this type of surgery including long needle drivers, long Allis clamps, a Bovie extender, and long scissors. Long narrow vaginal retractors such as the long Heaney or Briesky-Navratil retractors and the Steiner-Auvard long weighted speculum are essential in cases of poor uterine descent and should be used liberally throughout the surgery. Additional lighting such as a head lamp or lighted retractor or suction device may also be of value.

Without uterine descent, the initial circumferential incision around the cervix can be challenging because it is hard to achieve the appropriate angle with a long straight scalpel. We have found that using the Bovie cautery with the tip bent at approximately 45 degrees makes this incision much easier in these cases. After making the initial incision, it is useful to begin with the posterior colpotomy and insertion of the long narrow weighted retractor. This should be followed by clamping and suture ligation of the uterosacral ligaments. Ligation of the uterosacral and cardinal ligaments generally increases the amount of uterine descensus considerably, often bringing the cervix into the distal half of the vagina with traction. If this occurs, then the hysterectomy will usually proceed easily thereafter. After ligation of the uterine arteries and entry into the anterior and posterior cul-de-sacs are accomplished, bivalving the uterus or intramyometrial coring can be helpful to complete the hysterectomy.

In patients with a very narrow vaginal opening or when additional vaginal room is required, a Schuchardt incision can be performed (Fig. 8-6). This variation on the mediolateral episiotomy was first described to facilitate the performance of radical vaginal hysterectomies as initially described by Schauta. Classically, this incision is carried into the ischiorectal fossa and well into the upper vagina, but this is rarely necessary in cases of benign hysterectomy with introital narrowing. Typically a small incision starting just above the hymen and carried mediolaterally through the perineal structures is all that is required. Care should be made to avoid the anus and rectum. It is often useful to infiltrate the area with hemostatic solution such as dilute vasopressin or 0.5% or 1% lidocaine with epinephrine (1:200,000) and to use elecrocautery to make the incision in order to reduce blood loss. If needed, the incision can be extended proximally into the vagina, deeper into the ischiorectal fossa and levator ani muscles, or even performed bilaterally, but this will increase the risk of morbidity and postoperative pain.

Figure 8-6 Schuchardt perineal incision. The incision is started behind the hymenal ring and continued posterolateraly to curve around the anus. This can be a superficial incision or can be extended all the way to a point midway between the anus and the ischial tuberosity as is necessary to achieve the proper exposure (**A**). The vaginal portion of the incision can be extended as high as is necessary to provide the desired exposure to the vaginal vault. If needed, the incision can be extended into the fat of the ischiorectal fossa and the pubococcygeus muscle which can also be divided if greater exposure is required as shown by dotted line (**B**).

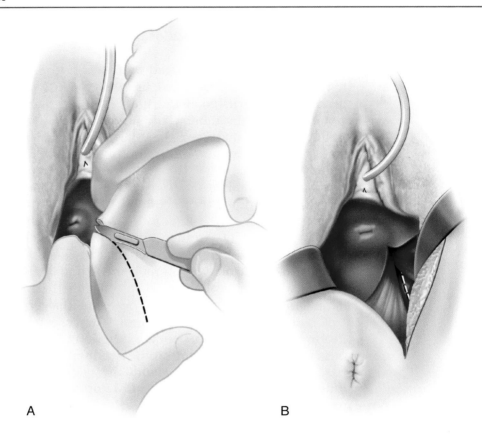

A   B

Case 3: Menorrhagia in a Patient with Multiple Prior Pelvic Surgeries

S.P. is a 38-year-old female gravida 3, para 3 with a 2-year history of worsening menorrhagia with menses lasting 8 to 9 days per month. She states that during the first several days she changes a pad every 1 to 2 hours, often having to "double up" on pads to avoid soiling her clothes. She has been using oral contraceptive pills in an attempt to control the bleeding for 12 months without success. A pelvic ultrasound reveals a uterus measuring 8 × 5 × 6 cm with a single 3.5-cm intramural fibroid distorting the uterine cavity. Office hysteroscopy confirms the distortion of the endometrial cavity and no intracavitary lesions are noted. Her obstetric history consists of one term vaginal delivery followed by two low transverse cesarean sections. Her surgical history is notable for a previous laparoscopic left salpingo-oophorectomy for ovarian torsion 18 years ago, tubal ligation performed at the time of her last cesarean section, and a laparoscopic left inguinal hernia repair with mesh performed 3 years ago. Physical examination reveals 6- to 8-week-size uterus that is mobile in all directions. An endometrial biopsy revealed secretory endometrium and her recent Pap smear is normal. Her laboratory studies are notable for a hematocrit of 28.5%. After discussing her treatment options in detail, she requests a vaginal hysterectomy.

Discussion of Case

Hysterectomy is a reasonable option in this patient with menorrhagia and anemia that is refractory to medical management. She has a history of several pelvic surgeries which will increase her risk of pelvic adhesive disease and may increase the technical difficulty of her hysterectomy. However, in general, prior pelvic surgery in and of itself should not be considered a contraindication to vaginal hysterectomy. Several large series have demonstrated that vaginal hysterectomy can be performed in most of these patients without increased morbidity. In general, the decision to proceed vaginally should be based on the same basic factors considered previously: uterine mobility and size, vaginal caliber, and shape of the bony pelvis independent of the history of prior pelvic surgery. A fixed, nonmobile uterus suggests severe pelvic adhesive disease and in this circumstance the hysterectomy should not be performed using the vaginal route. In contrast, the presence of a mobile uterus minimizes the risk of severe adhesive disease that would prevent the successful completion of a vaginal hysterectomy. Thin, filmy adhesions may still be present, but with the proper surgical technique these present a minimal obstacle to the vaginal approach.

Case 3: Menorrhagia in a Patient with Multiple Prior Pelvic Surgeries—cont'd

Adhesion formation after surgery is largely unpredictable and varies considerably from patient to patient. That being said, the nature of the previous operation(s) plays an important factor in determining the location and, to a lesser extent, the severity of potential pelvic adhesions, and can be a useful guide to when and where technical challenges may occur during surgery. Previous pelvic surgery can roughly be divided into three categories: those involving the adnexal structures, surgery on organs other than the genital tract, and those involving the uterus. As a general rule, prior surgery to the adnexal structures such as tubal ligation, ovarian cystectomy, surgery for ectopic pregnancy, and salpingo-oophorectomy do not pose a significant barrier to the vaginal approach. However, if the adnexal surgery was performed for severe endometriosis or pelvic inflammatory disease, then hysterectomy by the vaginal route may be unsafe. Similarly, in most circumstances prior pelvic surgery for nongynecologic indications should not prevent the successful completion of a vaginal hysterectomy. In fact, in certain cases such as the vertical midline incision or ventral hernia repair where anterior abdominal wall adhesions are common, the vaginal route may be the preferred approach because the uterus is typically uninvolved in these cases and gaining access to the pelvis via laparotomy or laparoscopy may be challenging. One exception where prior pelvic surgery to nongynecologic pelvic organs should preclude the vaginal route for hysterectomy is previous surgery for a pelvic inflammatory process such as diverticulitis, inflammatory bowel disease, or ruptured appendicitis. On the other hand, several large series have demonstrated that history of appendectomy for appendicitis in which the appendix has not ruptured is not a contraindication to vaginal hysterectomy. When available, it is often useful to review the prior operative notes and consider the nature and extent of any disease process noted at the previous surgery when making the decision about the appropriate route of hysterectomy.

Prior surgery to the uterus including cesarean section, myomectomy, and uterine suspension procedures has the greatest likelihood to result in adhesive disease that will impact the technical difficulty of any hysterectomy regardless of the route chosen. With the current cesarean section rate in the United States above 30%, previous cesarean section is by far the most likely previous surgery that the pelvic surgeon is likely to encounter. As has been noted throughout this text, prior low transverse cesarean section should not be considered a contraindication to vaginal hysterectomy. A scarred vesicovaginal space can make dissection more difficult whether the approach is abdominal, vaginal, or performed laparoscopically. As noted by Rooney and coworkers (2005) in a

series of 5092 hysterectomies, a history of previous cesarean section increases the risk of bladder injury during hysterectomy regardless of type (odds ratio [OR] 2.0; 95% confidence interval [CI] 1.2–3.5). In this series, the risk of injury in the presence of a prior cesarean section was not significantly different between abdominal and vaginal hysterectomy (1.8% vs. 3%), however LAVH was associated with an increased risk of injury (7.5%, $P = .005$). Thus, given the other benefits of the vaginal approach and the fact that the risk of bladder injury is not increased compared to other approaches, vaginal hysterectomy in this circumstance should remain the procedure of choice when feasible. With repeat cesarean sections, there is an increased risk of adhesions in the vesicovaginal space. However, there is no absolute upper limit to the number of cesarean sections beyond which the vaginal approach should be routinely avoided; the route of surgery in cases of multiple previous cesarean sections should be largely determined by the findings of the preoperative examination and the surgeon's skill and preference. When performing a hysterectomy in a patient with a prior cesarean section by whatever route, the surgeon should use careful and precise surgical technique in an attempt to minimize the risk of lower urinary tract injury. In these cases, we freely assess the integrity of the bladder using cystoscopy or similar techniques so that any injury that occurs can be identified and repaired intraoperatively, as unrecognized bladder (and ureter) injuries have substantially greater morbidity than those recognized and repaired at the time of the initial surgery.

In contrast to the low transverse cesarean section, uterine surgeries in which an incision is made in the uterine body rather than the lower uterine segment, such as some myomectomies and classical cesarean sections, are particularly prone to pelvic adhesive disease. In these circumstances, a careful preoperative examination with an assessment of uterine mobility is essential. It would be reasonable to consider a laparoscopic assessment for pelvic adhesions at the time of hysterectomy in these circumstances. When the uterine incision is on the anterior surface of the uterus or the fundus it is possible for adhesions to form between the uterus and the anterior abdominal wall, which would usually prevent successful vaginal hysterectomy. In this situation, the uterus will likely have little or no descent and may have decreased mobility in the other planes during preoperative pelvic examination or EUA. In some instances, traction on the uterus will cause a notable depression or dimpling of the anterior abdominal wall in the area of the previous incision (cervicofundal sign). When this is present any attempt at the vaginal approach should be abandoned.

Difficult Anterior Entry (See Video 8-2 🎥)

Even in routine vaginal hysterectomies, entry into the anterior cul-de-sac is often the most difficult step for many surgeons. As is emphasized in Chapter 7, there is no benefit to rushing this step; patience is key. Typically, with careful dissection and appropriate countertraction on the cervix and anterior vaginal incision, the bladder is mobilized off the cervix and, after 1 to 2 cm of dissection, the distal peritoneal reflection is identified by its characteristic look and feel and then safely entered. However, a number of conditions might cause difficult anterior cul-de-sac entry, including anterior adhesions from a previous cesarean section or other surgery, an anterior myoma in the lower uterine segment, previous bladder surgery, or an anterior cul-de-sac that is abnormally high. When difficulty is encountered, there are a number of general principles that the surgeon can follow to gain anterior peritoneal entry:

Enter the posterior cul-de-sac and proceed extraperitoneally. If not already performed, the posterior cul-de-sac should be entered and the uterosacral ligaments ligated. This will improve uterine descent and allow easier dissection and identification of the anterior peritoneum. In fact, as long as the bladder is protected, it is acceptable to continue dissection and subsequent pedicle ligations extraperitoneally as long as is necessary to gain the mobility and exposure required to secure anterior entry.

Sharp dissection. When scarring is present in the vesciovaginal space, sharp dissection is required. Firm traction of the uterus toward the surgeon and gentle traction of the vesicovaginal tissues anteriorly should be employed to generate maximal traction-countertraction in order to aid with dissection. Forcible blunt dissection, whether with a finger or retractor, should be avoided, as this will increase the risk of bladder injury (Fig. 8-7B). As noted in Chapter 7, no blind attempt should be made to enter the anterior cul-de-sac until the vesicouterine space has been developed and the peritoneum visualized in order to minimize the risk of bladder injury (see Video 7-2 🎥).

Use posterior access to identify the anterior peritoneal fold. If the uterus is normal size, it is often possible to identify the anterior peritoneal fold through the posterior cul-de-sac incision. If uterine prolapse is present, the surgeon can often reach the anterior cul-de-sac freely with one or more fingers from behind the uterus and identify the anterior peritoneal fold to aid in dissection (see Fig. 8-7C and Video 8-2 🎥). If prolapse is not present or space is not adequate to permit the insertion of the surgeon's hand, a uterine sound bent in the shape of a U can be inserted through the posterior peritoneal opening and over the uterine fundus. The tip can be palpated and dissection beneath the tip will expose the peritoneum of the anterior cul-de-sac which can be opened safely (Fig. 8-8). In some cases, uterine debulking may be required to allow adequate posterior access to assist with anterior entry. Intramyometrial coring is particularly useful in this circumstance because the dissection is maintained within the body of the uterus minimizing risk of bladder or other visceral injury.

Use a sound or retrograde filling to demarcate the bladder (see Video 8-2 🎥). If the location of the bladder is not clear, a uterine sound can be bent at an angle and passed per urethra into the bladder to demarcate the lower boundary of the bladder in the area of dissection. Alternatively, the bladder can be filled with fluid via the transurethral catheter to identify the bladder edge and then drained prior to proceeding with the dissection. Some surgeons advocate

Figure 8-7 Adhesions between the bladder and cervix from a previous cesarean section are noted. These are best taken down with sharp dissection (**A**). Blunt dissection may lead to inadvertent cystotomy, as the finger will pass into the area of least resistance (**B**). Passing a finger through the posterior peritoneal incision around the uterus, when possible, can facilitate dissection in the appropriate plane (**C**); Video 8-2

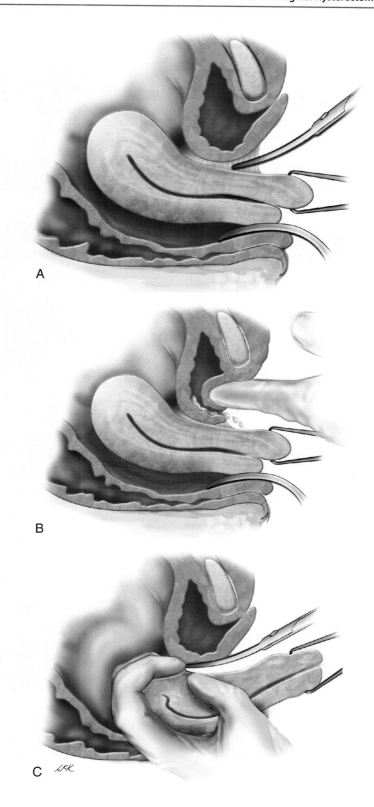

A

B

C

leaving 50 to 100 mL of saline or dilute indigo carmine in the bladder during the anterior dissection in order to help identify when a bladder injury has occurred.

Evaluate bladder integrity at the end of surgery. After a difficult anterior dissection, the bladder should be carefully inspected to identify any injury. Cys-

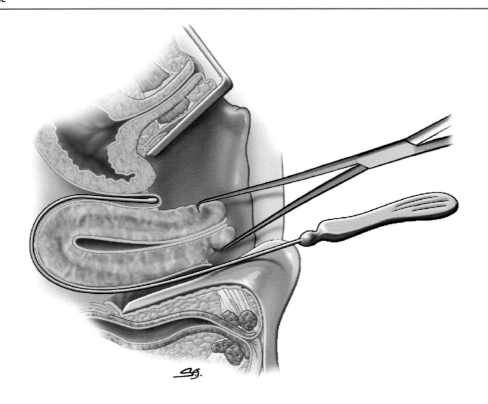

Figure 8-8 In cases of difficult anterior entry, a uterine sound bent in the shape of a U can be inserted through the posterior peritoneal opening and over the uterine fundus. The tip can be palpated and dissection beneath the tip will expose the peritoneum of the anterior cul-de-sac, which can be opened safely.

toscopy is particularly valuable in this regard because it also allows evaluation of ureteral patency if intravenous indigo carmine is administered. Alternatively, the bladder can be filled with dilute indigo carmine and the surgical site carefully inspected to identify any bladder injury. If a cystotomy occurs during a difficult anterior cul-de-sac dissection, it will almost always be located in the supratrigonal region of the bladder dome, typically in the midline. It is generally recommended that if a bladder injury is identified during the dissection, the area of injury should be marked with one or more sutures for easy identification and that repair be delayed until after the hysterectomy is complete. It is often easier to identify the correct plane of dissection to gain anterior peritoneal entry with the cystotomy open as the bladder can be directly palpated. Additionally, it is easier to identify the full extent of the injury and there will be more room to perform the cystotomy repair after the uterus is removed. Care should be taken however not to enlarge the cystotomy with a retractor during the rest of the hysterectomy. Any injury should be repaired in two layers using No. 2-0 or 3-0 absorbable suture ensuring that the closure is watertight followed by prolonged bladder drainage. See Chapter 11 for further discussion of identifying and repairing bladder injuries.

In some cases, anterior entry can be impeded by a fibroid in the anterior cervix or lower uterine segment. In these cases, completion of the anterior colpotomy might require posterior delivery of the uterus and removal of the fibroid. See the earlier Myomectomy section for a description of the surgical technique.

Difficult Posterior Entry (See Video 8-3 📹)

Difficulty entering the posterior cul-de-sac occurs less frequently than with anterior entry. Conditions that may result in difficult posterior cul-de-sac entry include endometriosis involving the rectovaginal septum; pelvic adhesive disease with small bowel in the cul-de-sac; a history of pelvic inflammatory disease, diverticulitis, previous anorectal surgery; and posterior cervical or lower uterine segment myomas. In patients with a history of endometriosis, it is useful to review the operative notes from the most recent prior surgery. In cases of mild or even moderate endometriosis that does not distort the cul-de-sac, vaginal hysterectomy is not contraindicated. However, in cases of severe endometriosis, particularly if it involves the rectovaginal septum or is associated with endometriomas, laparoscopy or laparotomy is recommended. During the preoperative bimanual examination or EUA, the presence of nodularity, thickening or decreased mobility on rectovaginal examination in a patient with endometriosis suggests rectovaginal involvement and hysterectomy by the vaginal route should be avoided.

The initial steps for gaining safe access to the posterior cul-de-sac when difficult posterior entry is encountered are similar to those described for difficult anterior entry: use of sharp dissection with good traction-countertraction, and continued dissection and suture ligation extraperitoneally until peritoneal entry is achieved. Dissection should be close to the uterus and the rectum protected posteriorly with retractors. In the face of particularly thick or difficult adhesions, it may be necessary to dissect within the posterior uterine serosa until more normal anatomy is encountered in order to avoid rectal injury. Rectal examination should be performed liberally throughout to assist in identifying the appropriate surgical plane and avoid rectal injury. Entry into the anterior cul-de-sac should be performed and can assist with posterior dissection. If the uterus is small, it may be possible to deliver the uterine fundus anteriorly or to access the posterior cul-de-sac digitally through the anterior peritoneal incision in order to better characterize the posterior adhesions and aid with dissection, but this is often more difficult than with the techniques described for anterior entry. If a posterior cervical myoma is impeding posterior cul-de-sac entry then a myomectomy should be performed using the techniques previously described. Intramyometrial coring or other uterine debulking techniques also may be employed if the uterus is enlarged in order to assist with delivery of the fundus or improve access for posterior peritoneal entry.

Another option to the traditional approach to posterior cul-de-sac entry that can be considered when posterior entry is anticipated to be difficult is transcervical access to the posterior cul-de-sac (see Fig. 8-9 and Video 8-3 🎥). This technique was originally described by Wertheim in 1906. In this approach, a retractor is placed over the posterior vaginal wall and the cervix is grasped with tenacula at 3 and 9 o'clock and pulled anteriorly with firm traction. After injecting posterior cervicovaginal tissue and the cervix itself with a hemostatic agent, a scalpel or heavy scissors with one blade inserted into the cervical canal are used to perform a full-thickness division of the posterior cervical wall in the midline. The incision is continued with small bites slowly dividing the overlying vaginal mucosa until the peritoneum of the cul-de-sac is entered. The initial peritoneal window is usually small and in the midline but is easily expanded digitally or with scissors to allow adequate posterior peritoneal access. The advantages of this approach are that it is relatively rapid and avoids extensive dissection in the rectovaginal space, and the peritoneum is entered in the most anterior aspect of the pouch of Douglas away from the rectum. Several authors have reported large series using this technique without rectal injury.

After a difficult dissection to obtain posterior peritoneal entry it is essential that the rectum be thoroughly examined to identify any injury. As with bladder

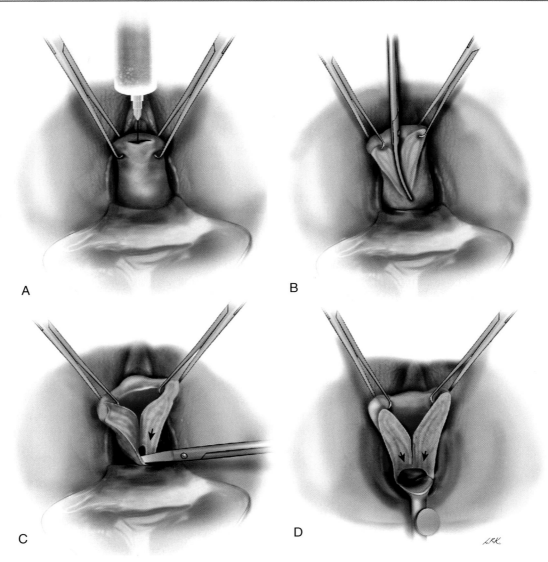

Figure 8-9 Cervicovaginal entry into the posterior cul-de-sac (see also Video 8-3 📹). **A,** Injection of a hemostatic solution into the posterior cervicovaginal tissues and intracervically to minimize blood loss. **B,** Using heavy scissors with one tip in the cervical canal, a cervicocolpotomy is performed. **C,** Small bites are made incrementally until the cul-de-sac is entered (*arrow*). **D,** The peritoneal opening is enlarged and a retractor inserted (*arrows*).

injury, unrecognized rectal injuries can have substantial morbidity, but a rectal injury that is identified and properly repaired rarely results in postoperative sequelae. A careful digital rectal examination will identify most rectal injuries. To identify small or even pinpoint rectal injuries, a bubble test can be performed. To perform a bubble test, the patient is placed in Trendelenburg position and saline (typically 50–100 mL) is put in the operative field so that it pools over the area of rectal dissection. A proctoscope is inserted just past the anal canal and air is inflated into the rectum. The pool of saline over the anterior rectal wall is then inspected for air bubbles which, if noted, indicate the presence and location of any rectal injury. Any identified rectal injury should be repaired in two layers using No. 2-0 or 3-0 absorbable suture. As most injuries that would occur at the time of posterior entry for hysterectomy will be extraperitoneal, bowel diversion is typically not necessary. Please refer to Chapter 11 for a more detailed discussion of rectal injury and its repair.

Uterine Adhesions

In a patient whose preoperative examination demonstrates good uterine mobility, it is unlikely that adhesions to the uterus will be encountered that will impair successful vaginal hysterectomy. Severe adhesions are more likely with previous surgery to the uterus or with a history of endometriosis or an inflammatory disease of the pelvis such as pelvic inflammatory disease, inflammatory bowel disease, or diverticulitis and this should be taken into account when planning the route of surgery as discussed previously. Pelvic adhesive disease is often unanticipated, however, and can occur in patients with uncomplicated histories and normal pelvic examinations. Adhesions that make anterior or posterior entry more difficult have already been discussed and usually can be managed successfully. However, adhesions to the uterine fundus pose greater uncertainty. It is good practice during any hysterectomy to regularly visualize and palpate the entire uterus or at least the portion of uterine fundus that is readily accessible throughout the surgery. If uterine adhesions are encountered, the surgeon should make every effort to characterize their nature and location by visualization or digital palpation. Adhesions to the uterine fundus typically involve the omentum, small bowel, or adnexal structures. The surgeon must assess whether there is adequate mobility and visualization to safely remove the adhesions and continue with the vaginal approach. Any attempts at adhesiolyis should always be made under direct vision, close to the uterus, and with meticulous surgical technique. Adhesions can be taken down as they are encountered during the progression of the hysterectomy to ensure maximum exposure. If the uterus is mobile, the fundus can be pulled to or through the anterior or posterior colpotomy incisions giving excellent exposure to the adhesions for removal. If the fundus cannot be delivered, intramyometrial coring is helpful as it will result in a decrease in the size of the uterine fundus while keeping dissection within the uterine body in order to avoid visceral injury. This will result in delivery of the fundus so that the adhesions can be removed under direct vision. If the adhesions are thick and impair the mobility of the uterus or the adhesions cannot be removed safely via the vaginal approach, then a laparotomy or laparoscopy should be performed.

Elongated Cervix

The size of the uterine cervix can vary significantly. As noted in Chapter 2, typically in the reproductive-aged female the uterine body is much larger than the cervix, while in prepubertal and postmenopausal females, the relative length of the uterine body and cervix is similar. In some cases, the cervix can become elongated, which can present a challenge during vaginal hysterectomy. Cases have been reported in which the cervix has measured as long as 10 to 15 cm. The cause of cervical elongation is largely unknown; however, it is more common in postmenopausal women. It can occur in isolation but is often associated with uterovaginal prolapse. For unknown reasons, it also seems to occur more frequently when the uterus is fixed and immobile from previous adhesive disease or from previous uterine fixation. On preoperative examination, cervical elongation is often characterized by the cervix extending well into the vagina, in some cases beyond the introitus (so-called pseudoprolapse); however, the posterior vaginal fornix is typically well supported and the uterine fundus is in a normal position within the pelvis which differentiates it from true uterine prolapse. With cervical elongation, the primary surgical challenge is entry into the anterior and posterior cul-de-sacs, as the anterior and posterior peritoneal folds are higher than usual. At the time of the EUA, the surgeon should carefully palpate the uterus and cervix in order to determine the cervical length and the location of the area of transition between the cervix and fundus at the lower uterine segment. The anterior peritoneal fold is usually located at or above this point. The posterior peritoneal fold may be more distal. It is useful to identify the distal extent of the bladder prior to making the initial anterior vaginal incision. Sometimes the bladder crease is readily apparent; when it is not, the bladder can be filled with fluid or a probe can be placed transurethrally to delineate this boundary. Similarly, the distal extent of the rectum can be determined by rectal examination. After identifying the distal extent of the bladder and rectum, the surgeon can make the initial circumferential vaginal incision distal enough to avoid visceral injury, but high enough to avoid unneeded dissection on distal aspect of the elongated cervix. This incision can be significantly higher than one would make when the cervix is normal length. Even with a more proximal initial incision, it is often necessary to perform dissection and sequential suture ligation extraperitoneally for several bites before the anterior and posterior peritoneal folds are encountered. After gaining posterior entry, it is often possible to digitally access the anterior cul-de-sac through the posterior peritoneal incision over the uterine fundus in order to aid in gaining anterior entry as has been previously described. Once anterior and posterior peritoneal entry are obtained, the remainder of the hysterectomy can proceed routinely. If necessary to gain more mobility or exposure during the remainder of the hysterectomy, the elongated cervix can be amputated.

Case 4: Uterovaginal Prolapse

A 67-year-old female gravida 3, para 3 presents with a 6-month history of "something bulging through her vagina." The bulging sensation has gradually worsened over the last several months and now she sees and feels a bulge that protrudes "several inches" beyond the vaginal opening. She also reports increased urinary frequency, nocturia, and feeling of incomplete bladder emptying. She has a 10-year history of mild stress urinary incontinence symptoms which resolved approximately 4 months ago. On physical examination, she is noted to have complete uterovaginal prolapse (stage IV) with the cervix protruding 6 cm beyond the hymen (Fig. 8-10). She desires surgical correction of her pelvic organ prolapse.

Discussion of Case

Uterine prolapse represents the most common indication for hysterectomy in postmenopausal women. Surgery is considered in patients with symptomatic prolapse who do not desire or have failed a pessary. Uterine prolapse is typically not an isolated event and is often associated with other pelvic support defects. A hysterectomy alone is never adequate treatment for prolapse; associated surgical repairs of vaginal support defects are necessary. This patient has uterine procidentia and by definition has defects of anterior, posterior, and apical support (see Fig. 2-31). Surgical correction of each of these support defects should be performed and can be accomplished by either a vaginal, abdominal, or laparoscopic approach. Although there are clinical trials demonstrating that prolapse surgery through the abdominal route (specifically, abdominal

sacral colpopexy) results in more durable anatomic correction than transvaginal prolapse surgery, overall outcomes of the abdominal and vaginal route including quality of life are relatively equivalent and vaginal surgery is associated with fewer serious perioperative complications, faster recovery, quicker return to work, and lower cost than abdominal prolapse repairs (Jelovsek et al, 2007). Given this, surgeons typically individualize the type and route of prolapse surgery for each patient, considering such factors as age, co-morbid conditions, and history of previous prolapse surgery. In the United States, approximately 80% to 90% of prolapse surgery is performed vaginally, but laparoscopic and robotic repairs are gaining some acceptance. There also are an increasing number of options for uterine preservation in women with uterovaginal prolapse, but few data exist on the efficacy of these options, so in the postreproductive woman hysterectomy remains the standard of care. In this older woman with complete uterine prolapse, surgical correction consisting of a vaginal hysterectomy with a vaginal vault suspension along with repair of her anterior and posterior vaginal prolapse is a good option. Preoperatively, she should receive at least a basic urodynamic evaluation with prolapse reduction in order to evaluate for stress urinary incontinence that may have become masked by urethral kinking resulting from her anterior vaginal wall prolapse. If stress incontinence is demonstrated, then an anti-incontinence procedure such as a midurethral sling is warranted. For a more detailed discussion of the anatomic aspects of this surgery please refer to Chapter 2.

Figure 8-10 Complete uterovaginal prolapse with two linear erosions of the posterior vaginal epithelium.

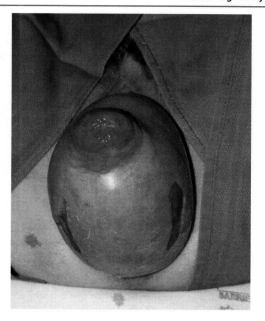

Surgical Technique for Uterovaginal Prolapse (See Video 8-4 🎥)

On the preoperative examination, it is important for the surgeon to fully characterize the support of the anteroposterior vaginal wall as well as the uterus. This is essential for planning the appropriate surgical repair. A reproducible prolapse grading system such as the pelvic organ prolapse quantification system (POPQ) is helpful in this regard. The surgeon should also carefully palpate the cervix and uterus to determine if cervical elongation is present, as this is not an uncommon finding in women with uterine prolapse. The basic steps for hysterectomy in the patient with complete prolapse are similar to those of the standard vaginal hysterectomy. The principal surgical challenge in these cases is the distortion of the normal anatomic relationships. In the absence of cervical elongation, the distal reflection of the bladder is 2 to 3 cm proximal to the cervix, so the initial vaginal incision should be made just proximal to the distal cervix. If cervical elongation is present, the surgical approach described previously for these cases should be followed. As noted in Chapter 2, eversion of the bladder trigone displaces the ureteral orifices distally so that they are approximately at the level of the distal bladder reflection. The course of the distal ureters is also significantly altered (see Fig. 2-32). As such, the surgeon should be sure to dissect close to the cervix and protect the bladder with retractors throughout the case. Posteriorly, the distal rectum often prolapses with the uterus and vagina, but not to the same degree as the bladder. Typically, the posterior cul-de-sac, which may contain prolapsing small intestine (i.e., enterocele), lies behind the upper half or so of the posterior vaginal wall and the distal rectum lies behind the distal posterior vaginal wall. As such, entry into the posterior cul-de-sac during hysterectomy in cases of uterovaginal prolapse is often easily accomplished but anterior entry can be more challenging. Once posterior entry occurs, it is often possible to pass a finger through the posterior cul-de-sac around the uterus to tent the anterior peritoneum to aid in anterior entry (see Fig. 8-7 and Video 8-2 🎥). In postmenopausal women, the uterine body is often small so that after ligation of the uterine arteries it usually does not require the ligation of more than two or three pedicles on either side before the uterus can be delivered through the vaginal incision.

Figure 8-11 McCall's culdoplasty. **A,** Placement of internal and external McCall sutures. **B,** Cross section of upper vagina and vaginal vault before and after tying sutures.

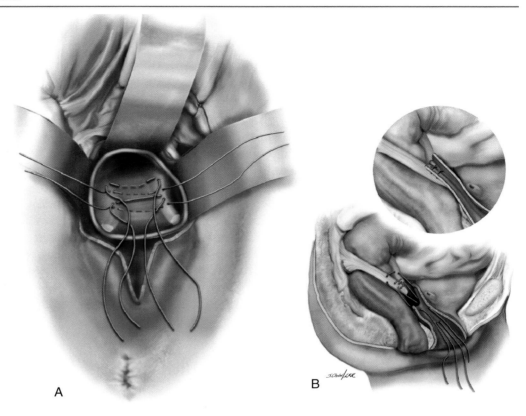

A

B

Once this is accomplished the utero-ovarian pedicles are ligated to complete the hysterectomy. Once the hysterectomy is completed, a vaginal vault suspension of some type always should be performed and repair of the anterior and posterior vaginal prolapse should be performed as necessary. Vaginal vault suspensions can be done intraperitoneally as in the McCall's culdoplasty (Fig. 8-11) and the uterosacral vaginal vault suspension or extraperitoneally such as the sacrospinous ligament fixation. For a broader discussion of the surgical correction of pelvic organ prolapse, please refer to *Pelvic Organ Prolapse* (Karram M, Maher C, eds.) in the *Female Pelvic Surgery Video Atlas Series*.

Conversion to Laparoscopy or Laparotomy

With any vaginal hysterectomy there is a chance that conversion to laparoscopy or laparotomy will be required in order to complete the operation safely, although the rate of this occurrence is rare (<1%) in uncomplicated cases. With increasing skill and experience using the techniques described in this chapter, the gynecologic surgeon will be able to successfully accomplish vaginal hysterectomy in more challenging cases and increase the proportion of hysterectomies he/she performs via the vaginal route. A natural consequence of taking on more challenging cases, however, is that the risk of conversion is likely to increase somewhat. Provided that the decision for conversion is made in a timely and controlled manner, there are no untoward consequences to the patient. Moreover, given the documented advantages of the vaginal route of hysterectomy in terms of patient outcomes and cost, increasing the proportion of hysterectomies performed vaginally is beneficial to patients and the health care system. Thus, assuming the patient was counseled appropriately and the decision for conversion from the vaginal approach to the abdominal approach was made in a controlled timely manner, the surgeon should not look at a conversion as a surgical failure, but rather as an exercise in good surgical judgment.

In some cases, such as uncontrolled hemorrhage, conversion to laparotomy should be performed emergently to prevent further blood loss and additional morbidity. In other situations, such as a difficult uterine morcellation, the presence of uterine adhesions or inability to gain safe entry into the anterior or posterior cul-de-sacs, the decision to convert from the vaginal approach can be more deliberate and is often made gradually after continued struggle. In both cases, it is important to maintain close communication with the anesthesia team and operating room staff. In nonemergent cases, when the surgery has become difficult and the surgeon begins to think that it might not be possible to safely complete the surgery vaginally, it is valuable to set a time limit on further vaginal surgery and communicate this with the operative team (for example: "If we do not make significant progress on this case in the next _____ minutes, we will be converting to laparotomy/laparoscopy"). This will allow the operating room team to start gathering the necessary equipment and setting up for the conversion should it prove necessary. Setting a time limit also will prevent a prolonged unnecessary struggle with the vaginal dissection that ultimately may harm the patient. It is often useful to have one of the assistants or the circulating nurse assume the role of the timekeeper because it is easy for the surgeon to lose track of time during a difficult case.

Once the final decision to convert has been made, the surgeon must decide whether to proceed with laparoscopy or laparotomy. In some situations, such as an unexpected adnexal mass or adhesions to the uterine fundus, laparoscopy is an excellent option as the patient can still benefit from a minimally invasive approach. In other situations, such as the emergent hemorrhage or severe adhesive disease, laparotomy is more prudent. Ultimately, the surgeon should base this decision upon the clinical situation at hand, his or her own particular set of surgical skills, and available operating room facilities. If the decision is made to convert to laparotomy and the situation is nonemergent, we have found it valuable to close the vaginal cuff vaginally before proceeding to the laparotomy. Invariably, it is quicker and easier to close the cuff from the vaginal route than it is abdominally. The cervix is pushed into the pelvis prior to closing or if necessary is amputated. Vaginal cuff closure can be done while the operating team is setting up for the laparotomy, further saving time. If a decision is made to proceed with laparoscopy, then the cuff should be left open to aid in removal of the uterus. To aid in peritoneal insufflation, the peritoneal incisions can be clamped or the vagina can be packed with a laparotomy sponge. At the completion of the surgery, the surgeon should have an open and honest dialogue with the patient and her family about the need to convert and the events that led to this decision.

Suggested Reading

Barber MD: Hysterectomy. In Sokol A, Sokol E (eds): Requisites in Obstetrics and Gynecology: General Gynecology. St Louis, Elsevier, 2007.

Benassi L, Rossi T, Kaihura CT, et al: Abdominal or vaginal hysterectomy for enlarged uteri: A randomized clinical trial. Am J Obstet Gynecol 2002;187:1561–1565.

Coulam CB, Pratt JH: Vaginal hysterectomy: Is previous pelvic operation a contraindication? Am J Obstet Gynecol 1973;116:252–260.

Darai E, Soriano D, Kimata P, et al: Vaginal hysterectomy for enlarged uteri, with or without laparoscopic assistance: Randomized study. Obstet Gynecol 2001;97:712–716.

Hoffman MS, Jaeger M: A new method for gaining entry into the scarred anterior cul-de-sac during transvaginal hysterectomy. Am J Obstet Gynecol 1990;162:1269–1270.

Hoffman MS, Spellacy WN: The difficult vaginal hysterectomy: A surgical atlas. New York, Springer-Verlag, 1995.

Hwang JL, Seow KM, Tsai YL, et al: Comparative study of vaginal, laparoscopically assisted vaginal and abdominal hysterectomies for uterine myoma larger than 6 cm in diameter or uterus weighing at least 450 g: A prospective randomized study. Acta Obstet Gynaecol Scand 2002;81:1132–1138.

Jelovsek JE, Maher C, Barber MD: Seminar on pelvic organ prolapse. Lancet 2007;369:1027–1038.

Johnson N, Barlow D, Lethaby A, et al: Surgical approach to hysterectomy for benign gynecological disease. Cochrane Database Syst Rev 2006;Issue 2:CD003677.

Karram MM: Vaginal hysterectomy. In Baggish MS, Karram MM: Atlas of Pelvic Anatomy and Gynecologic Surgery, 2nd ed. Philadelphia, WB Saunders, 2006.

Kovac SR: The difficult vaginal hysterectomy. In Sheth S, Studd J (eds): Vaginal Hysterectomy. London, Martin Dunitz, 2002.

Lash AF: A method for reducing size of the uterus in vaginal hysterectomies. Am J Obstet Gynecol 1941;42:452–459.

Lethaby A, Vollenhoven B, Sowter MC: Pre-operative GnRH analogue therapy before hysterectomy or myomectomy for uterine fibroids. Cochrane Database Syst Rev 2001;Issue 2:CD000547.

Le Tohic A, Dhainaut C, Yazbeck C, et al: Hysterectomy for benign uterine pathology among women without previous vaginal delivery. Obstet Gynecol 2008;111:829–837.

Nichols DH, Randall CL (eds): Vaginal surgery, 4th ed. Philadelphia, Lippincott Williams & Wilkins, 1996.

Raffi A, Samain E, Levardon M, et al: Vaginal hysterectomy for benign disorders in obese women: A prospective study. Br J Obstet Gynaecol 2005;112:223–227.

Rooney CM, Crawford AT, Vassallo BJ, et al: Is previous cesarean section a risk factor for incidental cystotomy at the time of hysterectomy? A case-control study. Am J Obstet Gynecol 2005;193:2041–2044.

Sesti F, Calonzi F, Ruggeri V, et al: A comparison of vaginal, laparoscopic-assisted vaginal and mini-laparotomy hysterectomies for enlarged myomatous uteri. Int J Gynaecol Obstet 2008a;103:227–231.

Sesti, F, Ruggeri V, Pietropolli A, Piccione E: Laparoscopically assisted vaginal hysterectomy versus vaginal hysterectomy for enlarged uterus. J Soc Laparoendosc Surg 2008b;12:246–251.

Sheth SS: Vaginal or abdominal hysterectomy? In Sheth SS, Sutton C (eds): Menorrhagia. Oxford, Isis Medical Media, 1999.

Sheth S, Studd J: Vaginal Hysterectomy. London, Martin Dunitz, 2002.

Wertheim E, Micholitsch T: Die technik der vaginalen bauchhölen—operationen. Liepzig, Verlag von Sittirzel, 1906;290–295.

Prophylactic Oophorectomy at Hysterectomy

James L. Whiteside M.D.
Rebecca S. Uranga M.D.

 Video Clips on DVD

9-1 Techniques in Vaginal Oophorectomy   **9-2** Vaginal Bilateral Salpino-oophorectomy

The fate of the ovaries in a woman considering an indicated hysterectomy is a common question in the practice of gynecology. The approximately 600,000 hysterectomies done annually in the United States attests to the number of times this decision is weighed by patient and physician. *The decision balances cancer prevention with surgical menopause* and varies with the woman's inherited and acquired risks for each of these issues. Risk assessment lies behind many of the choices made by patient and provider in the matter of oophorectomy. The decision to remove or not remove ovaries at hysterectomy should not be made lightly. For the patient, risk (and fear) of cancer and repeat surgery is contrasted with surgical menopause and the associated quality of life, bone, cardiovascular, and other risks. For the provider the method and risk of operative complications are contrasted between abdominal, laparoscopic, and vaginal approaches to hysterectomy. Fear may sway decision making by patient (in the form of inflated cancer fears) and physician (in the form of overstated risks). The good physician practices medicine with competence and compassion; hence, it is requisite that the best evidence for and against oophorectomy in a given patient be known and *communicated to the patient in an unbiased manner*. That evidence, however, is often inadequate and nearly always incomplete. Passions therefore will often carry the patient to her final decision.

Patient Case Presentations

It is worthwhile to consider three women facing the question of prophylactic oophorectomy at the time of hysterectomy. The first woman is 37 years old and has had three vaginal deliveries, the last of which left her with stage III uterovaginal prolapse. The woman reports significant bowel, bladder, and sexual issues related to her pelvic organ prolapse. Having tried and disliked a pessary, the woman now seeks a definitive surgical prolapse repair. As part of her repair a hysterectomy is planned and the woman asks about the fate of her ovaries.

Next is a 72-year-old woman who, having used a pessary for 5 years to manage her stage IV uterovaginal prolapse, develops significant vaginal ulcerations prompting her, among other reasons, to seek a definitive surgical repair. Like the 37-year-old woman, this woman is scheduled to have a hysterectomy and also ponders the fate of her ovaries.

Finally, a 47-year-old woman with a 3-year history of distressing menorrhagia, failing all conservative managements, is considering a hysterectomy. She has no personal or family

Table 9-1 Criteria for Referral for *BRCA* Testing*

For non–Ashkenazi Jewish women
- Two first-degree relatives with breast cancer, one relative in whom breast cancer was diagnosed before the age of 50 years
- A combination of three or more first- or second-degree relatives with breast cancer at any age
- A combination of both breast and ovarian cancer among first- and second-degree relatives
- A first-degree relative with bilateral breast cancer
- A combination of two or more first- or second-degree relatives with ovarian cancer at any age
- A first- or second-degree relative with both breast and ovarian cancer at any age
- A male relative with breast cancer

For women of Ashkenazi Jewish heritage
- Any first-degree relative with breast or ovarian cancer
- Two second-degree relatives on the same side of the family with breast or ovarian cancer

*Based on the U.S. Preventive Services Task Force recommendations for genetic risk assessment and *BRCA* mutation testing for breast and ovarian cancer susceptibility.
Data from Nelson HD, Huffman LH, Fu R, et al: Genetic risk assessment and *BRCA* mutation testing for breast and ovarian cancer susceptibility: Systematic evidence review for the U.S. Preventive Services Task Force. Ann Intern Med 2005;143:362–379.

Patient Case Presentations—cont'd

history of ovarian disease. Her medical history is unremarkable; however, she has had two prior cesarean sections. Her body mass index is 28 and on physical examination she has a 10-week-size anteverted, smooth, mobile uterus with no remarkable uterine prolapse.

Discussion of Cases

These three women could be seen to span the decisional spectrum for prophylactic oophorectomy. All things being equal, the first two women have somewhat more obvious decision processes to consider. For the youngest woman the scale tips sharply toward keeping her ovaries while for the much older woman the reverse is true. Either woman, however, may weigh the evidence differently and choose contrary to scales of evidence. It is further recognized that present neoplasm, family history, pelvic pain, endometriosis, or history of significant pelvic infection could modify the certainty of keeping the ovaries in the younger woman. Oophorectomy does increase the operative risk for the older woman, although the magnitude of this risk is unknown and variable between patients and hysterectomy approach. Beyond this operative risk there are few clear benefits to keeping the ovaries at age 72. Therefore, it is often the patient risks that drive the decision for oophorectomy in the younger woman and surgical risks that drive the decision against

oophorectomy in the older woman. More to the point, surgeon skill may often dictate ovary removal in the older woman (particularly in this 72-year-old woman who should have a vaginal hysterectomy for her stage IV uterovaginal prolapse).

The decision regarding the 47-year-old woman more delicately balances the risks and benefits of oophorectomy. For the 47-year-old woman age, family history, surgical history, habitus, and uterine support all impact the decision and technique of oophorectomy. Given that the mean age of menopause for U.S. women is approximately 51 years, this woman has approximately 4 years of remaining ovarian function. The patient's family history (with or without Ashkenazi Jewish heritage) renders no mandate to remove the ovaries or to test for high-risk genetic factors (Table 9-1). The patient's cesarean history should cause the physician to pause in considering the vaginal approach to hysterectomy but this too is debatable. On prophylactic oophorectomy, the American College of Obstetricians and Gynecologists (ACOG Practice Bulletin No. 89, 2008) offers no mandate on whether this woman's ovaries should be removed nor how best to remove them. In what follows we will consider this woman intermittently and discuss how her situation might be approached as to both the decision and potential techniques of prophylactic oophorectomy.

Surgical Technique

Planned removal of the ovaries at the time of hysterectomy considerably influences the route of surgical access. In a study by Davies and associates (1998) over 40% of abdominal hysterectomies appeared to have been justified on the basis of planned oophorectomy. This is not a surprising finding. Yet there does not appear to be any credible evidence to support the decision to pursue an

Figure 9-1 Grading system to estimate ovarian descent and accessibility of the ovary for vaginal removal (Modified from Kovac SR, Cruikshank SH: Guidelines to determine the route of oophorectomy with hysterectomy. Am J Obstet Gynecol 1996;175:1483–1488.)

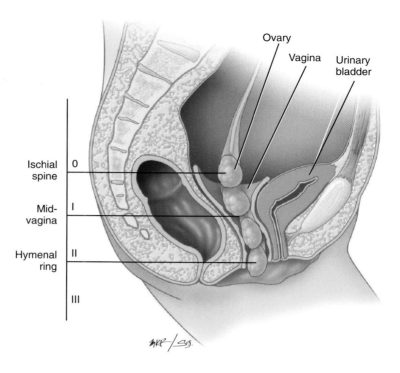

abdominal approach solely on the basis of the need to remove ovaries. Indeed, Agostini and associates (2006), in a randomized study comparing vaginal versus laparoscopically assisted hysterectomy, both with concurrent prophylactic bilateral oophorectomy, concluded the laparoscopic approach resulted in more injury. The complications noted to be higher among the laparoscopic group included blood loss greater than 500 mL, hematoma at the trocar and vaginal cuff sites, and postoperative fever. Irrespective of the evidence, surgeon skill and confidence will undoubtedly influence whether the ovaries will be pursued vaginally. Kovac and Cruikshank (1996) devised a system to grade the accessibility of the ovaries based on their relative proximity to the ischial spines, midvagina, and hymen (Fig. 9-1). The system is largely valuable only to testify that the lower the grade (closer to the ischial spines; higher in the pelvis), the lower the incidence and lower the success rate with vaginal ovarian removal.

Abdominal Approach to Oophorectomy

Abdominal removal of the ovaries can be performed during laparotomy or laparoscopy and the latter may include robotic assistance. The steps to remove the ovaries from this vantage are the same irrespective of surgical approach. Avoidance of ureteral injury is always paramount when operating in the pelvis. Understanding the course of the ureters and their relation to the ovarian blood supply is essential for safe resection of the ovary. Ligation of the ovarian blood supply can be accomplished using a variety of techniques including suture, electrocautery (e.g., bipolar vessel sealing), and stapling. Each of these techniques is used with obvious differentials in cost and with minimal (but unknown) differences in operative risk.

Once the surgeon has entered the abdominal cavity the ovaries and fallopian tubes should be inspected and any abnormalities noted and recorded in the operative dictation. With the ipsilateral ureter identified, the infundibulopelvic ligament is put on tension and the overlying peritoneum between the round

Figure 9-2 The uterus and ovary are retracted medially putting the infundibulopelvic ligament on tension. The overlying peritoneum is cut exposing the ureter, ovarian vessels, and iliac vessels. *Inset:* The ovarian vessels are clamped, cut, and ligated.

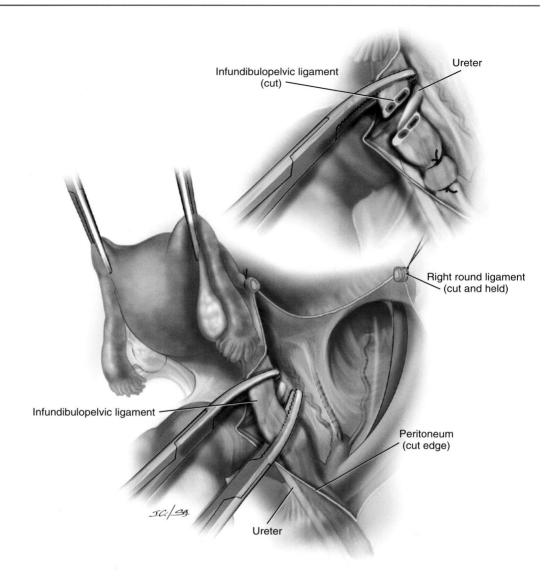

and broad ligament cut (Fig. 9-2). Next, careful dissection isolates the ovarian blood supply for ligature or vessel sealing, taking care to assure that the ipsilateral ureter is not within the surgical field. The ligated infundibulopelvic ligament with the ovary and tube are next reflected toward the uterus; and visually away from the ureter. Ultimately the line of dissection incorporates the round ligament and opening the opposing leaves of the broad ligament to begin the hysterectomy. Of note: some surgeons do not fully expose the blood supply of the infundibulopelvic ligament, choosing instead to ligate these vessels through the peritoneum. This practice is quicker and may reduce blood loss encountered with the more extensive dissection but potentially puts the ureter at increased risk. This difference may be less in laparotomy or robotic surgery possibly attesting more to surgeon skill and confidence than to any real differences in surgical approach. Irrespective of abdominal surgical approach, injury to the ureter in association with oophorectomy is most often encountered with the first pedicle across the infundibulopelvic ligament as all abdominal techniques (open, laparoscopic, and robotic) remove the ovaries from the pelvic brim toward the uterus.

Vaginal Approach to Oophorectomy

The most challenging and necessary task in vaginally removing the ovaries is securing the ovarian vessels contained within the infundibulopelvic ligament. There are several basic techniques used to accomplish this task (see Videos 📹). Both techniques follow transvaginal removal of the uterus. The first technique identifies the infundibulopelvic ligament by downward traction on the ovary (via Babcock or Allis clamp) prior to clamping and ligation (Fig. 9-3; Video 9-1 📹). Packing the bowel free of the operative field is recommended. Exposure of the operative field is facilitated with placement of retractors at 12 and 6 o'clock and either 3 or 9 o'clock, depending on the ovary being removed. Gentle downward traction on both the ovary and fallopian tube is necessary to safely pass a heavy clamp (e.g., Heaney clamp) across the blood supply of the infundibulopelvic ligament (see Fig. 9-3). The ovary and tube are removed and the ovarian vessels ligated with a free tie if desired, and then a second suture ligature is placed inside the free tie. Stapling devices or bipolar vessel sealing

Figure 9-3 With the uterus removed, the ovary, tube, and infundibulopelvic ligament are gently pulled downward with aid of a Babcock clamp for clamping and ligation.

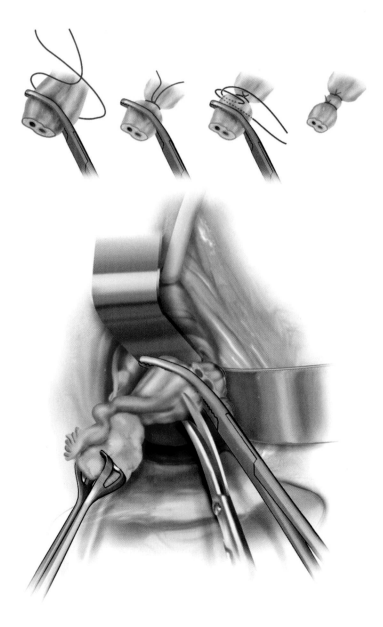

technologies such as Ligasure (Valleylab, Boulder, CO) can also accomplish the above tasks. In those cases in which the infundibulopelvic ligament is not easily accessible from the vagina an Endoloop (Ethicon, Somerville, NJ) ligature can facilitate isolation and ligation of the infundibulopelvic ligament (see Video 9-1). The Endoloop is passed through an ovary-suspending clamp onto the isolated infundibulopelvic ligament allowing ligation and ultimately division and removal of the ovary.

In the second technique for vaginal oophorectomy described by Ballard and Walters (1996) and Sheth (1991; 2005) and featured in Video 9-2, stepwise dissection between the round ligament and the infundibulopelvic ligament isolates the ovarian vessels for ligation and division (Fig. 9-4A to C; see Video 9-2). In this technique the uterus need not be completely severed prior to the oophorectomy on one side. On the other side, however, the uterus is divided from the adnexa. The round ligament is clamped separately, cut, and ligated and the suture is held long and retracted laterally for better visualization (see Fig. 9-4A, B). An alternative technique featured in Video 9-1 is to use electrocautery to cut away the round ligament from the infundibulopelvic ligament. Care must be taken in using electrocautery to keep the plane of dissection in the broad ligament between the round ligament and the ovarian vessels and to avoid large veins. Following these steps the infundibulopelvic ligament on one side tethers the uterus with the tube, ovary, and mesovarium. An angled Sheth adnexal clamp (Fig. 9-5), or a Heaney or long Kelly clamp, is applied to include only the infundibulopelvic ligament. Gentle handling of tissue is essential at this time to prevent tearing and bleeding in the broad ligament or ovarian vessels. The operative field is carefully inspected (to assure that bowel or the gauze pack is not in the clamp), the tube and ovary are removed, and sutures are placed (see Fig. 9-4C). The infundibulopelvic ligament is singly or doubly ligated with No. 0 absorbable suture. With exposure and isolation of the contralateral round ligament, the contralateral ovary is removed in the same manner, without the uterus present. Retraction of the bladder and vaginal walls during the oophorectomy can be accomplished with Heaney, Deaver, Breisky-Navratil, or other similar retractors. Trendelenburg patient positioning is recommended at the start, both to improve exposure and to limit bowel injury.

Outcomes and Complications

Surgical outcomes for prophylactic oophorectomy largely fall into predictable categories. The clinical significance of potentially more blood loss and longer operative times with oophorectomy may be insignificant but it does pose the usual risk dichotomy—immediate operative risk versus long-term outcomes. The long-term outcomes include the matters of cancer prevention and menopause and will be considered later in this chapter. In Table 9-2 from Sheth (1991) the complications listed between vaginal hysterectomy with and without vaginal oophorectomy are similar, but tubal tear and fallopian tube prolapse can occur only with and without oophorectomy, respectively. Surgical time was longer among women undergoing a vaginal oophorectomy by about 45 minutes and no differences were noted in length of hospitalization or rate of blood transfusion. Inability to remove the ovaries vaginally was associated with obesity, nulliparity, reduced pelvic space, and absent uterine descent, but not uterine size.

With regard to abdominal and laparoscopic hysterectomy with and without oophorectomy the complication rates are probably similar, although reliable

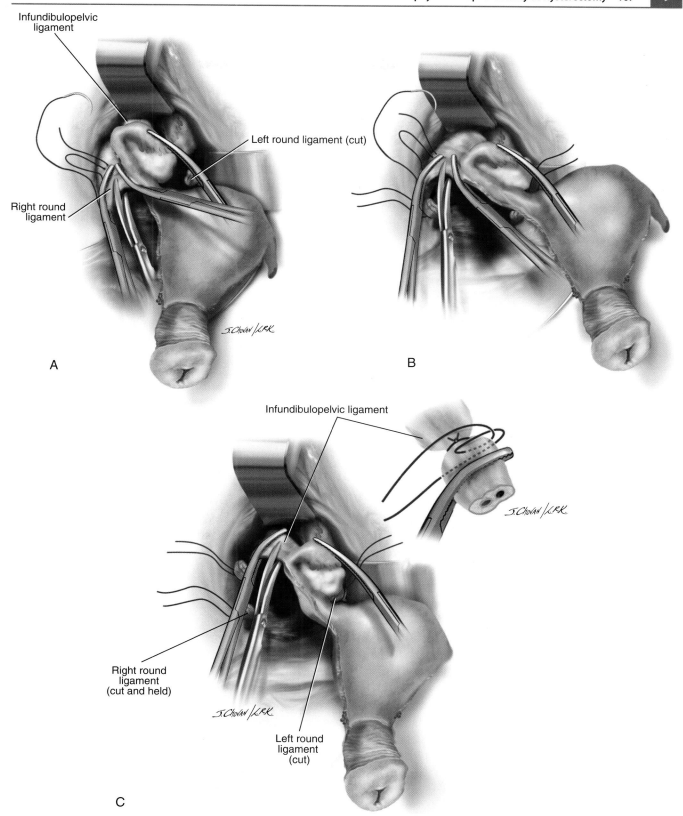

Infundibulopelvic ligament

Left round ligament (cut)

Right round ligament

A

B

Infundibulopelvic ligament

Right round ligament (cut and held)

Left round ligament (cut)

C

Figure 9-4 A, With the adnexal pedicle pulled downward, the round ligament is clamped, cut, and ligated. **B,** With the round ligament pulled laterally, subsequent bites continue along the broad ligament and mesosalpinx laterally and cephalad toward the infundibulopelvic ligament. **C,** The ovarian vessels are isolated and then clamped close to the ovary. The vessels are cut, removing the ovary and tube, and the pedicle singly or doubly ligated.

Figure 9-5 Heaney clamp and Sheth's adnexal clamp.

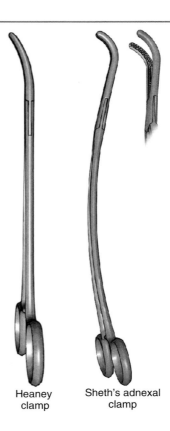

Heaney
clamp

Sheth's adnexal
clamp

Table 9-2 Complications of Surgery in Patients Undergoing Vaginal Hysterectomy with or without Oophorectomy

Complication	Number of Affected Patients (%)	
	With Oophorectomy (*n* = 740)	**Without Oophorectomy** (*n* = 700)
Pyrexia	32 (4)	34 (5)
Urinary tract infection	224 (30)	214 (31)
Wound sepsis	9 (1)	7 (1)
Primary hemorrhage	7 (1)	8 (1)
Paralytic ileus	1 (<1)	1 (<1)
Secondary hemorrhage	0 (0)	1 (<1)
Granulation tissue	40 (5)	86 (12)
Fallopian tube prolapse	24 (3)	92 (13)
Peritonitis	1 (<1)	1 (<1)
Resuturing of wound	0 (0)	1 (<1)
Shock	10 (1)	8 (1)
Tubal tear	226 (31)	—
Blood transfusion	30 (4)	26 (4)

From Sheth SS: The place of oophorectomy at vaginal hysterectomy. Br J Obstet Gynaecol 1991;98:662–666.

data demonstrating this are scarce. Ureter injury could be expected to be higher for oophorectomy at either abdominal or laparoscopic hysterectomy particularly if a cautery technique is used to ligate the ovarian blood supply. Indeed several studies have documented higher rates of lower urinary tract injury among laparoscopic-assisted hysterectomy, some of which undoubtedly reflect injury at the ovarian blood supply. The infundibulopelvic ligament is a common site of ureteral injury.

Regarding the long-term outcomes of oophorectomy, the data supporting the decision to remove or keep the ovaries during hysterectomy can largely be grouped into oncologic and nononcologic categories with cardiovascular, sexual, musculoskeletal, and cognitive factors prominent among the nononcologic category. We will consider each of these factors separately; however, these factors do not exist in isolation. Further, how each patient weighs these outcomes will differ and largely determine how any individual will regard the question of prophylactic oophorectomy. The importance a patient applies to a category of oophorectomy outcomes might balance quantity of life (cancer, future surgeries) versus quality of life (menopause, heart disease, sexual function, cognition). On oophorectomy, the American College of Obstetricians and Gynecologists (ACOG Practice Bulletin No. 89, 2008) cites other short-term factors that may sway the decision to keep or remove the ovaries at the time of hysterectomy. For example, pain, severe endometriosis, and pelvic inflammatory disease are cited as reasons to favor oophorectomy. The rationale for this recommendation is obvious but the evidence is thin and the physician must individualize each clinical situation.

Oncologic Outcomes Related to Oophorectomy

Ovarian Cancer

The American Cancer Society estimated that 21,650 new cases of ovarian cancer would be diagnosed in the United States in 2008, with an estimated 15,520 deaths (Jemal et al, 2008). Ovarian cancer is the seventh leading cancer in the United States, accounting for 3% of all female cancers. The lifetime risk of ovarian cancer in the general female population is 1.8%. This risk, however, is increased to 6.5% with any first-degree relative with ovarian cancer and to 7.5% with an affected mother (Sightler et al, 1991). Mortality rate from ovarian cancer is estimated to be 67% (Parker et al, 2005).

It is estimated that approximately 1000 cases of ovarian cancer could be prevented each year in the United States if all women undergoing hysterectomy at 40 years or older had elective salpingo-oophorectomy performed (Sightler et al, 1991). The most significant health benefit of prophylactic oophorectomy is reduced ovarian cancer risk. *Prophylactic* oophorectomy should be distinguished from *risk-reducing* oophorectomy. In both cases the ovaries are normal at the time of surgery; however, in the latter case some increased cancer risk (i.e., background ovarian cancer risk is > 1.8%) is being ameliorated, and in the former no background risk is implied (i.e., background ovarian cancer risk is 1.8%) and the ovaries are being removed at the time of another indicated procedure (usually hysterectomy).

Beyond familial-imparted risk, acquired risks for ovarian cancer include nulligravidity, decreased fertility, and increasing age. Concerning family history, cancer at young age, in a first-degree relative, in multiple generations, bilateral metachronous or synchronous cancer in one individual, and clustering of cancer on one side of the family all confer higher risk. Postmenopausal hormone replacement therapy appears to be a newly recognized though controversial risk for both acquiring and dying from ovarian cancer. According to the Women's Health Initiative (WHI) study (Anderson et al, 2003), women taking estrogen plus progestin were diagnosed as having invasive ovarian cancer at a rate of 42 per 100,000 person-years, 15 per 100,000 person-years more than the placebo group rate. An increase in ovarian cancer mortality rate was also noted.

Approximately 5% to 12% of invasive ovarian carcinomas stem from an inherited predisposition. *BRCA1/2* has the greatest influence on the risks of acquiring ovarian cancer followed by women with hereditary nonpolyposis colorectal cancer (HNPCC). Women with HNPCC have an 8% to 10% lifetime risk of ovarian cancer (Aarnio et al, 1999). Women with deleterious mutations in the *BRCA1* or *BRCA2* genes have a 9- to 36-fold increased risk of breast cancer and a 6- to 61-fold increased risk of ovarian cancer compared with the general population (Antoniou et al, 2003). At age 70 the estimated lifetime risk for ovarian cancer in a *BRCA1* carrier is 63% (Sightler et al, 1991). Given the limitations of ovarian cancer screening on reducing morbidity or mortality rate in the general population and in particular among women with *BRCA1/2* mutations, a risk-reducing oophorectomy is recommended once childbearing is complete.

Factors that reduce the risk of ovarian cancer include bilateral tubal ligation, hysterectomy with and without ovarian preservation, pregnancy, later onset of menarche, breastfeeding, and the use of oral contraceptives. Ovulation suppression with decreased mitotic stimuli and decreased exposure of the ovary to persistently high circulating levels of pituitary gonadotropins are two traditional hypotheses of why pregnancy and oral contraceptive use reduce the risk of epithelial ovarian cancer. However, in a case-control study to evaluate the impact of contraceptive methods on ovarian cancer development, 727 virgin women recently diagnosed with ovarian cancer were compared with 1300 control women (Ness et al, 2001). All methods of birth control, including oral contraceptives, intrauterine devices (IUDs), barrier methods, tubal ligation, and vasectomy, were found to reduce the risk of ovarian cancer. This finding implies that other mechanisms beyond hormonal or ovulatory factors impart protection from ovarian cancer. It was noted that term pregnancies were more protective than failed pregnancies and each additional pregnancy after the first confers the same percent reduction in risk of invasive cancer, estimated to be about 14% (Whittemore et al, 1992). The impact of tubal sterilization on reducing ovarian cancer risk was demonstrated in a 1993 prospective study wherein a strong inverse association was seen between tubal ligation and epithelial ovarian cancer with a risk ratio of 0.33 (Hankinson et al, 1993). This effect persisted after adjusting for age, oral contraceptive use, parity, and other ovarian cancer risk factors. The risk-reducing effect of tubal sterilization has been proposed to work by blocking potential carcinogens to ovarian epithelium, altering ovarian blood flow and changing ovulation, or by the "healthy screen effect" (Irwin et al, 1991).

The level of cancer risk reduction associated with prophylactic oophorectomy has been estimated from historical or cross-sectional population data to be as high as 95%. However, Finch and associates (2006) reported only an 80% reduction in ovarian cancer risk following prophylactic oophorectomy based on a multicenter cohort trial. Meijer and van Lindert (1992) attempted to quantify ovarian cancer risk reduction with prophylactic oophorectomy using data from the literature and a mathematical model. They calculated the lifetime risk of ovarian cancer at age 40, with no imparted familial risk, was 1.6%. Following a hysterectomy *with ovarian preservation*, this risk decreased to 0.62%. It was proposed that this effect stemmed from the opportunity to screen for visible premalignant ovarian disease at the time of hysterectomy (Meijer and van Lindert, 1992). However, it is unknown if this "protection" persists beyond 20 years. Further clouding the matter, Piver and Wong (1997) reported that 5% to 10% of women with ovarian cancer had had a previous hysterectomy at age 40 or older.

Other Gynecologic Cancers

Hereditary nonpolyposis colorectal cancer (HNPCC) or Lynch syndrome was mentioned as a hereditary risk factor for development of ovarian cancer; these women also have a 40% to 60% lifetime risk of endometrial cancer. Mutations in *BRCA1* and *BRCA2* also increase the risk for fallopian tube and peritoneal cancer. The rate of fallopian tube and peritoneal cancers among women without a hereditary risk has been considered very low. Recently, however, at the 2008 Annual Meeting of the American Association for Cancer Research, Keren Levanon, working out of the Dana-Farber Cancer Institute in Boston, reported that the fallopian tube fimbria, rather than ovarian surface epithelium, may be the origin for greater than 50% of sporadic and hereditary serous "ovarian" carcinomas (Levanon K, et al, 2008). The distinction between ovarian, fallopian tube, and peritoneal cancers can be difficult both clinically and pathologically and in light of this new research the distinction may be getting less clear. Hence, even though oophorectomy reduces the risk for nonovarian serous carcinomas, the risk is not eliminated, particularly if the fallopian tubes are not removed with the ovaries. Underlying the persistent (albeit low) risk for peritoneal cancer following prophylactic oophorectomy is either (1) clinically undetectable ovarian cancer cells remain in the peritoneum following removal of the ovaries, and (2) a "field defect" is present in the peritoneum as the epithelial covering of the ovary. The woman considering prophylactic oophorectomy should know that her risk for "ovarian" cancer is reduced but not eliminated. For the surgeon there may be growing impetus to remove the fallopian tubes at the time of oophorectomy to maximize the cancer risk reduction.

Breast Cancer

Bilateral oophorectomy has a role in breast cancer prevention, at least among women with a hereditary influence such as *BRCA1/2*. There is a 50% to 70% risk reduction in breast cancer among women with *BRCA1/2* who undergo bilateral oophorectomy (Rebbeck, 2002). The reverse association is also true: among *BRCA1/2*-positive women with breast cancer, the risk of developing ovarian cancer is higher. In one study the ovarian cancer risk at 10 years in women with breast cancer was 13% for the *BRCA1* mutation carrier and 7% for *BRCA2* carrier (Finch et al, 2006). This sort of evidence is unknown to exist outside the hereditary influence, although it is recognized that breast cancer can metastasize to the ovary.

Nononcologic Outcomes Related to Oophorectomy

Although the postmenopausal woman is not menstruating and believing her ovary is nonfunctional, the postmenopausal ovary does continue to have endocrine function. A longitudinal Australian study demonstrated that from 5 years before to 7 years after menopause, the circulating levels of testosterone did not change (Burger et al, 2000). In premenopausal women, testosterone is produced at about 300 μg/day with equal amounts derived from the ovaries and adrenal glands. Following natural menopause, serum testosterone and estradiol concentrations ultimately decline by 25% and 75%, respectively. In contrast, among women who undergo bilateral oophorectomy before menopause, serum testosterone and estradiol concentrations immediately decrease by approximately 50% and 80%, respectively (Guzick and Hoeger, 2000). Unlike the gradual decline in hormonal function seen with natural menopause that occurs over years, surgical menopause results in an abrupt cessation of all ovarian hormone production. The significance of this persistent ovarian hormone production after natural menopause is a matter of debate. Ultimately this debate has relevance only in how a woman's quality and quantity of life are affected. Indeed epidemiologic studies suggest that premature menopause, by any means, *without estrogen therapy,* is associated with an increased risk of cognitive impairment, heart disease, bone fractures, and shorter long-term non–cancer-related survival.

Cardiovascular Risk

Heart disease is the leading cause of death among U.S. women, accounting for over 50% of overall mortality. Heart disease in women is underdiagnosed and undertreated, and public awareness of this fact is under-recognized. Following menopause the risk of cardiovascular disease dramatically increases. *Indeed a women undergoing hysterectomy for benign disease is approximately 50 times more likely to die of heart disease than ovarian cancer.* This rise in cardiac disease has been attributed to the change in estrogen status that occurs naturally and surgically; yet, a distinction is made in the cardiovascular risk associated with surgical and natural menopause. This connection between estrogen and cardiovascular disease is based on large population studies such as the Nurses' Health Study. Colditz and associates (1987) conducted a 6-year cohort trial of 121,700 U.S. female nurses, 30 to 55 years old, beginning in 1976. After controlling for age and cigarette smoking, naturally menopausal women with or without hormone replacement therapy (HRT) had no appreciable increased risk of cardiovascular disease. In contrast, women having undergone bilateral oophorectomy and no HRT had increased risk for cardiovascular disease (relative risk [RR] 2.2, 95% confidence interval [CI], 1.2–4.2). Use of HRT in the oophorectomized woman appeared to eliminate this increased risk (RR, 0.9; 95% CI, 0.6–1.6). The conclusion of this study was that bilateral oophorectomy increased the risk of coronary heart disease; use of HRT appeared to ameliorate this risk.

Recently, Parker and associates (2009) published a 24-year follow-up analysis of the Nurses' Health Study. Compared with ovarian conservation, bilateral oophorectomy at the time of hysterectomy for benign disease is associated with a decreased risk of breast and ovarian cancer but an increased risk of all-cause death, fatal and nonfatal coronary heart disease, and lung cancer. In no analysis or age group was oophorectomy associated with increased survival.

Parker and colleagues (2005) also used a Markov decision-analysis model to estimate if the ovaries of women at least 40 years of age should be removed during a hysterectomy for benign disease. Using this model, ovarian conservation demonstrated a net benefit in overall survival probability at age 80, in terms of reduced heart disease and hip fracture, offsetting any adverse effects of new cases of ovarian and breast cancer. The conclusions drawn from this model are not surprising given a high base rate of cardiovascular disease. The model accounted for the age-varying mortality estimates with the two notable age-associated mortality rates of cardiovascular disease and ovarian cancer. When examining the survival curves between women with and without ovaries there was a convergence at age 65 leading the authors to recommend ovarian conservation up to this age.

Since the cardiovascular disease estimates draw from the Nurses' Health Study there is trouble with leaning too heavily on the conclusions of this model. The Nurses' Health Study was not a randomized trial and bias could have influenced the results. Further, a recent systematic review failed to find conclusive evidence of a link between coronary heart disease and bilateral oophorectomy (Jacoby et al, 2009a). Despite these inconsistencies, these and future studies are valuable tools to engage women in a serious discussion about the benefits and risks of oophorectomy, as it draws sharp attention to the real matter of cardiovascular disease among women.

Musculoskeletal Outcomes

Fifty percent of all white women will experience an osteoporotic fracture at some point in their lifetime. Osteoporosis is characterized as low bone mass and microarchitectural bone tissue deterioration. Androgen and estrogen receptors are found in bone cells and have positive roles in bone mass. Both estrogens and androgens inhibit bone resorption and androgens increase bone formation. In a cohort study of over 9000 women 65 years or older, baseline serum hormone concentrations were compared between 271 women who subsequently had hip and vertebral fractures and matched control subjects (Cummings et al, 1998). Those women with undetectable serum estradiol concentrations (<5 pg/mL) were 2.5 times more likely to have hip and vertebral fractures. In a 16-year longitudinal study of women, those who had undergone an oophorectomy *during their postmenopausal years* had 54% more osteoporotic fractures than women with intact ovaries (Melton et al, 2003). This study raises the issue of worsening osteoporosis in the discussion of whether to remove the ovaries in a postmenopausal woman who is not taking estrogen replacement.

Sexuality/Neurologic Outcomes

Between the ages of 45 and 55, at the peak rate for hysterectomy and vis-à-vis oophorectomy, major life events are occurring in women. Aziz and colleagues (2005a, 2005b) found that, among women in this age group who are adequately estrogenized with HRT, prophylactic bilateral oophorectomy did not negatively affect psychological well-being at 1 year. Indeed in this study, both hysterectomy-only and hysterectomy-oophorectomy had a positive effect on psychological well-being. Given that most aspects of sexuality are correlated to psychological well-being, this also improved. Likewise, a recent analysis of the Maryland Women's Health Study by Rohl and associates (2008) showed that bilateral oophorectomy was not associated with adverse effects on mood after hysterectomy, compared with unilateral or no oophorectomy.

Sex steroids are assumed to play a central role female sexual function. Estrogen insufficiency contributes to vaginal dryness and thinning of the vaginal epithelium with resulting decreased sensation. Although estrogen insufficiency can be amended, there is no standard replacement therapy for androgen deficiency that is also affected by oophorectomy. In a survey aimed at determining the prevalence of female hypoactive sexual desire disorder, Western European women having undergone surgical menopause were compared with premenopausal and naturally menopausal women (Dennerstein et al, 2006). Surgically menopausal women were more likely to meet the diagnostic criteria for hypoactive sexual desire disorder relative to the premenopausal or naturally menopausal women (OR 2.1, P = .001). This finding suggests that other endocrine functions, not replaced by standard HRT, could affect female sexual function. The possibility of sexual dysfunction should be discussed when considering prophylactic oophorectomy.

Rocca in three studies (Rocca et al, 2007; 2008a; 2008b) of the same cohort of Minnesota women documented an increased risk for cognitive impairment and parkinsonism among women who underwent oophorectomy before menopause. The younger the women who underwent oophorectomy, the greater the risk for these adverse cognitive outcomes. Based on laboratory evidence for a neuroprotective effect of estrogen, as well as this clinical research documenting worse neurologic outcomes among women undergoing oophorectomy before menopause, cognitive effects should be considered in the discussion of oophorectomy at the time of hysterectomy in a premenopausal woman. It is worth noting that among woman 65 to 79 years of age, use of conjugated equine estrogen for HRT was associated with a slightly higher risk of cognitive impairment and dementia compared to women who did not use this HRT (Shumaker et al, 2004).

Discussion

At this point we have attempted to cull the data relevant to the question of whether our 47-year-old woman facing an indicated hysterectomy should remove her ovaries. When balancing all the factors for a normal-risk woman, the ACOG (ACOG Practice Bulletin No. 89, 2008) recommendation to use menopausal status as the chief indicator for who should and should not consider prophylactic oophorectomy is sound (Fig. 9-6). In our 47-year-old woman, she has no personal family history that would sway the various adverse heart, bone, sexual, and cognitive impacts of premenopausal oophorectomy. Based on the relevant evidence, our 47-year-old woman *should favor keeping* her ovaries. However, the woman may weigh the evidence differently and, bowing to patient autonomy, the physician may be compelled to perform an oophorectomy if she desires this. Indeed, it appears that many women weigh the evidence differently given that bilateral oophorectomy is performed in 80% of women 45 to 54 years of age and in about 50% of hysterectomies in women 40 to 44 years of age (Lepine et al, 1997). Further, there is significant nationwide variation in the practice of bilateral oophorectomy, and nonclinical factors such as race, insurance status, and geographic location significantly influence this practice. These findings could suggest that women are swayed into a decision by incomplete or biased information and overstated risks.

Possibly the issues discussed so far complicate the bottom-line considerations that women most want to consider. These questions may be: (1) Which option renders the longest life? (2) Which option renders the best quality of life? (3) Are these two options mutually exclusive? Later menopause, natural or surgical, is associated with decreased cardiovascular risk but increased breast and endometrial cancer risk. On a population level, several investigators have studied this balance of acquired and cancer mortality rates. Ossewaarde and associates (2005) concluded that an older age of menopause was associated with a lower age-adjusted mortality rate, tipping the balance away from the cancer risks. This statistic is contrasted against a population-based study that found that overall mortality was not increased in surgically menopausal women

Figure 9-6 The decision-making process in considering oophorectomy at the time of hysterectomy in a woman without remarkable hereditary or acquired risks. Asterisks (*) indicate points of potential conflict. The accessibility of the ovaries and the feasibility of vaginal or laparoscopic surgery is dependent on surgeon skill. LAVH, Laparoscopic-assisted vaginal hysterectomy.

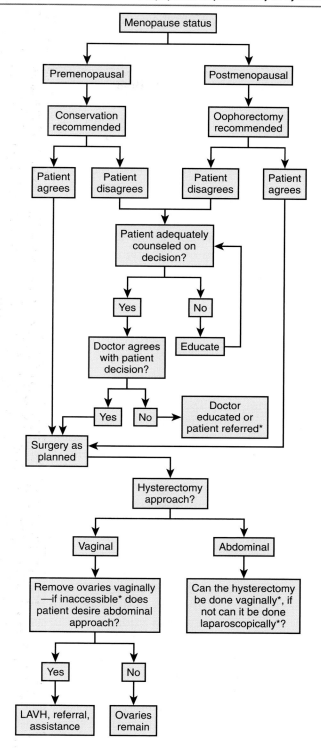

(Rocca et al, 2006). However, mortality rate was higher among women who had had their ovaries removed before the age of 45, with the increase mainly in women who had not received estrogen up to the age of 45 (Rocca et al, 2006). These findings echo those described earlier by Parker and colleagues (2005), wherein surgically menopausal women had an estimated mortality rate of 8.6% *more* than those who had ovarian conservation when the surgery was done before age 55 years, and 3.9% *more* for patients who had oophorectomy done before age 59 years. In fact, based on the most recent analysis by Parker and associates (2009), with an approximate 35-year lifespan after hysterectomy, one additional death would be expected for every nine oophorectomies performed.

Hereditary cancer risks will influence the balance of acquired and cancer mortality rates but a woman's awareness of her family cancer risks may not be so easy to appreciate for either the patient or physician. Difficulty in assessing the risk in women with a family history of ovarian cancer includes small family size, families with predominately male offspring, unknown paternity, difficulties in obtaining medical records, death of a relative at an early age before genetic expression of ovarian cancer, patient refusal to give information, physician noncooperation, misclassification of ovarian cancer as not ovarian, and patient ignorance of family members' causes of death. It would appear that in reference to the bottom-line questions, notwithstanding hereditary cancer risks, life expectancy would be optimized with ovarian conservation at least up to the age of menopause.

Quality of life is a difficult topic; one woman's quality of life may be better if she feels her risk of dying from cancer is reduced following oophorectomy irrespective of her potential risks of dying from heart disease. Nevertheless, Teplin and associates (2007) found scores using the Medical Outcomes Study Short Form 36 Quality-of-Life Survey did favor ovarian conservation at the time of hysterectomy. The difference was evident at 6 months following surgery but by 2 years this difference evaporated. It is reassuring that there do not appear to be any remarkable long-term differences between women who do and do not keep their ovaries with hysterectomy in regard to overall quality of life.

A consideration in managing the acquired risks of oophorectomy is HRT. Speroff and associates (1991) described a risk-benefit analysis of elective oophorectomy. A feature not appreciated in other such analyses was the matter of patient compliance with use of the HRT. Taking into account the risks of coronary heart disease, breast cancer, and osteoporotic fracture, and the influence of estrogen on these processes, the Speroff study illustrated that when compliance with estrogen therapy is *perfect*, oophorectomy yields longer life expectancy than retaining ovaries (Speroff et al, 1991). However the Women's Health Initiative (WHI) studies place this conclusion in doubt. On the matter of coronary heart disease in the WHI, among women aged 50 to 79 conjugated equine estrogen offered no overall protection against myocardial infarction or coronary death (Hsia et al, 2006). Given the tenuous and diminishing support for using HRT in the midst of the prevailing evidence, HRT should not be seen as a means to ameliorate the acquired risks of oophorectomy.

Returning to our 47-year-old woman, examining the individual health considerations, overall life span, and quality of life we still arrive at the conclusion she should keep her ovaries. Should this patient still like to remove her ovaries, citing she can use HRT to offset her risk, this too appears to rest on shaky evidence. If this patient remains undecided, are there unaccounted for differences between women who do and do not wish to have their ovaries removed with hysterectomy? In regard to this question, Aziz and coworkers (2005a) found that personality, sexuality, and the nature and severity of preoperative symptoms differed markedly among women who pursued prophylactic oophorectomy at elective hysterectomy. Such women appeared to be more anxious, less sexual and less emotionally attached to their partners. This group was also characterized by more episodes of irregular bleeding, a greater prevalence of climacteric symptoms, and more extensive use of hormonal replacement therapy (Aziz et al, 2005a). Thus, among women who pursue oophorectomy, values and personality issues also appear to influence the decision process.

In conclusion, in normal-risk women having hysterectomy, menopause status is a reasonable reference to make recommendations about oophorectomy; conserving ovaries before menopause and possibly removing them afterward. There is a growing body of literature suggesting that ovaries should be conserved even after menopause, but this remains controversial. Hereditary and acquired risk factors exist for cancer and benign ovarian disease, and it is imperative that physicians be aware of these factors and be able to apply them to their patients such that the patient can make an informed decision. Once the decision to perform bilateral oophorectomy at hysterectomy has been made, the gynecologist should remove the ovaries by the same route as the hysterectomy if possible, taking special care to avoid damage to the ureter. In counseling patients, physicians should be aware of their own biases and how these beliefs might influence both the decision to do oophorectomy and its surgical approach.

Selected Readings

ACOG Committee Opinion No. 385. The limits of conscientious refusal in reproductive medicine. Obstet Gynecol 2007;110:1203–1208.

ACOG Practice Bulletin No. 89. Elective and risk-reducing salpingo-oophorectomy. Obstet Gynecol 2008;111:231–241.

Aarnio M, Sankila R, Pukkala E, et al: Cancer risk in mutation carriers of DNA-mismatch-repair genes. Int J Cancer 1999;81:214–218.

Agostini A, Vejux N, Bretelle F, et al: Value of laparoscopic assistance for vaginal hysterectomy with prophylactic bilateral oophorectomy. Am J Obstet Gynecol 2006;194:351–354.

Anderson GL, Judd HL, Kaunitz AM, et al: Effects of estrogen plus progestin on gynecologic cancers and associated diagnostic procedures: The Women's Health Initiative randomized trial. JAMA 2003;290:1739–1748.

Antoniou A, Pharoah PD, Narod S, et al: Average risks of breast and ovarian cancer associated with BRCA1 or BRCA2 mutations detected in case series unselected for family history: A combined analysis of 22 studies. Am J Hum Genet 2003;72:1117–1130.

Aziz A, Bergquist C, Brännström M, et al: Differences in aspects of personality and sexuality between perimenopausal women making different choices regarding prophylactic oophorectomy at elective hysterectomy. Acta Obstet Gynecol Scand 2005a;84:854–859.

Aziz A, Bergquist C, Norolholm L, et al: Prophylactic oophorectomy at elective hysterectomy. Effects on psychological well-being at 1-year follow-up and its correlations to sexuality. Maturitas 2005b;51:349–357.

Ballard LA, Walters MD: Transvaginal mobilization and removal of ovaries and fallopian tubes after vaginal hysterectomy. Obstet Gynecol 1996;87:35–39.

Bhavnani V, Clarke A: Women awaiting hysterectomy: A qualitative study of issues involved in decisions about oophorectomy. Br J Obstet Gynaecol 2003;110:168–174.

Bhavnani V, Clarke A, Dowie J, et al: Women's views of two interventions designed to assist in the prophylactic oophorectomy decision: A qualitative pilot evaluation. Health Expect 2002;5:156–171.

Burger HG, Dudley EC, Cui J, et al: A prospective longitudinal study of serum testosterone, dehydroepiandrosterone sulfate, and sex hormone–binding globulin levels through the menopause transition. J Clin Endocrinol Metab 2000;85:2832–2838.

Colditz GA, Willett WC, Stampfer MJ, et al: Menopause and the risk of coronary heart disease in women. N Engl J Med 1987;316:1105–1110.

Cummings SR, Browner WS, Baver D, et al: Endogenous hormones and the risk of hip and vertebral fractures among older women. Study of Osteoporotic Fractures Research Group. N Engl J Med 1998;339:733–738.

Davies A, Vizza E, Bournas N, et al: How to increase the proportion of hysterectomies performed vaginally. Am J Obstet Gynecol 1998;179:1008–1012.

Dennerstein L, Koochaki P, Barton I, et al: Hypoactive sexual desire disorder in menopausal women: A survey of Western European women. J Sex Med 2006;3:212–222.

Finch A, Beiner M, Lubinski J, et al: Salpingo-oophorectomy and the risk of ovarian, fallopian tube, and peritoneal cancers in women with a BRCA1 or BRCA2 mutation. JAMA 2006;296:185–192.

Guzick DS, Hoeger K: Sex, hormones, and hysterectomies. N Engl J Med 2000;343:730–731.

Hankinson SE, Hunter DJ, Colditz GA, et al: Tubal ligation, hysterectomy, and risk of ovarian cancer. A prospective study. JAMA 1993;270:2813–2818.

Hoffman MS: Transvaginal removal of ovaries with endoloop sutures at the time of transvaginal hysterectomy. Am J Obstet Gynecol 1991;165:407–408.

Hsia J, Langer RD, Manson JE, et al: Conjugated equine estrogens and coronary heart disease: The Women's Health Initiative. Arch Intern Med 2006;166:357–365.

Irwin KL, Weiss NS, Lee NC, et al: Tubal sterilization, hysterectomy, and the subsequent occurrence of epithelial ovarian cancer. Am J Epidemiol 1991;134:362–369.

Jacoby VL, Grady D, Sawaya GF, et al: Oophorectomy as a risk factor for coronary heart disease. Am J Obstet Gynecol 2009a;200:140.

Jacoby VL, Vittinghoff E, Nakagawa S, et al: Factors associated with undergoing bilateral salpingo-oophorectomy at the time of hysterectomy for benign conditions. Obstet Gynecol 2009b;113:1259–1267.

Jemal A, Siegel R, Ward E, et al: Cancer statistics, 2008. CA Cancer J Clin 2008;58:71–96.

Kovac SR, Cruikshank SH: Guidelines to determine the route of oophorectomy with hysterectomy. Am J Obstet Gynecol 1996;175:1483–1488.

Lepine LA, Hillis SD, Marchbanks PA, et al: Hysterectomy surveillance—United States, 1980–1993. MMWR CDC Surveill Summ 1997;46:1–15.

Levamon K, Crum C, Drapkin R: New insights into the pathogenesis of serous ovarian cancer and its clinical impact. J Clin Oncol 2008;26:5284–5293.

Lewis CE, Groff JY, Herman CJ, et al: Overview of women's decision making regarding elective hysterectomy, oophorectomy, and hormone replacement therapy. J Women's Health Gend Based Med 2000;9(Suppl 2):S5–S14.

Meijer WJ, van Lindert AC: Prophylactic oophorectomy. Eur J Obstet Gynecol Reprod Biol 1992;47:59–65.

Melton LJ III, Khosla S, Malkasian GD, et al: Fracture risk after bilateral oophorectomy in elderly women. J Bone Miner Res 2003;18:900–905.

Nelson HD, Huffman LH, Fu R, et al: Genetic risk assessment and BRCA mutation testing for breast and ovarian cancer susceptibility: Systematic evidence review for the U.S. Preventive Services Task Force. Ann Intern Med 2005;143:362–379.

Ness RB, Grisso JA, Vergona R, et al: Oral contraceptives, other methods of contraception, and risk reduction for ovarian cancer. Epidemiology 2001;12:307–312.

Ossewaarde ME, Bots ML, Verbeek AL, et al: Age at menopause, cause-specific mortality and total life expectancy. Epidemiology 2005;16:556–562.

Parker WH, Broder MS, Liu Z, et al: Ovarian conservation at the time of hysterectomy for benign disease. Obstet Gynecol 2005;106:219–226.

Parker WH, Broder MS, Chang E, et al: Ovarian conservation at the time of hysterectomy and long-term health outcomes in the Nurses' Health Study. Obstet Gynecol 2009;113:1027–1037.

Piver MS, Wong C: Prophylactic oophorectomy: A century-long dilemma. Hum Reprod 1997;12:205–206.

Rebbeck TR: Prophylactic oophorectomy in BRCA1 and BRCA2 mutation carriers. Eur J Cancer 2002;38(Suppl 6):S15–S17.

Rocca WA, Bower JH, Maraganore DM, et al: Increased risk of cognitive impairment or dementia in women who underwent oophorectomy before menopause. Neurology 2007;69:1074–1083.

Rocca WA, Bower JH, Maraganore DM, et al: Increased risk of parkinsonism in women who underwent oophorectomy before menopause. Neurology 2008a;70:200–209.

Rocca WA, Grossardt BR, de Andrade M, et al: Survival patterns after oophorectomy in premenopausal women: A population-based cohort study. Lancet Oncol 2006;7:821–828.

Rocca WA, Grossardt BR, Maraganore DM, et al: The long-term effects of oophorectomy on cognitive and motor aging are age dependent. Neurodegener Dis 2008b;5:257–260.

Rohl J, Kjerulff K, Langenberg P, et al: Bilateral oophorectomy and depressive symptoms 12 months after hysterectomy. Am J Obstet Gynecol 2008;199:22.

Sheth SS: The place of oophorectomy at vaginal hysterectomy. Br J Obstet Gynaecol 1991;98:662–666.

Sheth SS: Vaginal hysterectomy. Best Pract Res Clin Obstet Gynaecol 2005;19:307–332.

Shumaker SA, Legault C, Kuller L, et al: Conjugated equine estrogens and incidence of probable dementia and mild cognitive impairment in postmenopausal women: Women's Health Initiative Memory Study. JAMA 2004;291:2947–2958.

Sightler SE, Boike GM, Estape RE, et al: Ovarian cancer in women with prior hysterectomy: A 14-year experience at the University of Miami. Obstet Gynecol 1991;78:681–684.

Speroff T, Dawson NV, Speroff L, et al: A risk-benefit analysis of elective bilateral oophorectomy: Effect of changes in compliance with estrogen therapy on outcome. Am J Obstet Gynecol 1991;164(1 Pt 1):165–174.

Teplin V, Vittinghoff E, Lin F, et al: Oophorectomy in premenopausal women: Health-related quality of life and sexual functioning. Obstet Gynecol 2007;109(2 Pt 1):347–354.

Whittemore AS, Harris R, Itnyre J, et al: Characteristics relating to ovarian cancer risk: Collaborative analysis of 12 U.S. case-control studies. II. Invasive epithelial ovarian cancers in white women. Collaborative Ovarian Cancer Group. Am J Epidemiol 1992;136:1184–1203.

Laparoscopic and Robotic-Assisted Total and Supracervical Hysterectomy

10

Marie Fidela R. Paraiso M.D.
Pedro F. Escobar M.D.

 Video Clips on DVD

10-1 Conventional Total Laparoscopic Hysterectomy
A: Sealing and Transection of Left Infundibulopelvic Ligament
B: Development of Bladder Flap
C: Uterine Vessel Ligation
D: Colpotomy

10-2 Robotic-Assisted Laparoscopic Supracervical Hysterectomy

A: Development of Bladder Flap and Sealing of Right Uterine Vessels
B: Transection of the Upper Pedicles on the Left Uterine Corpus
C: Transection of the Uterine Corpus from the Cervix
D: Closure of the Cervical Os

Approximately 40% of hysterectomies in the United States are performed by minimally invasive routes, including laparoscopic hysterectomy with or without vaginal or robotic assistance and vaginal hysterectomy (see Chapter 7). Since laparoscopic-assisted vaginal hysterectomy was introduced by Reich in 1989, laparoscopic surgery for hysterectomy has gained popularity but has not resulted in widespread conversion of abdominal hysterectomies to minimally invasive procedures as initially predicted. Reasons for this include the steep learning curves associated with advanced laparoscopic techniques (laparoscopic suturing and knot-tying, difficult bladder dissection, ureterolysis, and difficult retroperitoneal dissection) and insufficient advanced laparoscopic training and experience in many residency programs. After Food and Drug Administration (FDA) approval of robotic-assisted laparoscopy for gynecologic surgery in 2005, increased adoption of minimally invasive surgery has ensued, especially in gynecologic oncology. Laparoscopic suturing and precise dissection for pelvic and para-aortic lymph node excision and radical hysterectomy have been revolutionized with robotic assistance, partly because of three-dimensional magnified views and endowrist instrumentation with seven degrees of freedom.

Types of laparoscopic hysterectomy include total laparoscopic hysterectomy (TLH; extirpation of the uterus and cervix) and laparoscopic supracervical or

Table 10-1 Staging of Laparoscopic Hysterectomy

Stage 0	Laparoscopy performed without additional laparoscopic procedures prior to vaginal hysterectomy
Stage 1	Laparoscopy including both laparoscopic adhesiolysis and/or excision of endometriosis prior to vaginal hysterectomy
Stage 2	Laparoscopic mobilization of either or both adnexa prior to vaginal hysterectomy
Stage 3	Laparoscopic dissection of bladder from uterus in addition to transection of all upper pedicles prior to vaginal hysterectomy
Stage 4	Uterine artery and all upper pedicles transected and bladder flap dissected laparoscopically
Stage 5	Anterior and/or posterior colpotomy or entire uterus freed laparoscopically
Subscript 1	One ovary excised laparoscopically
Subscript 2	Both ovaries excised laparoscopically

subtotal hysterectomy (LSH; removal of the uterine corpus with preservation of the cervix). All steps of TLH are performed by the laparoscopic route whereas laparoscopic-assisted vaginal hysterectomy (LAVH) encompasses the laparoscopic portions of the procedure (ligation and transection of the utero-ovarian or infundibulopelvic ligaments, broad ligament, and possibly the uterine vessels) with the remaining steps completed by vaginal route (colpotomy, bladder dissection, ligation and transection of the uterosacral and cardinal ligaments). Staging of the various types of laparoscopic hysterectomy is shown in Table 10-1. According to the Cochrane review, the term "laparoscopic hysterectomy" should be applied to any hysterectomy in which all vessels are occluded laparoscopically. When no portion of the procedure is performed vaginally, the term "total laparoscopic hysterectomy" should be employed. This chapter will discuss total and supracervical laparoscopic hysterectomies, LAVH, and robotic-assisted laparoscopic hysterectomy, and will briefly summarize single-port laparoscopic hysterectomy.

Case 1: Abnormal Uterine Bleeding and Endometrial Hyperplasia

A 48-year-old gravida 3, para 3 woman presents with complaints of heavy, prolonged, frequent uterine bleeding for the last 9 months. Her menses are not associated with cramping or pelvic pain. Gynecologic history includes regular Papanicolaou (Pap) smears, which are all normal, and no history of sexually transmitted diseases. Past medical history is significant only for hypertension. She is taking a beta-blocker, multivitamin, and calcium; does not exercise regularly; and has no other medical problems. Family history is significant only for a maternal grandmother with history of breast cancer. She does not smoke, drink, or take drugs. On examination her vital signs are within normal limits, and her body mass index is 25 kg/m². On speculum examination there is some blood at the vaginal vault, no lesions on the bladder base or vaginal walls, and cervix is appears normal. Her uterus is 6 to 8 weeks in size and nontender; rectovaginal examination reveals no parametrial thickening or cul-de-sac nodularity. Ultrasound evaluation revealed a thickened endometrial lining and normal uterus and ovaries. An endometrial biopsy and endocervical sampling demonstrated endometrial glands (back-to-back architecture) with luminal outpouching, and minimal intervening stroma lined by atypical cells. A diagnosis of complex hyperplasia with atypia was made.

Discussion of Case: Total Laparoscopic Hysterectomy
Abnormal uterine bleeding (AUB) can be caused by many different conditions. The specific diagnostic approach will depend on whether the patient is premenopausal, perimenopausal, or postmenopausal. In the perimenopausal female normal hormonal cycling begins to change, a decrease in progesterone secretion coupled with continued estrogen secretion can cause the endometrium to grow and produce excess tissue. This histologic change in the endometrium (endometrial hyperplasia) can potentially cause abnormal

Figure 10-1 A, Egg crate mattress and positioning for laparoscopic hysterectomy cases. **B,** Chest taping for steep Trendelenburg position.

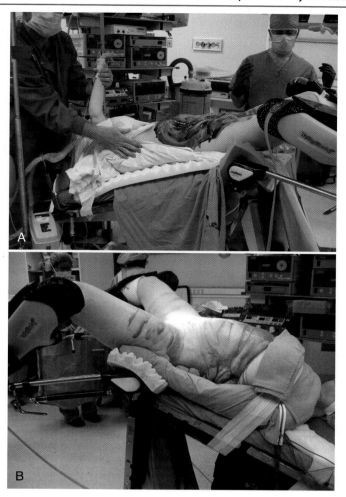

Case 1: Abnormal Uterine Bleeding and Endometrial Hyperplasia—cont'd

bleeding. Also, the obese woman has high levels of endogenous estrogen due to the conversion of androstenedione to estrone and the aromatization of androgens to estradiol, both of which occur in peripheral adipose tissue (Potischman et al, 1996). The presence of nuclear atypia is a worrisome finding in this case and puts the patient at risk to develop carcinoma. More important, the rate of endometrial carcinoma found at hysterectomy in women with a biopsy diagnosis of atypical endometrial hyperplasia is 42.6% according to a study by The Gynecologic Oncology Group (Trimble et al, 2006) . A similar rate, 45.6%, was reported at

John Radcliffe Hospital, Oxford, UK, by Pennant and associates (Pennant et al, 2008). When considering management strategies for women who have a biopsy diagnosis of atypical endometrial hyperplasia, clinicians and patients should take into account the considerable rate of concurrent carcinoma. This patient was amenable to minimally invasive surgery, had a normal-sized uterus and thus required no morcellation of the uterus. Cancer staging with prehysterectomy, pelvic washings, and para-aortic and pelvic lymph node dissection can be performed by conventional or robotic-assisted laparoscopy.

Surgical Technique: Total Laparoscopic Hysterectomy
(See Video 10-1 📹)

1. The patient is positioned directly on an egg crate mattress or beanbag cushion, which has been taped to the surgical bed (Fig. 10-1A). In cases in which a steep angle of Trendelenburg positioning is required, we work with our anesthesia colleagues to tape the patient's chest to the bed without

restricting ventilation (see Fig. 10-1B). These maneuvers prevent slippage of the patient toward the head of the bed while in steep Trendelenburg position. The legs are placed into Allen or Yellofin stirrups (Allen Medical Systems, Acton, MA) with the heel resting easily into the back of the boot, ascertaining that no lateral pressure on the calves, internal rotation of the knees, nor hyperflexion of the hips is present. Arms are tucked bilaterally with hands protected by pieces of egg crate or similar material. The hands must be checked intermittently to make sure that changing positions of the stirrups or foot of the bed do not result in inadvertent injury to the tucked hand. If the patient with tucked arms is wider than the bed, padded sleds are used to keep the arms in place. A three-way catheter facilitates retrograde filling of the bladder during difficult bladder dissection.

2. Uterine manipulators include the RUMI or ZUMI with Koh colpotomizer and balloon occluder (CooperSurgical Inc., Trumbull, CT), VCare (Conmed Corporation, Utica NY), the reusable Valtchev uterine manipulator (Conkin Surgical Intruments, Toronto, Canada), and the Pelosi uterine manipulator (Apple Medical, Bolton, MA). Placement of the uterine manipulator is performed concomitant with setup of laparoscopic equipment. More recently, the Koh uterine manipulator has been adapted with an independently standing bedside attachment, specifically for, but not limited to, robotic-assisted surgery (Fig. 10-2A and B). This minimizes the need for a vaginal assistant. One or two held stitches placed in the cervical parenchyma at 3 and 9 o'clock via vaginal route are threaded through the grooves of the snugly fitting Koh colpotomizer cup, easing placement of the RUMI manipulator. The VCare (Fig. 10-3) and Valchev manipulators do not require stay sutures. Choice of uterine manipulator is a matter of surgeon preference. The RUMI arm and associated colpotomizer cups and Valtchev and Pelosi uterine manipulators are reusable alternatives.

3. Our technique employs a 5-mm laparoscope inserted into a 5-mm optical trocar introduced through an intraumbilical incision for most laparoscopic hysterectomies whether conventional or robotic-assisted. Alternatively, a left upper quadrant port placement (two fingerbreadths below the subcostal margin in the midclavicular line) is performed to gain peritoneal access if infraumbilical adhesions are anticipated. For enlarged uteri, the laparoscope port is placed cephalad of the umbilicus. Distance away from the umbilicus depends on uterine size and whether concomitant para-aortic lymph node dissection is performed. Accessory ports are placed in the bilateral lower quadrants and lateral of the umbilicus as desired (Fig. 10-4). Size of the accessory ports depends on instrumentation. One or two 5 to 12 mm trocars with conical valves are used for introduction of CT-1 or CT-2 needles. The conical valve minimizes escape of pneumoperitoneum during extracorporeal knot tying. The 5 to 12 mm port is easily enlarged to 15 mm for introduction of a uterine morcellator. Insufflation of CO_2 through an upper-quadrant port and plume evacuation through one of the lower quadrant ports optimizes visual clarity and allows movement of gas upward when the patient is in steep Trendelenburg position.

4. Once all ports are placed, the entire perintoneal cavity is inspected. The same principles of countertraction and exposure in open and vaginal surgery apply to laparoscopy except when utilizing electrosurgical instruments. The instrumentation is longer; the incisions are smaller; and the field is magnified in two dimensions on the screen for conventional laparoscopy. We apply the same surgical techniques for laparoscopic hysterectomy as for

Figure 10-2 Uterine manipulators. Koh colpotomizer system: **A,** The Koh cup attached to the RUMI uterine manipulator causing acute anteversion of the uterus. **B,** Close-up of the Koh uterine manipulator.

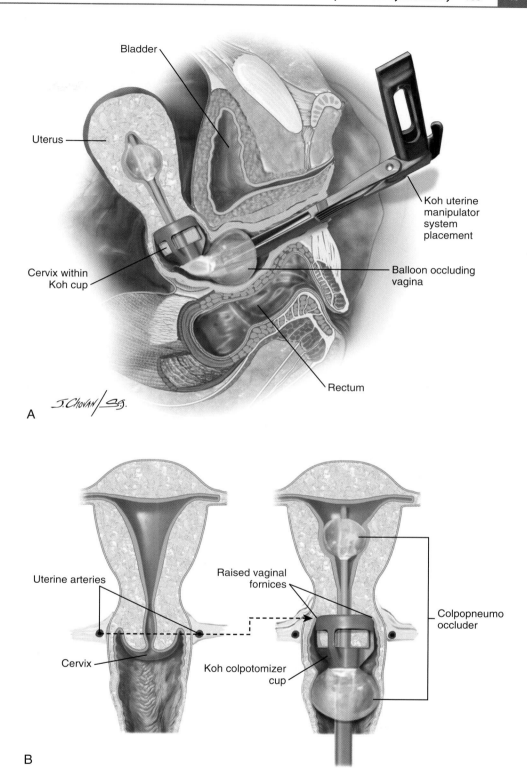

Bladder

Uterus

Cervix within Koh cup

A

Koh uterine manipulator system placement

Balloon occluding vagina

Rectum

J. Chovan

Uterine arteries

Cervix

Raised vaginal fornices

Koh colpotomizer cup

Colpopneumo occluder

B

abdominal hysterectomy with the exception of suture ligation of pedicles (vessel-sealing devices instead of suture ligation, although many surgeons use vessel-sealing devices via laparotomy). Adhesions, which obscure the operative field or port-site areas, are lysed. Excision of superficial cul-de-sac or pelvic sidewall endometriosis is easiest when all organs and sidewall

Figure 10-3 VCare uterine manipulator.

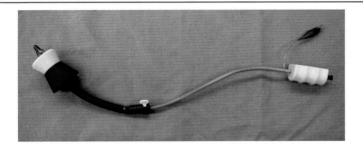

Figure 10-4 Port placement for conventional operative laparoscopy.

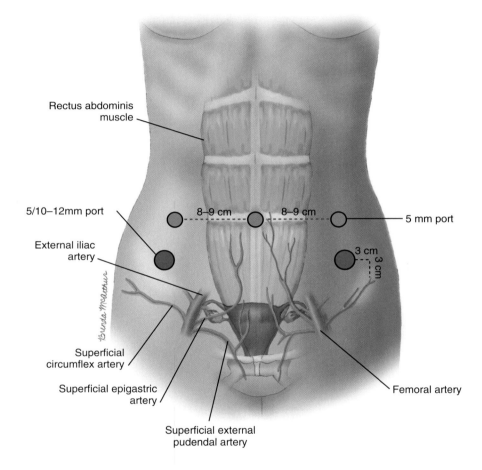

attachments are intact. We emphasize that most "smart" bipolar and ultrasonic devices must be utilized with little or no tension on the tissues to ensure vessel sealing (see the discussion of electrosurgical intruments later in the chapter). This "no-tension" principle is counterintuitive to maximizing countertraction to gain exposure but results in less blood loss.

5. We commence the hysterectomy by manipulating the uterine fundus away from the operative site to enhance exposure. The ipsilateral round ligament is electrosurgically or ultrasonically ligated and cut. This allows easy access for dissection of the retroperitoneal space and exposure of the ureter. The anterior broad ligament peritoneum is incised inferiorly to the bladder flap and superiorly toward the infundibulopelvic ligaments (see Video 10-1B ▶). The bladder flap is dissected with simultaneous upward traction of the cervix and retroflexion or midplane uterine placement. The

areolar tissue is incised to a level 1 cm below the colpotomizer cup. The ureter is visualized transperitoneally or through retroperitoneal dissection, where it courses in the medial leaf of the broad ligament toward its path beneath the uterine vessels.

6. When we perform concomitant salpingo-oophorectomy, we dissect a window in the medial leaf of the broad ligament above the ureters and ligate and cut the ovarian vessels (see Video 10-1A 🎥). Alternatively, the utero-ovarian ligament is sealed and cut prior to dissecting and incising the broad ligament and skeletonizing the ipsilateral uterine vessel (see Video 10-1C 🎥). Once the uterine vessel is sealed, the same pedicles are ligated on the contralateral side. Division of the uterine vessels after they are sealed bilaterally minimizes uterine back-bleeding. The cardinal ligaments are sealed and incised bilaterally prior to or after colpotomy depending on surgeon preference (see Video 10-1D 🎥). The uterosacral ligaments are incised as part of the colpotomy incision but can be tagged with suture for concomitant uterosacral ligament vaginal vault suspension or culdoplasty.

7. Colpotomy is performed with either a monopolar, bipolar, or ultrasonic hook. Another option is the monopolar tip of a recently introduced dual purpose instrument (Ligasure Advance, Covidien Inc., Boulder, CO). Alternatively, the ultrasonic energy scissors (Harmonic Ace, Ethicon Inc., Cincinnati, OH) or monopolar scissors may be utilized. The superior border of the colpotomizer or cervical rim of the VCare manipulator cup delineates the incision line for the colpotomy. A tight-fitting colpotomizer or cup around the cervix provides the greatest amount of upward countertraction to ensure that the bladder is thoroughly dissected away for safe colpotomy and results in optimal vaginal length. Once the cervix is incised from the vagina, the uterus is pulled through the vagina and sent for pathologic examination. A balloon occluder or tied-off glove is introduced into the vagina to maintain pneumoperitoneum. Alternatively, the uterus may be placed into the vagina to maintain pneumoperintoneum. Large myomatous uteri are morcellated in total or to a size suitable for delivery through the vagina.

8. Closure of the vaginal cuff can be done with simple or figure-of-eight interrupted No. 0 delayed absorbable sutures or a running suture using a Lapra-Ty (Ethicon, Inc., Cincinnati, OH) at each end. When closing the vaginal cuff we utilize laparoscopic needle holders and tie our knots with a open- or closed-ended knot pusher. A cautionary note is that increasing rates of dehiscence of the vaginal apex have been reported (Kho et al, 2009) and that interrupted delayed absorbable sutures for closure and use of ultrasonic or bipolar energy cutting devices, which minimize lateral thermal damage of tissue (as opposed to monopolar energy cutting devices) for colpotomy may help to circumvent vaginal cuff dehiscence.

9. We recommend reattachment of the uterosacral ligaments to the vaginal cuff in all cases to decrease risk of postoperative vaginal apex prolapse. In cases of mild uterine prolapse, the uterosacral ligaments are attached to the vaginal cuff with No. 0 absorbable or delayed absorbable sutures with or without reefing the cul-de-sac peritoneum. For greater amounts of uterine prolapse, multiple stitches are placed, bilaterally suspending the vagina high on the uterosacral ligaments. We recommend a peritoneal incision to release the ureters lateral of the uterosacral ligaments if necessary (Fig. 10-5). We also recommend routine use of cystoscopy to evaluate upper and lower urinary tract injury.

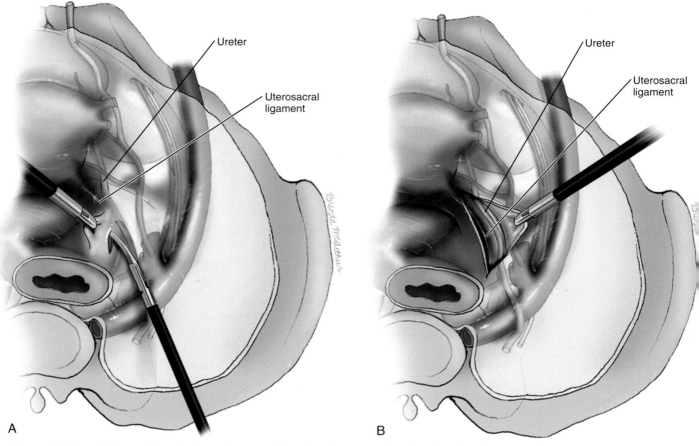

Figure 10-5 A and **B,** Ureterolysis with relaxing incision medial to the right ureter on the right pelvic sidewall.

10. When concluding a laparoscopic case, we routinely inspect all pedicles with decreased insufflation. All port incisions that are greater than 8 mm in diameter are closed en bloc with a fascial closure device, such as the Carter-Thomason CloseSure System (Inlet Medical, Inc., Eden Prairie, MN).

Case 2: Symptomatic Uterine Fibroids Refractory to Medical Therapy and Desires Preservation of the Cervix

The patient is a 42-year-old gravida 1, para 0 female who presents for consultation regarding hysterectomy for menometrorrhagia and dysmenorrhea for the past 2 years and known uterine fibroids. She reports daily bleeding for the last 2 months. She had an intrauterine device (IUD) in the past that was removed 6 months ago. She failed medical management with oral contraceptives and nonsteroidal anti-inflammatory drugs (NSAIDs). Past medical and surgical histories are unremarkable. Physical examination shows an anteverted globular uterus which is 10 weeks in size. Her laboratory studies are unremarkable except a borderline low hematocrit of 32.4%. A Pap smear showed no malignant cells. Saline infusion sonogram was benign-appearing without polyps but confirming two transmural uterine fibroids (largest 2.5 cm in

diameter), and an office endometrial biopsy was benign. She is not interested in future fertility or conception. She is an equestrian and manages a horse farm. She desires definitive management with hysterectomy and would like to discuss robotic-assisted laparoscopic hysterectomy with preservation of her cervix.

She was counseled regarding all options, including conventional LSH versus robotic-assisted LSH and chooses to proceed with robotic-assisted LSH. See Rationale for Supracervical Hysterectomy section later in this chapter.

Discussion of Case: Supracervical Hysterectomy

Abnormal uterine bleeding, specifically heavy menses and intermenstrual bleeding, can occur within a histologically

Case 2: Symptomatic Uterine Fibroids Refractory to Medical Therapy and Desires Preservation of the Cervix—cont'd

normal uterus or can be associated with uterine fibroids, adenomyosis, or neoplasia. Menometrorrhagia can present with mild anemia, as in this case, or be so severe that some women even require iron supplements or transfusions. This patient continued to have symptoms despite medical management, and experienced a lower health-related quality of life; thus, it is reasonable to consider hysterectomy as part of her treatment plan. Although treatments such as endometrial ablation or levonorgestrel intrauterine devices are effective in many women, hysterectomy has been shown to have a very high satisfaction rate in women with menometrorrhagia and an excellent cure rate for abnormal uterine bleeding,

dysmenorrhea, and cramping. This patient desires preservation of her cervix and was informed that she may continue to have cyclic vaginal bleeding and will require routine Pap smears. After a careful informed consent with review of the alternatives, risks, benefits, and outcomes, and documentation that no further childbearing is desired, a supracervical hysterectomy was chosen. In general, unless she has a strong desire for ovarian removal or is at high risk for ovarian cancer, we do not favor prophylactic removal of ovaries in a premenopausal woman having a hysterectomy by any route. Review Chapter 9 for an in-depth discussion of prophylactic oophorectomy.

Surgical Technique: Laparoscopic Supracervical Hysterectomy
(See Video 10-2)

Steps 1 to 6 described for total laparoscopic hysterectomy are the same for supracervical hysterectomy. See Videos 10-2B and 10-2D for transection of upper uterine pedicles .

Dissection of the bladder flap for LSH is not as extensive as that for TLH unless the patient is undergoing concomitant laparoscopic sacral cervicopexy (see Video 10-2A). Transection of the cervix at or below the level of the internal os is performed after both uterine vessels are sealed (see Video 10-2C). We recommend either a monopolar, bipolar, or ultrasonic hook for transection of the uterine corpus from the cervix. Another option is the monopolar tip of a recently introduced dual purpose instrument (Ligasure Advance, Covidien Inc., Boulder, CO). Alternatively, the ultrasonic energy scissors (Harmonic Ace, Ethicon Inc., Cincinnati, OH) or monopolar scissors may be utilized. A monopolar lasso-like instrument is also available but has not been widely adopted. When transecting the cervix, we recommend excising the upper portion of the endocervical canal in the shape of a cone and cauterizing the remainder of the endocervical canal to minimize the risk of postoperative cyclic bleeding in the premenopausal patient.

The top of the cervix is either closed with 1 to 2 figure-of-eight or simple stitches of No. 0 absorbable suture to reapproximate cervical parenchyma or the cervical stump is reperitonized with the bladder flap (see Video 10-2D). Our preference is to suture the cervical stump closed because we usually reattach the uterosacral ligaments to the cervix.

We recommend reattachment of the uterosacral ligaments to the posterior cervix in most cases to decrease risk of postoperative vaginal apex prolapse. In cases of mild uterine prolapse, the uterosacral ligaments are attached to the posterior cervix with No. 0 absorbable or delayed absorbable sutures with or without reefing the cul-de-sac peritoneum. For greater amounts of uterine prolapse, multiple stitches are placed bilaterally suspending the cervix high on the uterosacral ligaments. As noted earlier, we recommend a peritoneal incision to release the ureters lateral to the uterosacral ligaments in order to prevent kinking the ureters.

Surgical Technique: Robotic-Assisted Total Laparoscopic Hysterectomy and Supracervical Hysterectomy (see Video 10-2A to D 🎬)

Port placement for robotic-assisted TLH and LSH is shown in Figure 10-6. Three to four robotic ports are placed in addition to an assistant port for introduction of sutures and needles. Once the robot is docked, a 10-mm port is used for introduction of the robotic arm housing the three-dimensional camera.

Depending on surgeon preference (dominant hand), the monopolar scissors or harmonic scalpel is placed in the right 8-mm robotic port. The bipolar or PK vessel-sealing forceps are placed in the left side 8-mm robotic port. A third robot port may be used for retracting instruments (bowel graspers and forceps or uterine tenaculum) and can be placed on either the right or left side. All robotic instruments, except the harmonic scalpel, have seven degrees of freedom with the ability to rotate and articulate. Because of the nature of ultrasonic energy, the instrument cannot bend at the wrist of the instrument.

The TLH and LSH steps are identical to those of conventional laparoscopy. However, exchange of instrumentation is minimized. We recommend using one source of energy (either bipolar or monopolar) on a vascular pedicle unless there is loss of control of bleeding. For example, the utero-ovarian vessels should be sealed with bipolar forceps and then cut with scissors without the application of monopolar energy.

The colpotomy for a TLH and cervical transection at the level of the internal os for LSH can be performed with either a monopolar hook or a monopolar scissor. A smoke evacuator or suction with the suction-irrigator device by the surgical assistant clears the visual field. The smoke evacuator should be placed on a port upstream from the insufflation port.

Figure 10-6 Port placement for robotic-assisted laparoscopy.

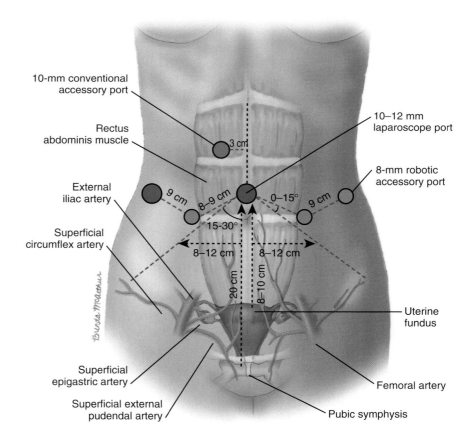

We close the vaginal cuff and cervical stump with figure-of-eight No. 0 polyglycolic acid suture on a CT-1 needle. At least one robotic needle holder should be used in the surgeon's dominant hand. Our preferred instrument is a suture-cut needle holder. Intracorporeal knots are thrown with either a smaller needle holder in the assisting hand or the larger needle holder in the dominant hand.

It is much easier to morcellate the uterine corpus or bulky uterus after undocking the robot; therefore, this is the final step prior to port closure.

Surgical Technique: Laparoscopic-Assisted Vaginal Hysterectomy

The surgical technique for LAVH is identical to TLH except that colpotomy, ligation of the lower uterine pedicles, and possibly bladder dissection are achieved by the vaginal route. Many surgeons seal and cut the round ligaments and utero-ovarian or infundibulopelvic ligaments, dissect the broad ligaments, and dissect the bladder flap by laparoscopic route and complete the additional steps by vaginal route.

The uterine vessels may be sealed and cut by laparoscopic route or cut or sealed and ligated via vaginal route.

See Chapter 7 for surgical technique of vaginal hysterectomy and Table 10-1 for staging of laparoscopic hysterectomy.

Surgical Rationale

Laparoscopic Supracervical Hysterectomy

Laparoscopic supracervical hysterectomy (LSH) has gained popularity over the last decade because of technical ease and purported benefits, including decreased complications, preserved pelvic organ support, and improved urinary and sexual function compared to hysterectomy involving removal of the cervix. This surgical procedure encompasses the extirpation of the uterine corpus at or below the internal cervical os and ablation of the endocervical canal after removal of the corpus. LSH is indicated in patients who are candidates for laparoscopic hysterectomy and have no history of cervical dysplasia, uterine hyperplasia, known or suspected malignancy, or cervical fibroids. Patients interested in supracervical hysterectomy must have normal and up-to-date screening for cervical cancer and a normal gross appearance of the cervix documented prior to surgery. Owing to the probable benefit of mesh erosion prevention at the vaginal apex, LSH is a favorable alternative in patients with uterovaginal prolapse, who desire or require hysterectomy and are undergoing concomitant laparoscopic sacral colpopexy (Griffis and Hale, 2005). In LSH, morcellation of the uterine corpus is required to facilitate its removal through the port site incisions; therefore, adequate preoperative evaluation of the uterine lining to exclude premalignant changes or malignancy is necessary. Finally, if the patient has a history suspicious for leiomyosarcoma (rapidly enlarging uterine fibroid associated with menometrorrhagia), laparotomy and possible staging should be recommended in lieu of laparoscopy.

The possible benefits of supracervical hysterectomy with regard to perioperative morbidity and postoperative sexual and urinary function are not substantiated by medical evidence. In three randomized controlled trials comparing open total and subtotal hysterectomies, there were no differences in complications including visceral or vascular injury, blood loss requiring transfusion, or postoperative infection. The incidence of postoperative cyclical vaginal bleeding ranged from 5% to 20% in women randomized to supracervical hysterectomy. Approximately 1.5% of participants required trachelectomy within 3 months. There were no differences in postoperative stress or urge urinary incontinence, urinary frequency, or incomplete bladder emptying in most studies. However, one European study did find a higher incidence of urinary incontinence after subtotal hysterectomy (see Lethaby et al, 2006). In regard to sexual function, there was no difference in any outcome in any of the prospective studies. Retrospective studies comparing outcomes between TLH and LSH demonstrate conflicting results. One large managed care organization study demonstrated longer operative time, but less blood loss, shorter hospital stay, and fewer major complications in LSH compared to total laparoscopic hysterectomy (ACOG Committee Opinion No. 388, 2007). Despite the lack of data supporting superior outcomes for supracervical hysterectomy, choosing between total and subtotal hysterectomy is a personal decision and some women may in fact have some alterations in sexual response if their cervix is removed. Detailed preoperative discussions are important because many patients have strong preexisting ideas about preserving (or removing) the cervix.

Robotic-Assisted Laparoscopic Hysterectomy

Trends in laparoscopic and robotic surgery among gynecologic surgeons, especially gynecologic oncologists, are evolving toward minimally invasive surgery (MIS), especially robotic-assisted laparoscopy. Minimally invasive surgical techniques have been utilized with increasing frequency in the management of endometrial cancer, the most common gynecologic malignancy in the United States. Numerous academic centers and practitioners have published their experience with this new technology. The use of MIS techniques does not appear to adversely affect survival for gynecologic malignancy, and quality of life is improved in the postoperative period. Robotic-assisted laparoscopy improves surgical precision in lymph node dissections compared to conventional laparoscopy and increases node counts. It also results in less blood loss and faster recovery. Nevertheless, the use of MIS is still limited owing to a prolonged learning curve, availability, and associated costs of robotic technology, with studies demonstrating a need of between 20 and 100 cases for optimal nodal counts and operating times (Abu-Rustum et al, 2003; Altgassen et al, 2000). Robotic-assisted TLH with the da Vinci Surgical System (Intuitive Surgical, Inc, Sunnyvale, CA) offers advantages over conventional TLH because of three-dimensional vision, wrist-like range of motion of instrumentation, and most likely, a shorter learning curve for suturing and intracorporeal knot-tying in comparison to conventional laparoscopy. A recent comparative study of three surgical methods for hysterectomy with staging for endometrial cancer (robotic assistance, laparoscopy, laparotomy) by Boggess and associates (2008) demonstrated that robotic assist with staging is feasible and preferable over laparotomy and perhaps may be preferable over traditional laparoscopy in women with endometrial cancer.

Single-Port Laparoscopic Hysterectomy

There has been recent interest in single-port laparoscopic hysterectomy with touted benefits of shorter hospitalization, decreased postoperative pain, and improved aesthetics. There are a variety of flexible single ports with multiple holes for insertion of various trocars or gelports, which allow placement of multiple trocars. The instrumentation ideal for single-incision surgery includes flexible scopes with operative flexible arms and flexible instruments with the ability to reticulate and articulate allowing triangulation of instruments. These emerging techniques for minimally invasive hysterectomy are evolving and will be greatly improved with new innovations and flexible robotics. Additionally, magnetically secured and controlled instruments are currently in development. This technique has not yet been widely adopted and results are preliminary. Most pioneers of single-port laparoscopy stress the advantages of improved cosmetic appearance of a single-umbilical incision and less postoperative pain in spite of longer operative times (early experience) and more expensive instrumentation compared to conventional laparoscopy.

Laparoscopic-Assisted Vaginal Hysterectomy

Laparoscopic-assisted vaginal hysterectomy (LAVH) was first introduced as an alternative to total abdominal hysterectomy in cases difficult to manage solely by vaginal route or when vaginal approach is contraindicated. Most of the indications for LAVH are the same as for TLH: endometriosis, significant pelvic adhesions, pelvic inflammatory disease, multiple cesarean sections, previous procedures involving the uterus (e.g., myomectomy), adnexal disease when hysterectomy is indicated, enlarged uterus, uterine hypomobility, and reduced vaginal access. Indications for LAVH over TLH include lack of proficiency with suturing skills for colpotomy closure by laparoscopic route, lack of technical feasibility of TLH due to instrumentation requirements, presence of significant bladder adhesions, medical indications, need to morcellate a bulky uterus by vaginal route, and surgeon preference (ACOG Committee Opinion No. 311, 2005). Many surgeons proficient in both TLH and vaginal hysterectomy see no indication for LAVH. Contraindications to LAVH include carcinoma or suspected carcinoma with need for morcellation of the uterus, large or suspicious adnexal masses, inability to use general anesthesia, inability to access the peritoneal cavity with ports, and lack of hip joint mobility for placement in lithotomy position.

Vessel-Sealing Technology

Choice of pedicle- and vessel-sealing instrumentation is based on surgeon preference. No tension should be used with application of vessel-sealing technology, which coagulates and divides pedicles.

The Harmonic Scalpel technology (Ethicon Endo-Surgery, Cincinnati, OH) uses ultrasonic energy for controlled coagulation and cutting. Coagulation occurs by means of protein denaturation when the vibrating blade couples with protein, denaturing it to form a coagulum that seals small vessels. When the effect is prolonged, secondary heat is produced that seals larger vessels. The active blade oscillates at approximately 55,000 cycles per second, which results in precise cutting without generating either smoke or char. The vibration of the ultrasonic scalpel is thought to generate low heat at the incision site with a reported 1 mm of thermal spread. The Enseal Device (Ethicon Endo-Surgery, Cincinnati, OH) combines mechanical pressure and energy to seal vessels and divide pedicles while closing the device. This high compression application uses low-energy voltage to control temperature and current flow, which results in 1 mm of thermal spread while minimizing char, stickiness, and smoke. Ligasure technology (Covidien, Boulder, CO) uses the combination of pressure and

Figure 10-7 Vessel-sealing devices **A,** Harmonic Ace. (Courtesy of Ethicon Endo-Surgery, Inc.) **B,** Enseal Device. (Courtesy of Ethicon Endo-Surgery, Inc.) **C,** Ligasure 5 mm Device. (Courtesy of Covidien, Inc.) **D,** Ligasure Advance with close-up of tip. (Courtesy of Covidien, Inc.) **E,** Gyrus cutting forceps (5 mm).

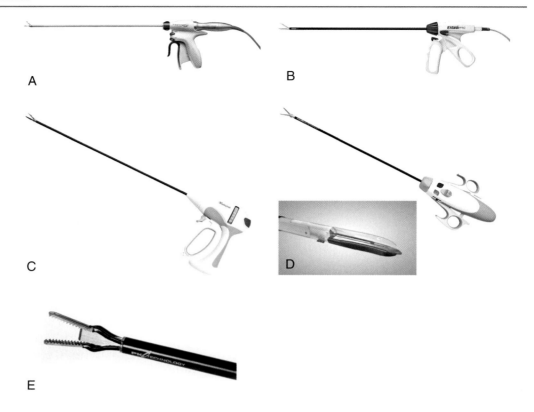

energy to create the vessel seal by melting the collagen and elastin in the vessel walls and re-forming it into a permanent, plastic-like seal. An internal blade subsequently divides the tissue. The instrument may also be used to mechanically divide tissue without the application of energy. The Ligasure instruments minimize thermal spread to approximately 2 mm and are available in 5-mm and 10-mm diameter sizes. The recently released Ligasure Advance combines 5-mm Ligasure vessel-sealing technology with a monopolar tip, touted to enhance laparoscopic surgery by decreasing instrument changes. Gyrus PK cutting forceps (Gyrus ACMI, Maple Grove, MN) use bipolar energy to coagulate pedicles and an internal blade to divide the pedicles. This internal blade can be used to cut tissue without applying energy. The Gyrus forceps allow intuitive blunt dissection of tissue, hence minimizing the need to exchange instruments. See Figure 10-7A through E to view a variety of vessel-sealing devices.

Staplers may also be used to achieve hemostasis and ligate tissue without cautery or suturing. The ENDO-GIA (Covidien Autosuture, Boulder, CO) is loaded with a cartridge that delivers rows of staples. The staples divide and an internal blade cuts the tissue in between the staples.

SUMMARY: Laparoscopic hysterectomy, including TLH and LSH, has become increasingly popular because of robotic technology and innovations in laparoscopic instrumentation. Single-port laparoscopic hysterectomy will also gain widespread adoption if surgical technique is feasible for the majority of surgeons and preliminary data show advantages over conventional laparoscopy. Generally, indications for laparoscopic hysterectomy are the same as for abdominal hysterectomy for benign disease, for endometrial cancers not requiring morcellation, and when vaginal hysterectomy is contraindicated or not feasible. The technique for hysterectomy depends on surgical indications, patient characteristics and preferences, and the surgeon's expertise.

Suggested Readings

ACOG Committee Opinion No. 311: Appropriate use of laparoscopically assisted vaginal hysterectomy. Obstet Gynecol 2005;105:929–930.

ACOG Committee Opinion No. 388: Supracervical hysterectomy. Obstet Gynecol 2007;110: 1215–1217.

Abu-Rustum NR, Gemignani ML, Moore K, et al: Total laparoscopic radical hysterectomy with pelvic lymphadenectomy using the argonbeam coagulator: Pilot data and comparison to laparotomy. Gynecol Oncol 2003;91:402–409.

Altgassen C, Possover M, Krause N, et al: Establishing a new technique of laparoscopic pelvic and para-aortic lymphadenectomy. Obstet Gynecol 2000;95:348–352.

Boggess JF, Gehrig PA, Cantrell L, et al: A comparative study of 3 surgical methods for hysterectomy with staging for endometrial cancer: Robotic assistance, laparoscopy, laparotomy. Am J Obstet Gynecol 2008;199:360.e1–9.

Falcone T, Walters MD: Hysterectomy for benign disease. Obstet Gynecol 2008;111:753–767.

Griffis K, Hale DS: Grafts in pelvic reconstructive surgery. Clin Obstet Gynecol 2005;48:713–723.

Jelovsek JE, Chen CCG, Roberts SL, et al: Incidence of lower urinary tract injury and the value of routine intraoperative cystoscopy at the time of total laparoscopic hysterectomy. J Soc Lap Surg 2007;11:422–427.

Johnson N, Barlow D, Lethaby A, et al: Methods of hysterectomy: Systematic review and meta-analysis of randomized controlled trials. BMJ 2005;330:1478.

Kho RM, Hilger WS, Hentz JG, et al: Robotic hysterectomy: Technique and initial outcomes. Am J Obstet Gynecol 2007;197:113.e1–4.

Kho RM, Akl MN, Cornella JL, et al: Incidence and characteristics of patients with vaginal cuff dehiscence after robotic procedures. Obstet Gynecal 2009;114(2 Pt 1):231–235.

Lethaby A, Ivanova V, Johnson NP: Total versus subtotal hysterectomy for benign gynaecological conditions. Cochrane Database Syst Rev 2006;(2):CD004993.

Nieboer TE, Johnson N, Lethaby, et al: Surgical approach to hysterectomy for benign gynaecological disease. Cochrane Database Syst Rev 2009;(3):CD003677.

Parker WH: Total laparoscopic hysterectomy and laparoscopic supracervical hysterectomy. Obstet Gynecol Clin North Am 2004;31:523–537.

Pennant S, Manek S, Kehoe S: Endometrial atypical hyperplasia and subsequent diagnosis of endometrial cancer: A retrospective audit and literature review. J Obstet Gynaecol 2008;28:632–633.

Potischman N, Swanson CA, Siiteri PK, Hoover RN: Reversal of relation between body mass and endogenous estrogen concentrations with menopausal status. J Natl Cancer Inst 1996;88: 756–758.

Ridgeway B, Falcone T: Indications and techniques for laparoscopic hysterectomy: Total and subtotal. In Falcone T, Goldberg JM (eds): Basic, Advanced, and Robotic Laparoscopic Surgery. Elsevier, Philadelphia, 2010.

Reich H: New techniques in advanced laparoscopic surgery. Baillieres Clin Obstet Gynaecol 1989;3:655–6581.

Trimble CL, Kauderer J, Zaino R, et al: Concurrent endometrial carcinoma in women with a biopsy diagnosis of atypical endometrial hyperplasia: A Gynecologic Oncology Group Study. Cancer 2006;106:812–819.

Complications of Hysterectomy

Mark D. Walters M.D.
Matthew D. Barber M.D., M.H.S.

 Video Clips on DVD

11-1 Transvaginal Cystotomy Repair
11-2 Intentional Cystotomy with Passage of Ureteral Catheters

As with all surgeries, complications related to hysterectomy should be carefully scrutinized to allow the surgeon and patient to better understand the risks (versus benefits) of this intervention for the patient's disease. Complications that occur can be directly related to the surgical technique, to the anesthesia, or to medical disorders in the perioperative period. The mortality rate from hysterectomy is estimated at 0.12 to 0.38 per 1000 surgeries, and is substantially higher when the hysterectomy is performed for an obstetric indication or for malignancy, or when significant co-morbidities exist.

The Maryland Women's Health Study, a prospective cohort study of 1299 women undergoing hysterectomy for benign disease, reported that 66.8% of patients had one or more mild complications, 11.1% had one or more moderate complications, and 0.7% had a serious complication (Kjerulff et al, 2000a). The hospital readmission rate for a reason related to the hysterectomy was 4% during the first year after surgery. The most common reasons for readmission were wound complications, surgery for adhesions, bowel obstruction, and urinary tract problems. McPherson and associates (2004) investigated the complication rate in 37,512 women undergoing hysterectomy for benign disease in the United Kingdom and found a 3% risk of severe complications including death, thromboembolic disease, myocardial infarction, stroke, hemorrhage, visceral injury, and end-organ failure. The risk of operative complications in this study increased in women undergoing hysterectomy for fibroids and decreased with increasing age. The highest risk groups were younger women who underwent laparoscopic hysterectomy for fibroids and those with a history of serious co-morbidities.

Race also may affect surgical morbidity; an analysis of 53,159 hysterectomies in Maryland from 1986 to 1991 found that, in comparison to white women, black women having hysterectomy had an increased risk of one or more complications of surgical or medical care (19.7% vs. 13%; odds ratio [OR] 1.4, 95% confidence interval [CI] 1.3–1.5) and higher in-hospital mortality rate (OR 3.1; 95% CI 2.0–4.8) (Kjerulff et al, 1993). Black women were more likely to have

Table 11-1 Major Complications of Hysterectomy in the eVALuate Trial

Complication	Abdominal Trial		Vaginal Trial	
	Abdominal Hysterectomy (%)	Laparoscopic Hysterectomy (%)	Vaginal Hysterectomy (%)	Laparoscopic Hysterectomy (%)
At least one major complication*	6.2	7.2	5.4	6.7
Intraoperative conversion to laparotomy		3.9	4.2	2.7
Major hemorrhage[†]	2.4	4.6	2.9	5.1
Bowel injury	1	0.2	0	0
Ureter injury	0	0.9	0	0.3
Bladder injury	1	2.1	1.2	0.9
Other[‡]	2.1	2.4	1.8	3.9

*Excluding intraoperative conversion to laparotomy.
[†]Major hemorrhage was defined as blood loss requiring a blood transfusion.
[‡]Includes pulmonary complications, anesthesia, return to the operating room, wound dehiscence, and hematoma.
Modified from Garry R, Fountain J, Mason S, et al: The eVALuate study: Two parallel randomized trials, one comparing laparoscopic with abdominal hysterectomy, the other comparing laparoscopic with vaginal hysterectomy. BMJ 2004;328:129–136.

had hysterectomies for fibroids and to undergo abdominal surgery, perhaps partly explaining the higher complication rate.

Rates of certain complications also vary by route of hysterectomy. The lowest complication rates are generally associated with simple vaginal hysterectomy, although the likelihood of complications increases somewhat if additional procedures are done to correct prolapse. Laparoscopic hysterectomy, like all laparoscopic procedures, has its own set of unique complications related to trocar insertion, energy sources, and peritoneal insufflation. The eVALuate study comprised two parallel randomized multicenter trials: one comparing laparoscopic with abdominal hysterectomy and the other comparing laparoscopic with vaginal hysterectomy for nonmalignant disease (Garry et al, 2004). A total of 1346 patients had surgery; patients with a uterine mass greater than 12-week size and those with stage II or greater prolapse were excluded. The primary endpoints were assessments of complications. Table 11-1 shows the complication rates, with the intraoperative conversion rate excluded as a major complication, but reported separately. All six ureter injuries occurred in the laparoscopic group. The overall urinary tract (ureter plus bladder) complication rate was higher in the laparoscopic group than in the vaginal or abdominal groups (abdominal 1%, vaginal 1.2%, laparoscopic 2.3%). A minor complication, mostly postoperative fever or infection, occurred in approximately 25% of patients in each group. If one *includes* conversion to laparotomy as a major complication, then more major complications were found in the laparoscopic hysterectomy group compared to abdominal hysterectomy (11.1% vs. 6.2%; OR 1.91, 95% CI 1.11–3.28). If one excludes conversion to laparotomy as a complication, then the complication rates are similar between all groups. This study also confirmed the advantages of less pain, shorter hospital stay, quicker recovery, and improved quality of life in the short term with the laparoscopic and vaginal groups. Laparoscopic surgery had longer operating room times compared with vaginal or abdominal surgery.

Table 11-2 Patient Safety Indicators Related to Hysterectomy

Complications of anesthesia
Accidental puncture or laceration
Death
Foreign body left during the procedure
Postoperative hemorrhage or hematoma
Postoperative physiologic or metabolic derangements
Postoperative respiratory failure
Postoperative pulmonary embolism or deep vein thrombosis
Postoperative sepsis
Postoperative wound dehiscence
Infections due to medical care
Transfusion reaction

Data from U.S. Department of Health and Human Services, Agency for Healthcare Research and Quality: Patient Safety Indicators Overview. Accessed at: http://www.qualityindicators.ahrq.gov/psi_overview.htm.

Medical co-morbidities are associated with mortality and complication rates after hysterectomy. Heisler and colleagues (2009) found that a history of congestive heart failure or myocardial infarction, prior thrombosis, perioperative hemoglobin decrease greater than 3.1 g/dL, or preoperative hemoglobin less than 12.0 g/dL were associated with increased perioperative complications. Quality improvement efforts should attempt to modify these variables to optimize outcomes. There are some general patient safety indicators that may help identify potentially preventable complications associated with the surgical event (Table 11-2). This chapter will specifically address certain surgical complications at hysterectomy: perioperative bleeding, surgical site infections, wound complications, lower urinary tract injury, fistula, bowel injury, vaginal cuff evisceration, and fallopian tube prolapse.

Perioperative Hemorrhage

Case Presentation and Discussion: Postoperative Hemorrhage

G.W. is a 47-year-old gravida 3, para 3 obese woman with a 5-year history of severe abnormal uterine bleeding in association with uterine fibroids approximately 12-week size. She has been treated medically for the last 5 years but has continued anemia with hemoglobin of 9.8 g/dL. She has been presented with the full range of treatment options including further medical therapy, myomectomy, uterine fibroid embolization, or hysterectomy, and she desires a hysterectomy. Her pelvic examination confirms a 12- to 14-week-size mobile, anteverted uterus with a large central fundal fibroid. She has adequate vaginal capacity and mobility with her cervix descending approximately 3 cm with gentle traction. She has no other significant prolapse of her vagina or stress urinary incontinence.

A vaginal hysterectomy with morcellation was done over the course of approximately 1 hour. The uterus weighed 260 g and was sent to pathology. Both tubes and ovaries were normal and were not removed. The estimated blood loss for the surgery was 350 mL and she was transferred to the recovery room in stable condition.

Approximately 4 hours after surgery the physician is called to the bedside with a report that the patient is developing hypotension and tachycardia and that she had an increase in vaginal bleeding that now appears bright red. On physical examination, she is a somewhat pale-appearing female with a pulse of 110 bpm and a blood pressure of 100/60 mm Hg that decreases to 90/palpable when she sits up. Her abdomen is somewhat distended and bright red blood is noted from the vagina. An urgent hemoglobin is sent and is 6.8 g/dL. She is given a bolus of intravenous fluids and 4 units of blood are ordered from the blood bank.

The gynecologist, while waiting for the blood transfusion to begin, is faced with a decision between two major interventions: immediately returning to the operating room to find and correct the source of the bleeding, or immediate consultation with an interventional radiologist for consideration of embolization of the bleeding vessel. If the patient is hemodynamically unstable and operating room facilities are available, then the most prudent and efficient treatment would be to return to the operating room. Once in the operating room the gynecologist

Case Presentation and Discussion: Postoperative Hemorrhage—cont'd

should perform a vaginal examination of the vaginal cuff to attempt to identify and ligate the bleeding vessel, probably a uterine or vaginal artery, or a branch of it. If the gynecologist is unable to identify the bleeding vessel vaginally and there are signs of bleeding within the peritoneal cavity, then a laparotomy needs to be performed to ligate the bleeding vessels.

If the patient is hemodynamically stable, especially with fluid and blood resuscitation, and if the gynecologist has

facilities to perform an immediate assessment by an interventional radiologist, then it might be reasonable to perform angiography to locate and embolize the bleeding vessel. This has been reported to be successful in multiple circumstances involving hemorrhage in gynecology and obstetrics and is an excellent and viable alternative in appropriate patients who are in hospitals with adequate facilities for this.

The most common serious intraoperative complications of hysterectomy are hemorrhage and lower urinary tract injury. Although the definition of hemorrhage is somewhat arbitrary, most would consider a blood loss of greater than 1000 mL or need for a blood transfusion as acceptable criteria. Using this definition, the risk of hemorrhage at hysterectomy is approximately 1% to 3%. Bleeding after surgery can occur from any of the vascular pedicles, especially the uterine and ovarian vessels. Arterial bleeding from the vagina is usually from the uterine artery that has slipped from its ligature. This would require reoperation for suture ligation or embolization by an interventional radiologist. Venous bleeding may result in a pelvic hematoma, which can be diagnosed by pelvic examination or imaging studies. Careful observation, with or without blood transfusion, usually is adequate, but the patient should be carefully followed for signs of anemia and pelvic infection.

The systematic review performed by the Cochrane collaboration found no differences in transfusion rate between the abdominal, vaginal, or laparoscopic approaches. Subtotal (supracervical) hysterectomy appears to have reduced blood loss during surgery compared to the other approaches. The risk of intraoperative bleeding is increased in the presence of extensive endometriosis, malignancy, a uterus enlarged by fibroids (>500 g), and large pelvic masses that obscure the operative field. A hysterectomy performed for an obstetric indication is also at increased risk of excessive blood loss. Last, hysterectomy in the presence of thrombocytopenia, coagulopathy, or use of anticoagulation would likely increase the risk of excessive intra- and postoperative bleeding and transfusion.

In situations in which excessive bleeding at hysterectomy is anticipated or expected, the patient's blood should be cross-matched and available in the blood bank. Appropriate blood products should be available in the presence of coagulopathy. A CellSaver® (Haemonetics Corp., Braintree, MA) for autologous blood transfusion and thrombin products to enhance hemostasis should be available during surgery. Specialists in areas such as vascular surgery, anesthesia, and interventional radiology could be alerted preoperatively in case they will be needed.

Fever and Perioperative Infections

Fever

The most common postoperative complication of hysterectomy is febrile morbidity which occurs in 10% to 20% of women. Fevers after hysterectomy can occur for the following reasons: (1) an operative site infection such as a vaginal cuff cellulitis, pelvic abscess, or abdominal wound infection; (2) an infection remote from the operative site, such as pneumonia or pyelonephritis; or (3) the fever may be unexplained and resolve without consequence (50% of all posthysterectomy fevers). Recent evidence suggests that most unexplained postoperative fevers are not due to pulmonary atelectasis, but are the result of an increase in interleukins and cytokines. Regardless of the cause, a postoperative fever after hysterectomy increases the hospital stay an average of 1 to 2 days. Fevers that persist and are associated with clinical signs, symptoms, and laboratory findings suggestive of a surgical site infection require appropriate treatment with antibiotics.

Infections with an associated abscess or fluid collection, such as an abdominal wound infection or pelvic abscess, require surgical drainage. In the case of the posthysterectomy pelvic abscess, drainage can sometimes be accomplished transvaginally; however CT (computed tomography)-guided drainage or surgical exploration is sometimes required. Pelvic abscesses also require a course of intravenous broad-spectrum antibiotics followed by 10 to 14 days of oral antibiotics after the fevers resolve. Vaginal cuff cellulitis is diagnosed in patients who have persistent postoperative fever, vaginal cuff induration, and purulent discharge, without evidence of abscess. Antibiotics are usually adequate therapy. Abdominal wound infections often do not require antibiotics unless there is an associated skin cellulitis. Urinary tract infections are relatively common after hysterectomy; however, they are rarely a source of fever unless the upper urinary tract is involved.

Surgical Site Infections

Although data vary widely, most case series cite surgical site infection rates of 3% to 5% after abdominal hysterectomy, and this rate can increase up to 12% in obese women. Patient-related factors that increase the risk for surgical site infections include obesity, advanced age, medical conditions, cancer diagnosis, malnutrition, smoking, alteration of cervicovaginal flora, and immunosuppression (Walsh et al, 2009; Boesch and Umek, 2009). Operative risk factors include length of surgery, length of postoperative stay, increased blood loss, and tissue trauma. Factors that predispose obese women to surgical site infections include decreased vascularity of subcutaneous tissues, increased intra-abdominal pressure causing increased tension on the wound closure, more bacterial growth on skin, higher prevalence of diabetes and poor gylcemic control, longer operations, and decreased tissue concentrations of prophylactic antibiotics (Walsh et al, 2009). The route of hysterectomy is also important: the most recent Cochran Review (Nieboer et al, 2009) reports that vaginal hysterectomy has fewer febrile episodes or infections than abdominal hysterectomy (OR 0.42), and laparoscopic hysterectomy has fewer wound or abdominal wall infections than abdominal hysterectomy (OR 0.31).

A number of strategies can be used in the perioperative period to lower the risk of surgical site infections, particularly in obese patients (Table 11-3). The use of prophylactic antibiotics to decrease the risk of surgical site infections is one of the most important perioperative techniques to lower morbidity rate after hysterectomy. The time of administration of the antibiotic is critical to lowering the frequency of surgical site infection. The antibiotics should be given preoperatively to achieve minimal inhibitory concentrations (MIC) in the skin and tissues by the time the incision is made. This typically means an intravenous injection within 60 minutes of incision with a first- (cephalexin)

Table 11-3 Operating Room Strategies to Prevent Surgical Site Infections in Obese Patients*

- Administer an adequate dose of an appropriate antibiotic within 0 to 60 minutes before surgery.
- Administer at least 80% oxygen during abdominal surgery.
- Maintain intraoperative core normothermia.
- Close the subcutaneous tissue.
- The method of incising the subcutaneous tissues does not matter significantly, nor does placing a subcutaneous drain at the time of initial surgery.

*Supported by level I evidence.
Modified from Walsh C, Scaife C, Hopf H, et al: Prevention and management of surgical site infections in morbidly obese women. Obstet Gynecol 2009;113:411–415.

Table 11-4 Recommended Antimicrobial Prophylactic Regimens for Hysterectomy*

Regimen	Dose (Single Dose)
Cefazolin[†]	1 g *or* 2 g[‡] IV
Clindamycin[§] *plus*	600 mg IV
Gentamicin *or*	1.5 mg/kg IV
Quinolone[‖] *or*	400 mg IV
Aztreonam	1 g IV
Metronidazol[§] *plus*	500 mg IV
Gentamicin *or*	1.5 mg/kg IV
Quinolone	400 mg IV

*As suggested by the American College of Obstetricians and Gynecologists (ACOG).
[†]Acceptable alternatives include cefotetan, cefoxitin, cefuroxime, and ampicillin-sulbactam.
[‡]A 2-g dose is recommended in women with a body mass index greater than 35 or weight greater than 100 kg (220 lb).
[§]Antimicrobial agents of choice in women with a history of immediate hypersensitivity to penicillin.
[‖]Ciprofloxacin or levofloxacin or moxifloxacin.
Adapted from ACOG Practice Bulletin No. 104. Antibiotic prophylaxis for gynecologic procedures. Obstet Gynecol 2009;113:1180–1189.

or second- (cefoxitin) generation cephalosporin. These antibiotics were chosen because the likely site infection pathogens for hysterectomies are gram-negative bacilli, enterococci, group B streptococci, and anaerobes. Several alternative regimens are suggested by American College of Obstetricians and Gynecologists (ACOG Practice Bulletin, 2009) if the patient is allergic to penicillin or cephalosporins (Table 11-4). Longer procedures require re-dosing; the recommended interval for cephalexin is 3 to 5 hours and cefoxitin is 2 to 3 hours (Bratzler and Houck, 2004). A recent large multicenter collaborative study confirms these observations of a consistent relationship between the timing of antimicrobial prophylaxis and surgical site infection risk, with a trend toward lower risk occurring when prophylactic antibiotics with cephalosporins and other antibiotics with short infusion times are given within 30 minutes prior to incision (Steinberg et al, 2009).

During surgery, good surgical technique, gentle tissue handling, and meticulous hemostasis probably help lower the risk of infectious morbidity. Closure and nonclosure of the visceral and parietal peritoneum have the same effect on inflammatory complications after vaginal hysterectomy and abdominal hysterectomy. The advantage of leaving the peritoneum open is the time-saving aspect, and there is a suggestion that fewer peritoneal adhesions will result. The thickness of the subcutaneous tissue layer in obese women is a strong risk factor for wound infection after hysterectomy. The bulk of evidence supports closing the subcutaneous tissue when the depth is greater than 2 cm, although not all studies support this conclusion. No difference in surgical site infections after incisions made with a cold scalpel or with electrocautery has been found. Likewise, placing a subcutaneous drain does not appear to lower the wound morbidity rate (Soper et al, 1995).

When abdominal wound infections do occur the wound usually assumes a reddish appearance associated with edema, warmth, and erythema. The wound may be somewhat tender and fever may or may not be present. If nonpurulent or bloody drainage occurs without wound erythema, it may represent a seroma or hematoma and would benefit from opening a small portion of the wound and evacuating as much fluid, blood, and clot as possible. If active bleeding is found, then the source of this must be determined and hemostasis achieved. It is usually important to gently probe the wound to determine the extent of the open space and to verify that the fascia is intact. The wound is then irrigated copiously and local wound care is instituted. If a cellulitis is also present with associated edema, erythema, pain, tenderness, or fever, then removal of staples or sutures from the area with more extensive drainage and débridement of the infected issue is the cornerstone of management. Again it is important to determine that the fascia is intact at the initial wound exploration. Antibiotics are not usually necessary but could be considered, especially when the patient is immunocompromised or a more serious infection such as fasciitis is suspected.

Dehiscence of the fascia with or without extrusion of the intra-abdominal contents is a serious complication that requires emergent surgery to replace the bowel contents, irrigate and débride the wound, and meticulously reclose the fascia. Necrotizing fasciitis is a dangerous synergistic bacterial infection involving the fascia, subcutaneous tissue, and skin. Patients with necrotizing fasciitis may exhibit signs of systemic infection with fever and leukocytosis, and have wound findings of severe pain, edematous skin, necrotic wound edges, and crepitus. Typical findings on CT imaging may also be found. Necrotizing faciitis constitutes a medical and surgical emergency and requires intravenous broad-spectrum antibiotics, wide surgical débridement of all affected skin and fascia, and cardiovascular and fluid support if necessary (Perkins and Pattillo, 2009).

Lower Urinary Tract Injury

Case Presentation and Discussion: Ureteral Obstruction after Surgery for Prolapse

The patient is an 81-year-old female with procidentia (Pelvic Organ Prolapse Quantification System's stage IV). She underwent a vaginal hysterectomy, uterosacral ligament colpopexy, and anterior and posterior colporrhaphy. The surgery was uncomplicated. Near the completion of the procedure, the patient was given 5 mL of intravenous (IV) indigo carmine, and a cystoscopy was performed. After 15 minutes of continuous observation, no dye could be seen to efflux from the right ureteral orifice.

This is a situation that can create substantial anxiety for the surgeon. Assessment of the bladder, urethra, and ureters requires competence with the use of a cystoscope. If the gynecologist does not perform cystoscopy and a ureteral obstruction is suspected, then an intraoperative urologic consultation would be necessary.

Ureteral obstruction after this type of hysterectomy and transvaginal repair of severe prolapse is usually due to ureteral kinking (not ligation or transection) and occurs after initial placement of sutures in 1% to 6% of patients. The main rule, in this case, is not to leave the operating room unless verification of kidney and ureteral function is accomplished. In an older woman, renal function may be somewhat delayed, or the anesthesiologist may be overcautious about volume replacement. Before taking further action, give 5 to 10 mg of IV furosemide. Call for ureteral stents to be brought to the operating room and use this time to recheck the chart to make sure that the blood urea nitrogen (BUN) and creatinine levels were normal. Were a previous renal ultrasound or intravenous pyelogram (IVP) obtained, review the results again at this time; however, use of radiologic studies, even in patients with total

Case Presentation and Discussion: Ureteral Obstruction after Surgery for Prolapse—cont'd

prolapse, is not routinely indicated. It is also useful to confirm that the patient has not had a previous nephrectomy and that the indigo carmine has actually been given.

After about 20 minutes, if blue dye has still not passed through one or both ureteral orifices, then start removing the vaginal vault suspension sutures in the uterosacral ligament on the offending side, which is the most likely source of the obstruction; this will relieve the obstruction about 85% of the time (Gustilo-Ashby et al, 2006). If there is still no flow, carefully examine the sutures near the right uterine artery and palpate for the ureter. Remove any offending sutures if necessary, and then remove the cystocele repair sutures. If still no flow, try to pass a right retrograde ureteral catheter. If it passes easily, remove it and postoperatively follow the patient closely. After prolapse repairs ureteral catheters are usually difficult to pass, however, even if the ureters are patent, because of the distortion of bladder base from the prolapse and repair. If the catheter did not pass, and there is still no blue dye efflux after suture removal, then obtain a one-shot IVP or retrograde pyelogram with an acorn-tip catheter in the operating room, if possible. The x-ray is to confirm that both kidneys are present and functioning and also to look for early hydronephrosis or ureteral obstruction. Consider obtaining an intraoperative Urology consultation by this time, depending on the operator's comfort with the management of this condition. Unrecognized renal tumors and nonfunctioning atrophic kidneys can occur in this situation, but they are rare.

If the IVP shows that both kidneys are functioning (or one is unable to get an IVP), there is no efflux of urine from one or both ureters despite removal of the sutures, and the surgeon is still unable to pass a ureteral stent, the next decision is more difficult. One would then have to decide whether to perform an immediate laparotomy or laparoscopy with ureteral reimplantation or to postoperatively place nephrostomy tubes to temporarily divert the urine. If the surgeon is reasonably certain that a ureter is damaged, and the patient is able to tolerate the additional time of surgery with its associated morbidity risk, some would prefer to proceed with laparotomy or laparoscopy and ureteroneocystostomy in consultation with a urologist. If not, nephrostomy tubes could be later placed, and then antegrade passage of a catheter into the bladder could be attempted and will sometimes pass through the ureteral obstruction. If this cannot be accomplished, then the patient would remain with nephrostomy tubes until she is able to tolerate reimplantation.

Case Presentation and Discussion: Ureteral Injury after Laparoscopic Hysterectomy

The 48-year-old para 3 female has a long history of symptomatic uterine fibroids that have failed all forms of conservative medical management. The uterus is approximately 14-weeks size with several lower uterine segment fibroids as seen on ultrasound. Her hematocrit is 32% and her Papanicolaou (Pap) smear is normal. After carefully discussing all of the treatment options she has elected to undergo total laparoscopic hysterectomy with removal of the cervix.

A laparoscopic hysterectomy is done using bipolar techniques to coagulate and cut the vascular pedicles. Because the lower uterine segment fibroid is near the uterine artery, visualization of the right uterine artery was difficult. Some bleeding was encountered during coagulation and cutting of the right uterine artery and right parametrial tissue. Ultimately good hemostasis was achieved and the hysterectomy was further completed without difficulty. Estimated blood loss was 450 mL.

She was discharged approximately 36 hours after surgery but called on the third postoperative day with a low-grade fever and some persistent nausea. She was seen in the emergency department and was found to have a temperature of 38.2° C with some right costovertebral angle (CVA) tenderness and mild abdominal distention with hypoactive bowel sounds. Her hematocrit was 28%, white blood cell count 11,000, and creatinine 1.2 mg/dL. An abdominal and pelvic CT scan showed no evidence of small bowel obstruction or bowel leak but revealed mild right hydronephrosis with a suggestion of fluid extravasation near the right distal ureter.

A urology consultation was obtained. The patient was admitted and scheduled for cystoscopy the following day. At cystoscopy, retrograde ureterograms and passage of ureteral catheters were attempted. The left ureter was completely patent and normal-appearing. The right ureter had no flow of urine and obstruction was found approximately 3 cm from the bladder in the distal ureter.

Later that day, a percutaneous nephrostomy was performed in the right kidney without difficulty. An antegrade nephrostogram was done showing mild hydronephrosis of the proximal ureter (Fig. 11-1). An obstruction and defect in the distal right ureter with extravasation of dye into the retroperitoneal space was noted suggesting a transection or leak in the distal ureter (Fig. 11-2). The percutaneous nephrostomy was left in place to drain the right kidney and the patient was scheduled for right ureteroneocystostomy over the next several days.

Figure 11-1 Right percutaneous nephrostomy with antegrade nephrostogram showing mild right hydronephrosis.

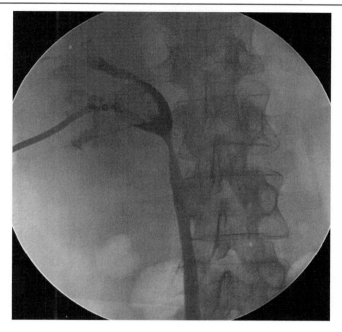

Figure 11-2 Right antegrade nephrostogram showing retroperitoneal extravasation of dye from a leak or transection of the distal right ureter.

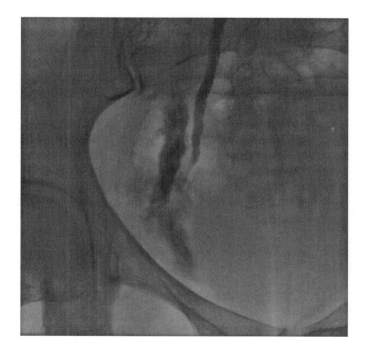

Incidence of Lower Urinary Tract Injury

Lower urinary tract injury, including bladder injury, ureteral injury, urethral injury, and vesicovaginal fistula, occurs in approximately 0.5% to 3% of hysterectomies. There is an increased risk of lower urinary tract injury in women with previous cesarean sections, severe pelvic adhesive disease, pregnancy, malignancy, and those undergoing concurrent urogynecologic procedures. A systematic review of 27 randomized trials found that laparoscopic hysterectomy has a 2.6 times greater risk of lower urinary tract injury than that of abdominal hysterectomy.

Bladder Injury

Bladder injuries occur during hysterectomy in about 0.5% to 2% of cases. Some studies have shown an increased risk of bladder injury with vaginal hysterectomy, while others have not. Bladder injury can take the form of sutures in the bladder, thermal injury from energy sources, or cystotomy. Cystotomies can occur with any route of hysterectomy and the principles of evaluation, recognition, and management are the same. Adhesions between the cervix and bladder, as after a prior cesarean delivery, probably increase the risk of cystotomy. Special care should be taken to avoid forcible blunt retraction of the bladder off the cervix. A gauze on a forceps may be especially prone to damaging the bladder (Fig. 11-3A to C) because of poor tactile sensation over these delicate tissues. We prefer sharp dissection of the bladder off the cervix using gentle traction-countertraction techniques. Other maneuvers to help dissect the bladder off the uterus in difficult cases are shown in Chapters 7 and 8.

Every effort should be made to recognize bladder injuries intraoperatively so that they may be immediately repaired. Immediate repair of cystotomy followed by bladder drainage has a high likelihood of success. Delayed repair is associated with increased morbidity including fever, prolonged hospital stay, ileus, vesicovaginal fistula, and additional surgery. If the surgeon suspects that a cystotomy may have occurred, careful visual assessment of the bladder muscularis is done to look for urine leaks. If still unsure, the bladder can be retrograde filled through a Foley catheter to again examine for leaks. Staining the fluid blue with indigo carmine may aid identification of small cystotomies. If a cystotomy occurs, the bladder should be dissected free from the uterus using sharp dissection (Fig. 11-4A and B). Visual examination of the ureters is done to assure that one or both ureters were not also damaged. Bladder injuries should be repaired without tension using two layers of small caliber absorbable suture, such as No. 2-0 or 3-0 polyglycolic acid (Fig. 11-4C). Closures should be water-tight and the bladder drained for 3 to 14 days depending upon the size and location of the injury. (See DVD Video 11-1 for video demonstration of transvaginal repair of cystotomy. 📹)

Ureteral Injury

The risk of ureteral injury is 0.2% to 0.8% after abdominal hysterectomy, 0.05% to 0.1% after vaginal hysterectomy, and 0.2% to 3.4% after laparoscopic hysterectomy. The most common location of ureteral injury at the time of hysterectomy is the distal 3 to 4 cm of the ureter as it passes under the uterine artery and travels through the cardinal ligament to enter the bladder. Injury can also occur at or below the infundibulopelvic ligament and along the pelvic sidewall just above the uterosacral ligament (Fig. 11-5). The ability to adequately identify ureteral injuries at the time of the initial operation is of paramount importance. Permanent renal damage can, in most cases, be avoided if the diagnosis of the ureteral injury is made at the time of surgery. Delay can put the patient at risk of permanent loss of renal function and ureterovaginal fistula. Studies have shown that intraoperative recognition and immediate repair decreases postoperative morbidity, minimizes loss of kidney function and need for nephrectomy, and decreases the incidence of ureterovaginal fistula development, when compared to postoperative diagnosis and delayed repair of ureteral injuries.

If a ureteral injury is suspected or if the patient is at high risk of a ureteral injury, intraoperative cystoscopy with IV indigo carmine dye is an effective method of confirming ureteral patency. In fact, some authors have advocated routine use of intraoperative cystoscopy for all hysterectomies. Visco and asso-

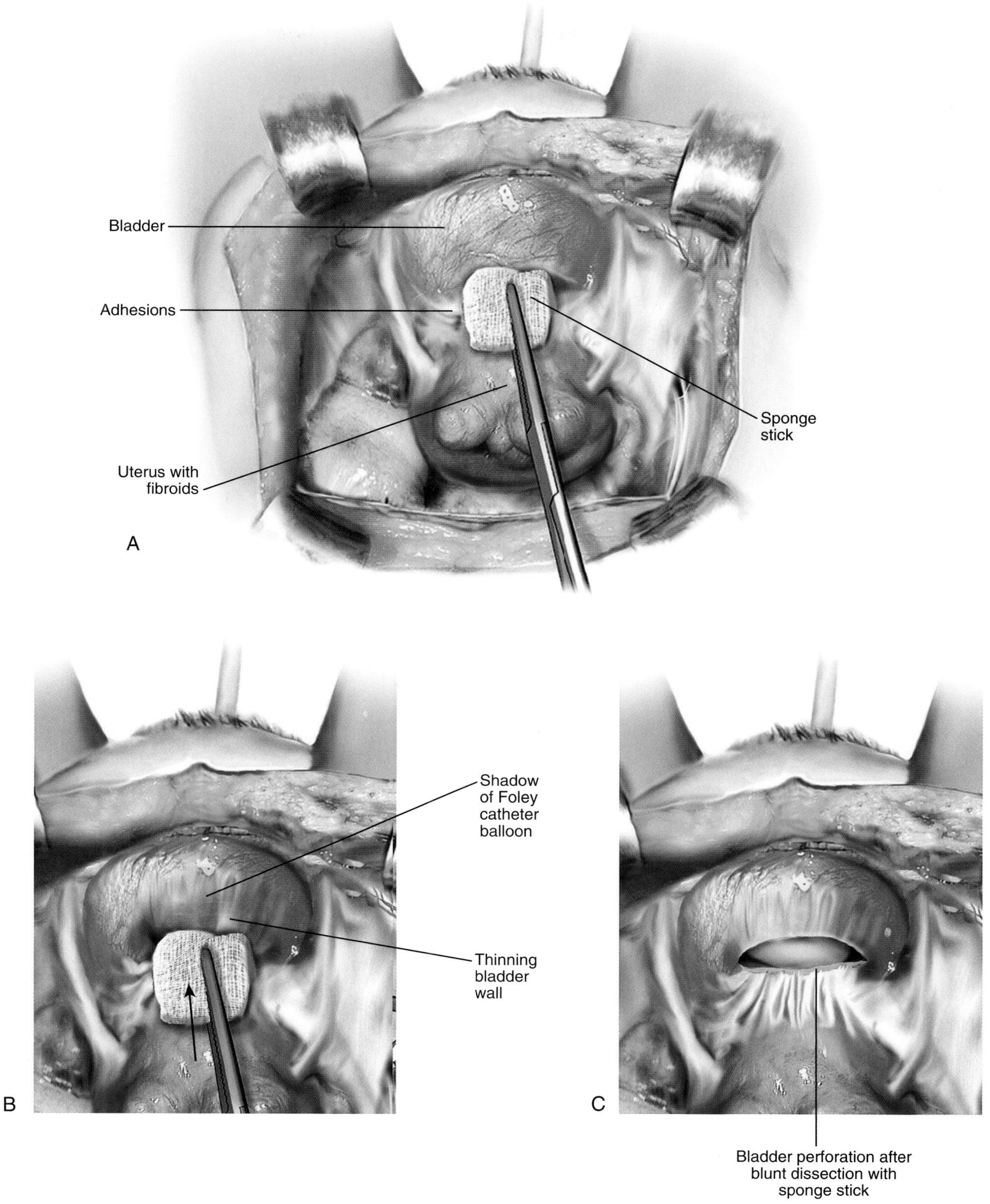

A

Bladder

Adhesions

Sponge stick

Uterus with fibroids

B

Shadow of Foley catheter balloon

Thinning bladder wall

C

Bladder perforation after blunt dissection with sponge stick

Figure 11-3 A, During abdominal hysterectomy with a prior cesarean delivery, a gauze on a forceps is used to forcibly separate the bladder from the cervix. **B,** Thinning of the bladder wall results from damage to the bladder muscularis. **C,** Cystotomy results.

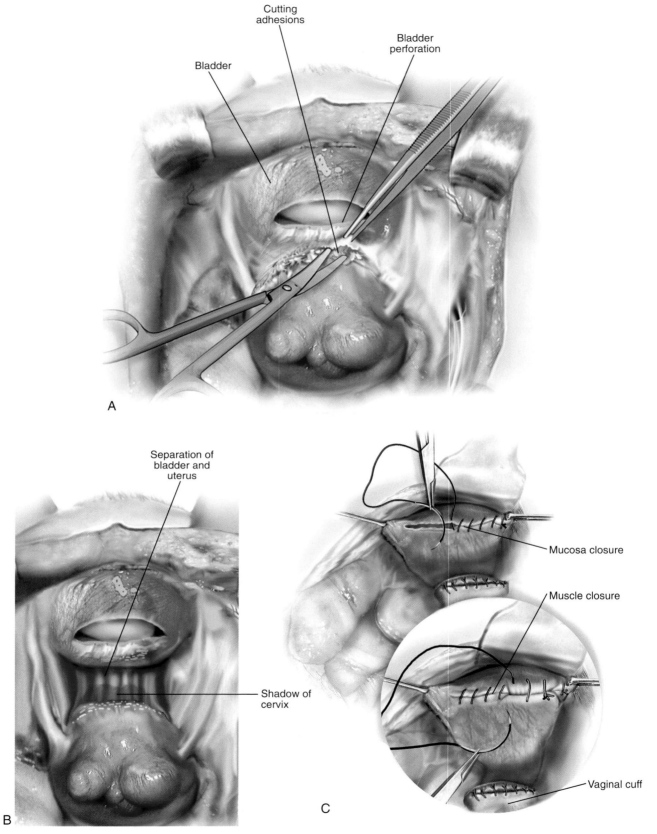

Figure 11-4 A, The entire cystotomy is examined and the bladder is sharply dissected off the cervix. **B,** The bladder edges are now free and mobile. **C,** The bladder laceration is closed in two layers.

Figure 11-5 Location of the three common sites of ureteral damage at hysterectomy: **A,** Near the infundibulopelvic ligament, **B,** passing under the uterine artery and vein, and **C,** at the ureterovesical junction. (Reprinted with permission of The Cleveland Clinic Center for Medical Art & Photography, copyright 2009. All rights reserved.)

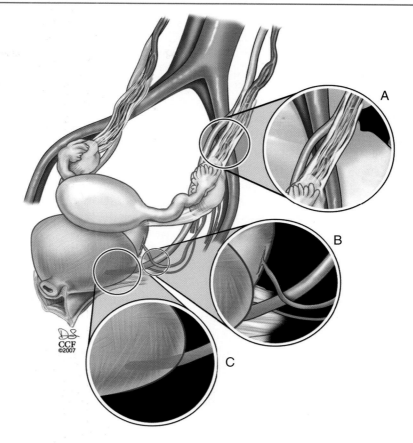

ciates (2001) evaluated the cost-effectiveness of this strategy and found that when the risk of ureteral injury was greater than 1.5%, routine cystoscopy at the time of hysterectomy resulted in a cost savings. For abdominal hysterectomies, where the average rate of ureteral injury is about 0.5%, 200 cystoscopies would need to be performed to diagnose one ureteral injury intraoperatively, and would cost a total of $16,600 for each ureteral injury diagnosed. The medicolegal costs associated with an unrecognized ureteral injury were not included in this analysis. Based on these data, it seems prudent to perform intraoperative cystoscopy routinely during procedures where the risk of lower urinary tract injury is high, such as during laparoscopic hysterectomy, where the average risk is approximately 1.5%, or during cases involving malignancy, severe adhesions, severe endometriosis, large pelvic masses or fibroids, pelvic organ prolapse, or distorted anatomy requiring extensive sidewall dissection. Ureteral catheters can be placed before surgery, although we do not recommend that this be done routinely, even before difficult cases. Catheters can also be placed intraoperatively to assess for possible ureteral injury during hysterectomy, especially if no flow of urine is seen. An intraoperative retrograde ureterogram is effective at localizing the site of ureteral damage and is helpful in planning maneuvers needed to re-establish patency of the affected ureter.

Other techniques to assess for potential ureteral injury include open or laparoscopic retroperitoneal dissection with ureterolysis with direct visualization of potential injury, ureteral catheterization intraoperatively either via a cystoscope or through a cystotomy incision (see DVD Video 11-2 for video demonstration of high cystotomy and passage of ureteral catheters), or radiologic techniques such as intravenous urography or retrograde ureterogram. In fact, the integrity of a single ureter can be demonstrated by injecting indigo carmine into the lumen of the ureter proximal to the surgical site to assess for resistance to dye injected (suggesting ureteral obstruction) or extravasations of dye (suggesting damage to the ureteral wall). These techniques are individualized to the surgery, the potential type of injury involved, and to the route of hysterectomy.

During laparoscopic or open surgery, if absence of ureteral flow is noted, then ureteral angulations and kinks should be released if they have caused significant obstruction. A ligated ureter should have the ligating suture removed. Minor ureteral crush injuries may be managed with ureteral stenting; significant crush injuries require resection of the damaged segment and ureteroneocystostomy or ureteroureterostomy. On occasion, partial lacerations of a ureter can be repaired by placement of several No. 3-0 absorbable or delayed-absorbable sutures to close the laceration over a ureteral catheter. Complete lacerations of the ureter and loss or devascularization of a segment of ureter require definitive surgical repair.

The surgical procedures recommended for ureteral repair vary according to the ureteral segment that is involved. Because most gynecologic injuries to the ureter involve the distal 4 to 5 cm, most can be repaired by simple repair of the ureteral laceration or ureteroneocystostomy. Injuries just below the pelvic brim, such as during ligation of the ovarian vessels, may be repaired by ureteroureterostomy or a psoas-hitch procedure.

Continuous bladder drainage, either transurethrally or suprapubically, should be initiated whenever there is a cystotomy, ureteroneocystostomy, or other ureteral repair. When only a ureteral repair has occurred and there is no cystotomy, the bladder catheter may be removed before the ureteral catheter or stent is removed. The repair of ureteral injuries should be followed by an intravenous urogram to determine the integrity of the repair and the presence or absence of a stenosis. This is done to detect fistulas or conditions that might cause renal damage. Ureteral catheters are usually left in 2 to 3 weeks and then removed after documentation of good healing is demonstrated radiographically.

Vesicovaginal Fistula

Vesicovaginal fistulas are a rare complication of hysterectomy with an incidence of 0.1% to 0.2%; hysterectomy is the most common cause of vesicovaginal fistula in the United States. Most posthysterectomy vesicovaginal fistulas occur after an apparently uncomplicated total abdominal or laparoscopic hysterectomy for benign disease. Steps to avoid fistula formation include identification of the proper plane between the bladder and cervix, use of sharp dissection to develop the bladder flap rather than blunt dissection or use of electrocautery, assuring that the bladder is dissected below the level that the cervix will be transected from the vagina, and intraoperative identification of any lower urinary tract injury using the techniques previously outlined. Animal studies suggest that vesicovaginal fistulas usually result from unrecognized bladder injuries. Unrecognized suture placement into the bladder at the time of cuff closure is unlikely to result in fistula formation in the absence of a concurrent bladder laceration. Patients who develop a vesicovaginal fistula typically have a difficult early postoperative course followed by development of watery drainage from the vagina 10 to 14 days after surgery. If not readily apparent on vaginal examination, the diagnosis can be made by cystoscopy or by instilling the bladder with dilute methylene blue or indigo carmine dye and placing a tampon into the vagina. If the dye is noted on the tampon then a bladder fistula is confirmed. If there is no dye apparent, ureterovaginal fistula must be ruled out by intravenous administration of indigo carmine dye or by radiologic evaluation of the ureter with an IVP or CT scan. Small fistulas may heal spontaneously after 6 to 12 weeks of continuous bladder drainage. For those that do not heal spontaneously, surgical repair is required.

Case Presentation and Discussion: Vesicovaginal Fistula

A 42-year-old female with symptomatic 14-week-size uterine fibroids underwent a laparoscopically assisted vaginal hysterectomy. The surgery and hospital course were uncomplicated and the patient was discharged from the hospital on postoperative day 1. Three days after discharge, the patient noted new onset urinary leakage and contacted her surgeon with this complaint. She was instructed to drop off a urine specimen to rule out a urinary tract infection as the source of her new symptoms. The urinalysis revealed 2+ blood but was otherwise normal. A urine culture eventually returned negative. Six days after discharge, the patient presented to clinic for evaluation of worsening urinary leakage. She described continuous leakage of urine throughout the day, particularly when standing, and also noted that her bed sheets were wet the last several mornings. Her only other complaint was "crampy" lower abdominal pain. On physical examination, she was afebrile and in no acute distress. Her abdomen was not tender or distended. Pelvic examination revealed pooling of clear fluid in the upper vagina and a healing vaginal cuff with

sutures present. A Foley catheter was placed and the bladder filled with 5 mL of indigo carmine diluted in 300 mL of normal saline. Visual inspection of the vaginal cuff revealed leakage of blue fluid in the middle of the vaginal cuff incision confirming a vesicovaginal fistula. Office cystoscopy was performed and revealed a 3- to 4-mm defect in the bladder mucosa above the trigone in the midline. No sutures or foreign bodies were noted. An intravenous pyelogram revealed normal upper urinary tracts with no evidence of a ureterovaginal fistula. A Foley catheter was placed and left to continuous drainage for 4 weeks. During this time, the patient reported a significant decrease in urinary leakage, but still noted daily urinary leakage associated with increasing activity. Repeat cystoscopy 5 weeks after surgery revealed a persistent 2- to 3-mm vesicovaginal fistula in the supratrigonal region in the midline. Speculum examination demonstrated a healed vaginal cuff with a 2-mm well-epithelialized midline tract consistent with a fistula. The patient subsequently underwent surgical repair of her vesicovaginal fistula using the Latzko technique with resolution of her urinary leakage.

Bowel Injury

Bowel injury occurs in 0.1% to 1% of hysterectomies. Injury to the small intestines occurs most commonly during entry into the abdomen at the time of abdominal or laparoscopic hysterectomy, typically in patients with abdominal wall adhesions. Small lacerations can be closed in two layers with small caliber sutures. For the first layer, No. 3-0 absorbable suture is used to approximate the mucosa. For the second layer interrupted No. 3-0 or 2-0 suture, often silk, is used to reinforce the serosa. Lacerations should be closed transversely in relation to the bowel lumen in order to avoid narrowing. Large lacerations or evidence of devascularization require small bowel resection.

Rectal injuries occur most often at the time of vaginal hysterectomy, at rectocele repair, during sacrospinous colpopexies, or in cases of an obliterated posterior cul-de-sac from malignancy or endometriosis. Rectal examination during the posterior wall dissection may help prevent and recognize rectal injuries. Small rectal lacerations are repaired with a two-layer closure and most heal without complications. Large lacerations may require rectal resection or diverting colostomy.

Vaginal Cuff Evisceration

Case Presentation and Discussion

L.M. is a 44-year-old para 1 woman who underwent a total robotic hysterectomy 21 days earlier for uterine fibroids. The cervix was removed laparoscopically and the vaginal cuff was closed with two transverse nonlocking sutures of No.1-0

polyglactin started at each cuff angle and run to the midline and tied. She had an uncomplicated postoperative course and was discharged the day after surgery. On the 21st postoperative day, while walking at her home, she noticed an

Case Presentation and Discussion—cont'd

increase in watery vaginal bleeding followed a few minutes later by a sensation of something in the vagina protruding to the introitus. She touched it and felt soft fleshy tissue, so she immediately laid down and called her physician. She was transported to the emergency room where she was found to be well-appearing and hemodynamically stable. Vaginal examination revealed apparent small bowel in the vaginal canal. The bowel appeared healthy without evidence of devascularization, bleeding, laceration, or intestinal content. A diagnosis of evisceration of small bowel from the vaginal cuff was made and she was taken to the operating room and, under general anesthesia, an examination was done verifying the diagnosis.

On examination under anesthesia, the bowel appeared healthy and was freely mobile in and out of the peritoneal cavity. There was no evidence of infection, intestinal contents, feces, or abscess. All of the bowel material that had prolapsed was carefully examined and no other abnormalities noted. The vaginal edges appeared healthy and not infected; and the defect in the vaginal cuff was approximately 3 cm. The patient was placed in Trendelenburg position and the small bowel fed back into the abdominal cavity. The vaginal cuff then was closed in two layers with No. O-PDS suture without complication. She was observed in the hospital for two nights until she was eating well and had a bowel movement, after which she was discharged and had a full recovery.

Dehiscence of the vaginal cuff, with or without evisceration of small intestine, is rare but may be increasing in incidence due to the more common use of total laparoscopic and robotic hysterectomy. Few risk factors for this have been identified due to its rarity; rare cases have followed vaginal intercourse or instrumentation either after hysterectomy or spontaneously.

In a review of over 7000 hysterectomies performed at one hospital over 6 years, the incidence of vaginal cuff dehiscence after total hysterectomy was 0.14%. Importantly, there was an increase in vaginal dehiscence later in the series in parallel with an increase in the use of total laparoscopic hysterectomy, and there was a strong statistical association of dehiscence with laparoscopic hysterectomy compared to vaginal or abdominal routes. The median time between initial hysterectomy to vaginal dehiscence was 11 weeks and 6 of 10 patients with this complication also had bowel evisceration. There were no recurrent dehiscences in this series, although this has been known to occur. Recently an analysis of 510 robotic simple and radical hysterectomies revealed a 4.1% incidence of postoperative vaginal cuff dehiscence, with bowel evisceration in about one third of cases (Kho et al, 2009). There is speculation that the use of thermal energy or perhaps fewer sutures to close the vaginal cuff may be responsible for this increase. A more meticulous closure of the vaginal apex or supracervical approach would decrease the risk of this complication (Hur et al, 2007).

After an examination under anesthesia, if the bowel appears healthy, the surgeon is faced with the choice of a transvaginal repair followed by observation versus a laparoscopic or open repair with closure of the vaginal cuff. If the bowel appears completely healthy and not damaged, reduction of the bowel and transvaginal closure of the vaginal apex followed by observation is a reasonable option. If there is any concern that there may be infection, abscess, or bowel damage, then an operative laparoscopy or laparotomy is necessary to carefully examine the bowel, then close the vaginal apex in two layers. It would probably be prudent to restrict the patient to limited activity and no sexual intercourse for 3 months after repair of a vaginal cuff evisceration.

Fallopian Tube Prolapse

Fallopian tube prolapse is a rare but unique complication of hysterectomy. Patients present with vaginal spotting, postcoital bleeding, and occasionally pelvic pain or dyspareunia. On examination, fallopian tube prolapse often appears as granulation tissue at the vaginal cuff but is usually very tender to direct touch. In patients who have vaginal cuff granulation tissue that does not resolve after several efforts of cauterization or removal, is exquisitely tender, or in patients in whom the diagnosis is unclear, an excisional biopsy should be performed. Fallopian tube prolapse is easily treated by transvaginal excision in the operating room with or without laparoscopic assistance.

Suggested Readings

ACOG Practice Bulletin No. 104. Antibiotic prophylaxis for gynecologic procedures. Obstet Gynecol 2009;113:1180–1189.

Barber MD: Hysterectomy. In Sokol A, Sokol E (eds): Requisites in Obstetrics and Gynecology: General Gynecology. St. Louis, Elsevier, 2007.

Boesch CE, Umek W: Effects of wound closure on wound healing in gynecologic surgery: A systematic literature review. J Reprod Med 2009;54:139–144.

Bratzler DW, Houck PM, for the Surgical Infection Prevention Guidelines Writers Workgroup: Antimicrobial prophylaxis for surgery: An advisory statement from the National Surgical Infection Prevention Project. Clin Infect Dis 2004;38:1705–1715.

Caceres A, McCarus SD: Fallopian tube prolapse after total laparoscopic hysterectomy. Obstet Gynecol 2008;112:494–495.

Carlson KJ, Miller BA, Fowler FJ: The Maine Women's Health Study: I. Outcomes of hysterectomy. Obstet Gynecol 1994;83:556–565.

Chan JK, Morrow J, Manetta A: Prevention of ureteral injuries in gynecologic surgery. Am J Obstet Gynecol 2003;188:1273–1277.

Croak AJ, Gebhart JB, Klingele CJ, et al: Characteristics of patients with vaginal rupture and evisceration. Obstet Gynecol 2004;103:572–576.

Dicker RC, Greenspan JR, Strauss LT, et al: Complications of abdominal and vaginal hysterectomy among women of reproductive age in the United States: The collaborative review of sterilization. Am J Obstet Gynecol 1982;144:841–848.

Falcone T, Walters MD: Hysterectomy for benign disease. Obstet Gynecol 2008;111:753–767.

Garry R, Fountain J, Mason S, et al: The eVALuate study: Two parallel randomized trails, one comparing laparoscopic with abdominal hysterectomy, the other comparing laparoscopic with vaginal hysterectomy. BMJ 2004;328:129–136.

Gustilo-Ashby AM, Jelovsek JE, Barber MD, et al: The incidence of ureteral obstruction and the value of intraoperative cystoscopy during vaginal surgery for pelvic organ prolapse. Am J Obstet Gynecol 2006;194:1492–1498.

Harris WJ: Early complications of abdominal and vaginal hysterectomy. Obstet Gynecol Surv 1995; 50:795–805.

Heisler CA, Aletti GD, Weaver AL, et al: Improving quality of care: Development of a risk-adjusted perioperative morbidity model for vaginal hysterectomy. Am J Obstet Gynecol 2010;202: 137.e1–5.

Hur H, Guido RS, Suketu M, et al: Incidence and patient characteristics of vaginal cuff dehiscence alter different modes of hysterectomies. J Min Invas Gynecol 2007;14:311–317.

Hurt WG: Gynecologic injury to the ureters, bladder, and urethra: Prevention, recognition, and management. In Walters MD, Karram MM (eds): Urogynecology and Reconstructive Pelvic Surgery, 3rd ed. Philadelphia, Elsevier (Mosby), 2007.

Johnson N, Barlow D, Lethaby A, et al: Surgical approach to hysterectomy for benign gynaecological disease. Cochrane Database of Syst Rev 2006;Issue 2:CD003677.

Juillard C, Lashoher A, Sweell CA, et al: A national analysis of the relationship between hospital volume, academic center status, and surgical outcomes for abdominal hysterectomy done for leiomyoma. J Am Coll Surg 2009;208:599–606.

Kho RM, Akl MN, Cornella JL, et al: Incidence and characteristics of patients with vaginal cuff dehiscence after robotic procedures. Obstet Gynecol 2009;114:231–235.

Kjerulff KH, Guzinski GM, Langenberg PW, et al: Hysterectomy and race. Obstet Gynecol 1993;82:757–764.

Kjerulff KH, Langenberg PW, Rhodes JC, et al: Effectiveness of hysterectomy. Obstet Gynecol 2000a;95:319–326.

Kjerulff KH, Rhodes JC, Langenberg PW, Harvey LA: Patient satisfaction with results of hysterectomy. Am J Obstet Gynecol 2000b;183:1440–1447.

McPherson K, Metcalfe MA, Herbert A, et al: Severe complications of hysterectomy: the VALUE study. Br J Obstet Gynaecol 2004;111:688–694.

Nieboer TE, Johnson N, Lethaby A, et al: Surgical approach to hysterectomy for benign gynaecological disease. Cochrane Database Syst Rev 2009;(3):CD003677.

Perkins JD, Pattillo RA: How to avert postoperative wound complication—and treat it when it occurs. OBG Management 2009;21:43–53.

Soper DE, Bump RC, Hurt WG: Wound infection after abdominal hysterectomy: Effect of the depth of subcutaneous tissue. Am J Obstet Gynecol 1995;173:465–469.

Steinberg JP, Braun BI, Hellinger WC, et al, for the Trial to Reduce Antimicrobial Prophylaxis Errors (TRAPE) Study Group: Timing of antimicrobial prophylaxis and the risk of surgical site infections: Results from the Trial to Reduce Antimicrobial Prophylaxis Errors. Ann Surg 2009;250:10–16.

United States Department of Health and Human Services, Agency for Healthcare Research and Quality: Patient safety indicators overview. Available at http://www.qualityindicators.ahrq.gov/psi_overview.htm. Retrieved March 22, 2010.

Visco AG, Taber KH, Weidner AC, et al: Cost-effectiveness of universal cystoscopy to identify ureteral injury at hysterectomy. Obstet Gynecol 2001;97:685–692.

Walsh C, Scaife C, Hopf H: Prevention and management of surgical site infections in morbidly obese women. Obstet Gynecol 2009;113:411–415.

Wingo PA, Huezo CM, Rubin MB, et al: The mortality risk associated with hysterectomy. Am J Obstet Gynecol 1985;152:803–808.

Alternative Treatments to Hysterectomy

Linda D. Bradley M.D.
Devorah R. Wieder M.D., M.P.H.

 Video Clip on DVD

12-1 Operative Hysteroscopic Myomectomy

Despite increasing medical and surgical options, the number of hysterectomies in the past decade has not decreased. Hysterectomy remains the second most common operative procedure performed in women only superseded by cesarean delivery. In 2003, the Nationwide Inpatient Sample of the Healthcare Cost and Utilization Project reported 538,722 hysterectomies were performed for benign conditions. Only 10% of hysterectomies were performed for genital malignancy. The most common indications for hysterectomy included uterine fibroids (33%) and menstrual disorders (17%). Approximately 5.8 hysterectomies per 1000 U.S. females are performed annually. Regional variations in hysterectomy are also reported; the highest rates of hysterectomy in the United States occur within the southern states and the lowest rates are in the western part of the country.

Hysterectomy for benign disorders has a number of drawbacks, not the least of which is an overall complication rate of 17% to 23%, regardless of approach—abdominal, transvaginal, laparoscopic, or robotic. Hysterectomy is not appropriate for women who wish to retain their fertility; moreover, the procedure may have a significant negative impact on psychosexual health.

Even though hysterectomy unequivocally solves fibroid-related symptoms (abnormal bleeding, dysmenorrhea, pelvic pain, leukorrhea, and bulk symptoms), increasingly patients and physicians are seeking alternatives to hysterectomy for the treatment of fibroids and menstrual disturbances. Open or laparoscopic myomectomy is a well-established alternative in select women. What other alternatives exist? The first report in 1995 demonstrated the benefits of uterine fibroid embolization (UFE) for the treatment of fibroid-related symptoms. The introduction of the operative hysteroscope has permitted treatment of intracavitary leiomyomas and polyps. There are women with abnormal bleeding and a normal uterine cavity or with intramural fibroids (<3 cm) that do not distort the endometrial cavity who may benefit from endometrial ablation. MRI-focused ultrasound also offers a subset of women with symptomatic uterine fibroids another treatment option. Recently, the Food and Drug Administration (FDA) approved the progesterone intrauterine system for heavy menstrual bleeding in women who also need contraception. Clinical reports of excellent efficacy outcomes demonstrate superior improvements in menorrhagia, abnormal uterine bleeding, and dysmenorrhea.

Physicians managing patients with uterine fibroids and abnormal bleeding must comprehend the risks and benefits of each of these treatment modalities. Future fertility is an important factor in determining the appropriateness or exclusion for many of these alternatives. A patient's ultimate choice among available fibroid therapies may depend upon the fibroid-related impact on her health-related quality of life (HRQOL), the length of convalescence that is acceptable to her, and the importance she assigns to tolerable invasiveness and symptom resolution.

Medical Management with Levonorgestrel-Releasing Intrauterine System

Case Presentation

A 33-year-old gravida 4, para 2, aborta 2 presents with a history of gradually developing menorrhagia without anemia. She describes regular menses during which she passes large clots. At the peak of her bleeding, these symptoms require changing her pad and tampon every 3 hours. Pad changes as well as soiling of her clothes interfere with her daily activities at work and home during her menses. She underwent sonohysterography with findings of a 9-cm uterus with a 2-cm intramural myoma and no intracavitary lesions. Her hematocrit and Papanicolaou (Pap) smear are normal. She relates that she and her husband would like to have another child and asks what her options are to control her heavy bleeding.

Indications

Newer safety data on the use of contemporary intrauterine systems (IUS) and the relaxation of eligibility criteria have expanded use of these devices for both contraceptive and noncontraceptive benefits. The progestin-impregnated IUS was introduced in the 1970s to increase contraceptive efficacy and reduce expulsion rates by decreasing uterine contractility. The progestin exerts a local suppressive effect on the endometrium rendering it unresponsive to the proliferative effects of estrogen. This results in a reduction in the number of days of bleeding and progressive decrease in mean blood loss, sometimes to amenorrhea. Owing to these endometrial effects, use for noncontraceptive benefits is increasing, although this does represent off-label usage. The use of the levonorgestrel-releasing intrauterine system (LNG-IUS) in women with fibroids is somewhat controversial, but the available data support its use in women with fibroids that do not distort the uterine cavity.

Patient Selection

Prior to recommending an IUS for control of menorrhagia a thorough interview is necessary to establish the patient's preference for medical management. The advantages and disadvantages of LNG-IUS are shown in Table 12-1. Often desire for future fertility plays a large role in the patient's decision. A complete medical and surgical history with a specific focus on gynecologic and obstetric events must be obtained to ensure that the patient is an appropriate candidate. A long history of menorrhagia as well as nongynecologic bleeding episodes may prompt evaluation for hematologic disorders, most commonly von Willebrand disease. Subsequently, a physical examination is needed to evaluate for any concerns, especially those relating specifically to IUS placement, such as cervical stenosis and the presence of fibroids. Transvaginal ultrasound or sonohys-

Table 12-1 Advantages and Disadvantages of Levonorgestrel-Releasing Intrauterine System (LNG-IUS)

Advantages	Disadvantages
Office-based, allowing for flexible scheduling	Requires replacement every 5 years
Immediate resumption of normal activities	Initially may result in erratic bleeding patterns
Fertility retained after removal	Risk of expulsion or perforation
Cost-effective if use continued for 5 years	Unsuitable for women with cavity-distorting fibroids
Improved bleeding profile, with possible amenorrhea	Cultural or personal taboos related to contraceptive
Decreased dysmenorrhea	effects or presence of foreign body
Favorable side effect profile	

terography may be needed for further evaluation of the uterine cavity if fibroids are suspected. Irregular bleeding patterns may require an endometrial biopsy. Routine screening for sexually transmitted infections is not supported by available evidence but may be appropriate in a high-risk patient. Documentation of a current normal Pap smear is also prudent. Thorough and effective patient counseling to dispel common myths and ensure appropriate expectations for the IUS can serve to increase acceptance among patients.

Per current American College of Obstetrics and Gynecology (ACOG) guidelines, contraindications for IUS use include current pregnancy, current or recent pelvic inflammatory disease, current cervicitis, current or recent postpartum endometritis or infected abortion, undiagnosed abnormal uterine bleeding, known or suspected genital tract malignancy, allergy to any component of the IUS, and known uterine anomalies or fibroids that distort the uterine cavity in a way incompatible with IUS insertion. The package insert for the LNG-IUS currently marketed in the United States includes additional restrictions such as untreated bacterial vaginitis; acute liver disease or liver tumor; history of multiple sexual partners in the woman or her partner; increased susceptibility to infections, leukemia, acquired immune deficiency syndrome (AIDS) and intravenous (IV) drug abuse; genital actinomycosis; a previously inserted IUS that has not been removed; known or suspected carcinoma of the breast; or a history of ectopic pregnancy or condition that would predispose to ectopic pregnancy. Even though many of these contraindications appear reasonable, most are not directly described in the literature. Use of the IUS in nulliparas may be associated with an increased rate of expulsion but is not contraindicated; however, cervical dilation may be required.

Use of the IUS may reduce symptoms and therefore reduce the rate of diagnosis of fibroids. Comparison of various case series describing both success and failure of the LNG-IUS in ameliorating menorrhagia in women with fibroids reveals that outcomes in these patients may be dependent on overall uterine dimensions, fibroid size, and size of the uterine cavity. Studies have shown decreased mean blood loss with type II fibroids, meaning intramural fibroids that may have a submucosal component. Use of the IUS does not routinely result in decreased fibroid or uterine size and expulsion is more common with cavity-distorting fibroids. The World Health Organization (WHO) criteria state that insertion of the IUS in women with cavity-distorting fibroids who desire contraception represents an unacceptable risk.

Insertion Techniques

After the appropriate evaluation and discussion, informed consent and a negative pregnancy test on the day of the procedure must be obtained. Product brochures and replacement reminder cards should be given to the patient.

Product packaging for the LNG-IUS recommends placement during menses to avoid insertion with unknown pregnancy. Timing the insertion on day 5 to 7 may result in easier passage; however, the IUS can be inserted at any time in the cycle that pregnancy can be excluded. Misoprostol has been shown to aid insertion, but the effect of this medication on expulsion rate is not known.

A bimanual examination prior to insertion can aid placement by assessing uterine size and position.

Lower pain scores have been noted with the use of 2% intracervical lidocaine gel. Many practitioners advise patients to pretreatment with nonsteroidal anti-inflammatory drugs (NSAIDs) prior to insertion or they perform a paracervical block, but there are no data on efficacy of these types of analgesia.

Aseptic techniques should be followed throughout insertion and after placement of a vaginal speculum. The cervix should be cleansed.

A tenaculum is used to grasp the anterior lip of the cervix and the uterus sounded to determine patency of the endocervical canal and internal os. Placement of the tenaculum on the posterior lip may be more helpful if the uterus is retroflexed. In some women, especially nulliparous or perimenopausal, the sound cannot be passed and cervical dilation may be necessary. The uterus should sound within 6 to 10 cm and the product should not be placed into a cavity that is less than 6 cm. If no intracavitary assessment has been performed, sweeping the sound laterally at the fundus has been advocated to assess the feasibility of high fundal placement. In patients with a markedly retroverted uterus, placement under ultrasound guidance can be helpful to decrease perforation and ensure correct placement.

The IUS package should only be opened after these preparatory steps have been completed to decrease costs related to an unused but opened IUS. The IUS then is loaded into the insertion tube and the IUS threads secured. The IUS flange is set to the sounded depth. The loaded insertion tube is then advanced into the uterine cavity until it is 1.5 to 2 cm from the fundus. The IUS arms are then deployed and the IUS is advanced gently to the fundus. The insertion tube is gently retracted without pulling on the IUS strings. The strings are cut to 3 cm in length, taking care not to cut at an angle and may be tucked under the cervix to minimize partner discomfort during intercourse.

After insertion, the need for analgesia is assessed and the patient is counseled on expected bleeding patterns over the next several months. She is instructed to watch for signs of expulsion, pregnancy, and infection. Re-evaluation of string placement after 4 to 12 weeks should be scheduled, at which time the strings may be trimmed if needed. She is also instructed on how to check the strings herself. The patient should be advised to call with any concerns including bleeding, abnormal discharge, pelvic pain, fever, or painful intercourse.

Complications

Difficulties that can occur during IUS insertion include vasovagal reaction, cervical stenosis requiring dilation, failed insertion, or uterine perforation. Uterine perforation occurs in less than 0.5% of women. This risk may be increased in postpartum and lactating women and may be minimized by proper insertion technique. Suspected uterine perforation must be confirmed by ultrasound and the IUS removed by laparoscopy; rarely is laparotomy required. Expulsion can occur in up to 5% of patients and is increased in nulliparas and with postpartum or postabortal insertion. Occasionally the IUS is noted to be present in the cervix on physical examination or ultrasound. Advancing the IUS can be attempted with caution but the procedure should be abandoned if not easily completed. Following advancement, a pelvic ultrasound should be ordered with an additional string check following the next menses.

Early studies showing a link between IUS use and pelvic inflammatory disease (PID) are now thought to be flawed. PID infections are now thought to be rare among IUS users although there has been some increase in those with active infection at the time of placement or within the first 30 days. Prophylactic antibiotics are not currently recommended but could be considered in a high-risk patient. Current data show no effect on parameters such as hypertension, glucose control, or lipids aside from possible increase in high-density lipoproteins (HDLs), although more studies are needed.

Pregnancy rates with the IUS are similar for perfect and typical use with 5-year failure rates less than 0.5%. Pregnancy rates can be minimized by high fundal placement with subsequent decrease in partial or complete expulsion. The overall pregnancy rate remains extremely low; however, the relative rate of spontaneous abortion and ectopic pregnancy are increased. No specific congenital anomalies are associated with pregnancies with an IUS in place. Preterm delivery is more common under these circumstances.

Outcomes

Early discontinuation rates are highly linked to menstrual abnormalities and this decision may be tempered by counseling for realistic expectations prior to placement. Additional side effects are usually mild but can include weight gain, bloating, acne or oily skin, nausea, and breast pain. The first studies describing the use of the LNG-IUS for menorrhagia were performed in the 1980s. Since then the device has been shown to control bleeding more effectively than other medical regimens including hormonal treatments, prostaglandin inhibitors, antifibrinolytic agents, and nonsteroidal medications such as mefenemic acid. Although bleeding patterns in the first 4 to 6 months may be variable, overall bleeding can decrease by up to 90%. At 1 year of use, 20% of women experience complete amenorrhea. The rate of amenorrhea increases to 50% to 75% in women with menorrhagia, and in anemic women hemoglobin rises by 2 to 3 g/dL at 1 year. Cost analysis reveals that the LNG-IUS is less expensive than other medical regimens, possibly due to decreased need for surgical management of bleeding, and results in increased quality-adjusted life-years. The use of the LNG-IUS in women with known bleeding disorders also results in decreased blood loss and the device may have the same effect in women with adenomyosis.

Transcervical endometrial ablation has been compared to the LNG-IUS and results in greater initial decrease in blood loss, but similar rates at 3 years with comparable patient satisfaction. Additionally, placement of the IUS after global ablation can further improve bleeding profiles. Although post-ablation placement may be theoretically logical, it represents off-label usage. Also, the development of intense fibrosis and Asherman syndrome after ablation may make the IUS difficult to remove. When the LNG-IUS was provided to women on the waiting list for hysterectomy because of menstrual dysfunction, at 6 months 64.3% of women had canceled their surgery and at 12 months 47% still continued its use. Five-year follow-up results from a randomized controlled trial of the LNG-IUS compared to hysterectomy revealed comparable improvement in quality of life, with 48% of women indicated continued use. Expenses related to hysterectomy were noted to be three times higher and the IUS was felt to be a cost-effective alternative to hysterectomy in the first year of use. Additional benefits of the LNG-IUS include retained fertility and no requirement for operative skills or surgical facilities.

Many studies have included dysmenorrhea as a secondary outcome with improvement in pain scores after IUS insertion. One study noted improvement in endometriosis staging after IUS insertion. The device is also under evaluation in clinical studies for the prevention of endometrial hyperplasia. Use of the LNG-IUS in high-risk women with known uterine cancer has been described in case reports. Thus, the LNG-IUS represents an effective office-based intervention to the patient with menorrhagia, although limited in its scope by the extent of uterine disease.

Hysteroscopic Myomectomy

Case Presentation

J.B. is a 51-year-old, gravida 7, para 6 who recently noted changes in her menstrual cycles. Previously her cycles were every 28 to 30 days and lasted 4 to 5 days. She changed her menstrual products (pads or tampons) three to four times daily. She did not have dysmenorrhea and her menstrual cycles did not interfere with her lifestyle. Within the past 6 to 9 months, her cycles are still monthly, but last for 8 to 10 days, requiring her to change her menstrual products every 1 to 2 hours, with night-time changing, soiling through clothing, and avoiding travel, sports, and leisurely activities during her cycles. On examination, her uterine size felt normal without adnexal masses. Recent laboratory findings included a normal Pap test and negative human papillomavirus (HPV) test. Anemia was detected: hemoglobin 8.0 g/dL and hematocrit 27%, normal platelet count. Her thyroid-stimulating hormone (TSH) level was normal. Saline infusion sonography revealed a posterior 3.3 cm intracavitary leiomyoma (Fig. 12-1). She was scheduled for operative hysteroscopic myomectomy.

Discussion of Case

The desire of many women to retain their uterus and return to normal activities quickly prompted the emergence of less invasive technologies for the treatment of symptomatic fibroids. In the early 1980s, the urologic resectoscope was first used to remove intrauterine polyps and fibroids. The development of a continuous flow hysteroscope resectoscope permitted distention of the uterine cavity with fluid and removal of blood and debris (Fig. 12-2). Ancillary wire loops, scissors, morcellators, and vaporizing electrodes permit numerous procedures (Fig. 12-3). Resectoscopy permits removal of endometrial polyps, submucosal fibroids, targeted and directed endometrial biopsy, division of uterine septa, and endometrial ablation. Further improvements in optics, video recording, and intrauterine distention systems provided additional safety features for operative hysteroscopic procedures.

Operative hysteroscopic myomectomy requires an understanding of fluid management; good hand–eye coordination; sound judgment about when to abandon the hysteroscopic approach; and a thorough preoperative evaluation including a detailed knowledge of the number, size, location, and depth of myometrial involvement of the fibroids.

Figure 12-1 Saline infusion sonography with intracavitary leiomyoma.

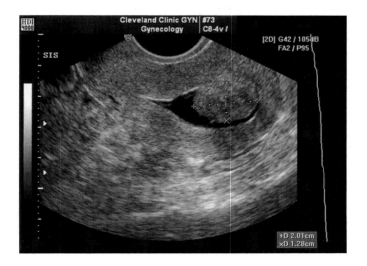

Figure 12-2 Handle of operative hysteroscope.

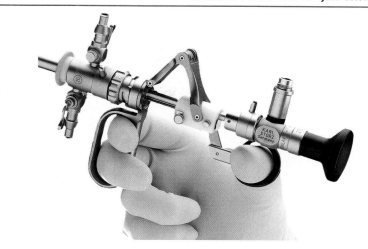

Figure 12-3 Operative hysteroscope and tips.

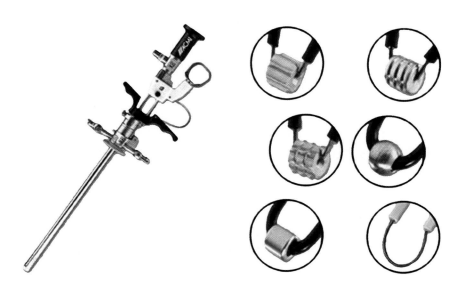

Preoperative Evaluation

Preoperative evaluation of the uterine cavity is important to determine the size, number, location, and depth of penetration of the leiomyoma. These factors will determine the surgical expertise necessary, risks, and surgical complications, as well as the ability to complete the procedure in one surgical setting. Most important, these factors determine whether a hysteroscopic surgical approach is indicated. Patient selection criteria for operative hysteroscopy are shown in Table 12-2.

There is no hysteroscopic classification system that is uniformly accepted. However, Wamsteker and associates (1993) and Lasmar and associates (2005) agree that the depth of myometrial involvement determines the degree of difficulty, surgical expertise, and risks of fluid overload. The European Society of Gynaecological Endoscopy (ESGE) classification considers only the degree of myometrial penetration, which is determined hysteroscopically. Type G0 myomas are completely within the endometrial cavity; type G1 myomas extend less than 50% into the myometrium; and type G2 have more than 50% of their volume within the myometrium. The ESGE system is derived hysteroscopically and therefore depth of myometrial involvement is subjec-

Table 12-2 Patient Selection for Operative Hysteroscopy

Indications for Operative Hysteroscopy	Contraindications to Operative Hysteroscopy
Removal of intracavitary fibroids and some intramural fibroids	Viable intrauterine pregnancy
Endometrial polypectomy	Active pelvic infection
Removal of endocervical lesions	Active or prodromal herpes infection
Retrieval of foreign bodies (e.g., laminaria tents, embedded intrauterine devices, displaced intrauterine systems, suture, retained products of conception)	Cervical cancer
Excision of intrauterine adhesions or septa	Uterine perforation
Targeted endometrial biopsies	
Ablation/resection of the endometrium	
Hysteroscopic sterilization	
Tuboplasty or cannualization	

tively obtained and may be influenced by intrauterine distending media and pressure.

The ESGE classification system recommends that resection of leiomyoma be limited to type 0 and type 1 myomas, unless a surgeon has expert hysteroscopic skills. Although the ESGE does not specify a size limitation, the physician should be aware of increasing complexity of surgery when the fibroid is greater than 4 to 5 cm. Limited operative views, narrower surgical spaces, and the accumulation of large leiomyoma chips can lead to increased operative time and subsequent volume overload. Increased physician experience is required in these cases to safely and successfully navigate hysteroscopic myomectomy.

The choice of anesthesia—local, regional, or general—depends upon many factors, such as surgeon's preference, patient's medical status, type and complexity of the procedure, facility capabilities, and patient preference.

Procedure for Hysteroscopic Myomectomy

Prior to hysteroscopy, inspection of the vulva and bimanual examination is necessary to determine uterine position and to exclude adnexal or pelvic tenderness. Knowledge of the uterine position will help orient placement of the hysteroscope and decrease the risk of uterine perforation. After the speculum is inserted, the cervix is visualized and then cleansed with an antiseptic solution. Hysteroscopy should not be performed in the presence of mucopurulent cervicitis, pelvic inflammatory disease, or herpetic infections.

Vaginoscopic or no-touch technique has increasingly has been advocated. Without use of a speculum, the hysteroscope is introduced in the lower vagina and cervix. Proponents advocate its use because it is associated with less pain, and decreases the need for premedication, analgesia, or anesthesia when used in office diagnostic hysteroscopy. It can also be used during operative hysteroscopy.

In the absence of infection, the distal end of hysteroscope is inserted into the cervix and panoramic inspection of the endocervix performed. The hysteroscope should be advanced under direct inspection with distention medium and without undue force into the uterine cavity. Once inside the uterine cavity the topography of the endometrial cavity and tubal ostia is assessed. When fluid is used for uterine distention, the maximal pressure is 100 mm Hg. Ideally the intrauterine pressure should be maintained at less than the mean arterial pressure. However, if higher pressures are needed for visualization, close monitoring of the fluid deficit is necessary.

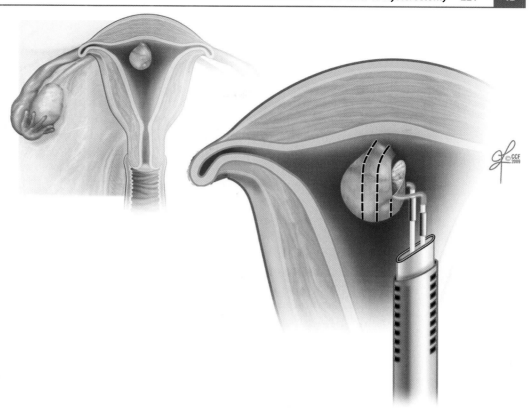

The operative resectoscope is an adaptation of the urologic resectoscope, with the added ability to provide continuous circulation of fluid. The continuous flow mechanism clears debris and mucus, permitting excellent visualization throughout the surgical procedure.

Hysteroscopic myomectomy is commonly performed using a resectoscope. Currently there are four hysteroscopic methods to remove intracavitary leiomyoma: wire loop resection, vaporizing electrode, hysteroscopic morcellator, and scissors. Once inside the endocervix, the exact location of the lesion(s) should be determined, the uterotubal ostia visualized, and size of the lesion(s) confirmed. These maneuvers map out the surgical procedure to provide the safest operative strategy for hysteroscopic removal. When multiple lesions are encountered, removal of the lesions nearest the cervix and posterior wall is advised, followed by resection of more fundal and lateral lesions.

The basic resection technique involves serial slicing or shaving of a lesion until it is flush with the endometrium (Fig. 12-4). The wire loop (monopolar or bipolar) is placed behind the lesion and drawn toward the physician when the electrode is activated. Cutting begins at the surface, with the trajectory always directed toward the operator, keeping the loop visible at all times. With each passage of the wire loop, crescent-shaped pieces of tissue will float into the uterine cavity. When visualization is obscured, the accumulated fibroid pieces should be removed with the wire loop, Corson graspers, or polyp forceps. When tissue chips are removed blindly, care must be taken to prevent uterine perforation. Although fibroid chips may pass spontaneously, leaving them within the uterus may result in colicky pain, persistent leukorrhea, adhesions, or intrauterine infection. Furthermore, pathologic examination of the tissue is essential. (See DVD Video 12-1 for video demonstration of Hysteroscopic Myomectomy. 📹)

Additional Techniques

Fibroids may have a myometrial attachment. Full enucleation requires expert hysteroscopic skills and identification of the surgical planes. To facilitate removal, intermittent uterine decompression, manual massage, injection of prostaglandin $F_{2\alpha}$, and wire loop mechanical resection techniques have been described. The use of preoperative Cytotec 200 to 400 µg, orally or vaginally taken at bedtime prior to hysteroscopic myomectomy, facilitates cervical dilation and may increase uterine contractions to assist in the enucleation of leiomyomas.

A variety of cutting and coagulating loops, barrels, or balls are available. Monopolar and bipolar operative hysteroscopes are currently available. When a monopolar operative hysteroscope is used, a dispersive pad must be placed on the patient and a nonelectrolyte, nonconducting, distending medium such as 1.5% glycine, 3% sorbitol, or 5% mannitol must be used. With a bipolar device, saline or Ringer lactate is used and the patient does not need a dispersive pad.

Recently, a Hysteroscopic Morcellation System (Smith & Nephew, Andover, MA) and MyoSure Tissue Removal System (Interlace Medical, Framingham, MA) were introduced that resect intracavitary lesions without electrical energy and utilizes saline as the distending medium. A recent modification of the traditional hysteroresectoscope, the Chip E-Vac system (Richard Wolf Corp., Vernon Hills, IL) is currently available in the United States as a bipolar system, and permits rapid resection of intracavitary lesions. The added benefit is that the resected fibroid "chips" are suctioned through the hysteroscopic sheath. This adaptation is beneficial because it reduces the number of fibroid "chips" within the uterine cavity, decreases the frequency of needing to remove the hysteroscope for fibroid chip retrieval, and keeps the operating field clear of debris. Additionally, saline is used as the distention medium. Most hysteroscopic sheaths have an outer diameter of 7 to 10 mm and include both inflow and outflow ports for distending media.

Historically, grasping forceps, such as Leahy clamps or Corson graspers, have been placed within the uterine cavity and in the hopes that blind grasping of an intracavitary lesion would lead to avulsion technique and retrieval of tissue. If this method is chosen, it is important to look hysteroscopically after attempts at blind retrieval have been undertaken to decrease the chances of incomplete removal or remnants of tissue left in situ. Blind attempts at grasping intracavitary lesions also can be associated with uterine perforation, bowel injury, or uterine inversion.

Targeted endometrial biopsies are indicated when focal lesions are noted. The endometrial surface may have focal irregularities, polypoid projections, and discrete lesions. Using the wire loop, hysteroscopic targeted biopsies with complete removal of lesions may be obtained and sent for histologic analysis.

Among women wishing to preserve fertility, some gynecologists empirically prescribe high-dose estrogen to aid in re-epithelization of the endometrium with the aim of decreasing the risk of intrauterine adhesions after hysteroscopic myomectomy. Typically, conjugated estrogen 1.25 daily or estradiol 1 mg twice daily is given for 30 days, followed by 12 days of progesterone (i.e., norethindrone 5 mg or medroxyprogesterone 10 mg). Alternatively, a pediatric Foley catheter, inflated with 5 to 10 mL of normal saline or sterile water is inserted for 7 to 10 days to prevent the juxtaposition of the uterine walls. If an indwelling pediatric is placed, prophylactic use of doxycycline 100 mg orally twice daily until the catheter is removed is advised. Repeat office hysteroscopy is performed within 7 to 14 days following extensive myomectomy to evaluate the endometrium for synechiae. We advocate office flexible hysteroscopy when the pediatric foley is removed. If detected early, the adhesions are filmy and easily lysed with the distal tip of a hysteroscope.

Electrocautery and Laser

Specially adapted loop electrodes, roller balls, and vaporizing electrodes can be used to resect, desiccate, or ablate endometrial tissue. When monopolar electrodes are used, a cutting current of 60 W to 100 W is utilized. When bipolar electrical energy is utilized the default settings are applied. Generally speaking wire loop resection is performed for procedures such as polypectomy, submucous resection, and endomyometrial resection ablation. Rollerballs are used for hysteroscopic endometrial ablation. The neodymium:yttrium-aluminum-garnet (Nd:YAG), argon, and potassium titanyl phosphate (KTP) lasers can be used for hysteroscopic surgery. Lasers can be used to perform endometrial ablation, lysis of adhesions, or desiccation of intracavitary lesions. Lasers are more expensive to maintain, require additional nursing and surgeon training, and have little advantage over electrosurgical resection techniques.

Distention Media

General Principles

The endometrial cavity is a potential space. It must be distended with fluid or CO_2. Operative hysteroscopy is generally performed with fluid. The type of electrical energy utilized determines the selection of fluids. Monopolar energy requires hypotonic, low-viscosity fluids such as glycine 1.5%, sorbitol 3%, or mannitol 5%. Bipolar energy requires isotonic solutions such as normal saline or Ringer lactate. Glycine, a low-viscosity fluid, is used with monopolar electrocautery because it is a poor electrical conductor, minimizes hemolysis during irrigation, and provides excellent optical images. If electrolytic solutions are inadvertently used during monopolar resectoscopy, there is diffusion of electrical current and the wire loop will not cut.

During hysteroscopy, the major mechanism of fluid loss is through systemic intravascular absorption. Very little fluid is lost via the fallopian tubes. When excessive absorption of electrolyte-free solution occurs systemically, hyponatremia may ensue. When the serum sodium level declines, there is an increase in the hypotonic solutes from the distention media causing a decline in serum osmolality. Glycine is a nonessential amino acid and is metabolized in the liver and kidney by oxidative deamination via glycine oxidase to ammonia and glycolic acid. Encephalopathy occurs as a result of ammonia toxicity. In the midbrain, spinal cord, and ganglion cells in the retina, glycine has an inhibitory effect. Transient blindness may be due to these mechanisms. The greatest risk of morbidity and mortality in operative hysteroscopy is due to fluid overload. Clinical symptoms from hyponatremia can occur when the serum sodium levels are below 120 mmol/L. Postoperatively, signs of hyponatremia include nervous system agitation, nausea, vomiting, headache, blurred vision, and seizures.

Factors that increase the risk of fluid intravasation include excessive intrauterine pressure, resection of large fibroids, prolonged operative times, deep myometrial resection, resection of septa, and treatment of Asherman syndrome. Close attention to fluid deficits are advised. Electronic fluid pumps or a dedicated nurse who calculates input and output are imperative for patient safety.

Bipolar energy requires normal saline or Ringer lactate. Isotonic solutions, by virtue of their serum osmolality and sodium content, prevent the development of hyponatremia and hypo-osmolality. The use of isotonic solutions does not decrease the risk of excessive intravasation. Excessive intravascular absorption of saline can be associated with congestive heart failure and pulmonary edema. Avoidance of preoperative overhydration and minimal intravenous hydration should be communicated with the anesthesiologist when complicated cases are anticipated.

Fluid Management

Fluid management systems (fluid pumps) play a vital role in the safety of operative hysteroscopy. Many fluid management systems are available; patient safety is increased when guidelines for managing fluid absorption are followed. These pumps provide an automated system with minute-to-minute calculation of inflow and calculation of the fluid deficit. The physician can preset the allowable fluid deficit, based on the patient's risk factors (age, cardiovascular reserve, and renal function). Automatic audible alerts will alert the surgeon when the maximal fluid deficit has been reached. An additional advantage to the fluid pump is the ability to determine intrauterine pressure and to easily adjust fluid pressures to control bleeding and decrease "false negative" views of the endometrial cavity that may occur with higher or constant endometrial pressure. Alternating the intrauterine fluid pressure may also help facilitate full resection of uterine fibroids by causing myometrial contraction, which helps enucleate the myoma. Automated fluid pumps are essential in modern operative hysteroscopy. Less desirable is the technique of elevating the bags above the patient and infusing by the force of gravity or placed in a large blood pressure cuff and infused by pressurizing the cuff. Because fluid can rapidly and unpredictably be absorbed, continuous deficit monitoring is essential. If fluid pumps are not available, a nurse dedicated to calculating the I/O's every 5 to 10 minutes is necessary.

Complications

Patients generally have minimal postoperative pain following hysteroscopic myomectomy. A serosanguinous discharge for 1 to 4 weeks is typical following the procedure. Mild cramping is easily alleviated with low-dose NSAIDs, and a few patients require narcotics for postoperative pain management. Patients typically resume normal activities within 24 to 48 hours after the procedure. Sexual activity can be resumed 1 week postoperatively. If an incomplete resection has occurred, some patients may pass pieces of fibroid tissue several weeks after the procedure or complain of leukorrhea and cramping.

Common intraoperative complications of resectoscopic surgery include uterine perforation and absorption of distending medium. Two ancillary medications, vasopressin and misoprostol, may decrease the risks associated with operative hysteroscopy. The most common complication of operative hysteroscopy is uterine perforation. Cervical stenosis and deep myometrial resection increase the risk of perforation and fluid absorption. A prospective double-blind study and randomized clinical trial demonstrated the benefits of dilute vasopressin (Phillips et al, 1996). Vasopressin decreases fluid absorption, decreases blood loss, decreases fluid intravasation, and induces smooth muscle contractions of the uterine capillaries, small arterioles, and venules. Its use is advocated when prolonged surgery, larger lesions, or deeper myometrial resection is anticipated, or when cervical stenosis is encountered.

To decrease the risk of uterine perforation due to cervical stenosis and difficult cervical dilation, misoprostol may be considered. Misoprostol is a prostaglandin PGE_1 analog used for cervical ripening. Misoprostol increases intracellular accumulation of free water, softens the cervix, and passively increases the diameter of the cervical os. These factors combined lead to easier cervical dilation, decreased risk of cervical lacerations, uterine perforation, and creation of false tracks during dilation. Various routes (oral, vaginal, rectal, and sublingual), dosages, and times of administration have been advocated. Alternatively a laminaria tent can be inserted the day before the surgical procedure.

Patients with postoperative fever, malaise, worsening pain, or escalating pain medication requirements should be carefully evaluated for bowel injury, bladder injury, and endometritis. Office evaluation must be undertaken including thorough abdominal and pelvic examination. Laboratory testing including electrolytes, complete blood count (CBC), sedimentation rate, ultrasound, and flat plate of the abdomen (kidney, ureter, bladder [KUB]/upright film) may be required, depending upon the clinical scenario. Sometimes a computed tomography (CT) scan of the pelvis/abdomen may be needed if perforation with bowel or bladder injury is suspected.

Conclusions

Patients now have an array of options available for the treatment of symptomatic uterine fibroids. Hysteroscopic myomectomy is a well-established treatment for women with hysteroscopically resectable uterine fibroids. Preoperative evaluation is essential to the success of the procedure. Appropriately triaged patients have excellent outcome, low morbidity rate, and resolution of menstrual aberrations. Additionally, intraoperative hysteroscopic techniques to facilitate complete removal and close attention to fluid management provide optimal safety and improved clinical outcome.

Endometrial Ablation

Case Presentation

A 41-year-old gravida 4, para 3 female reports a long history of heavy regular periods without associated dysmenorrhea. Her past medical history is notable for multiple deep venous thromboses (DVT) and she is now on lifelong anticoagulation. Her past surgical history is significant for one prior cesarean section with tubal ligation. On examination, she is not obese and has a normal 10-week size anteverted uterus. On saline infusion sonography, she is noted to have a 10-cm uterus with a single 2-cm submucus fibroid. Evaluation of her prior lower uterine segment uterine scar reveals normal thickness (>10 mm) in this area. She denies symptomatic pelvic organ prolapse or incontinence. Previous attempts to manage her bleeding included Depo-Provera, that caused irregular bleeding, and a Mirena Intrauterine Device (Bayer Health Care Pharmaceuticals, Montville, NJ), was declined by the patient. Recent endometrial biopsy and cervical cytologic findings are normal. She would like to avoid hysterectomy if possible due to her history of DVT and use of anticoagulation.

Endometrial ablation plays a unique role in the spectrum of treatment for menorrhagia. Treatment is indicated for women who have primary menorrhagia disruptive to quality of life, have failed or cannot tolerate medical therapy, and have completed childbearing. For most women, ablation results in marked improvement in bleeding with 65% to 70% experiencing hypomenorrhea. Between 5% and 19% of women fail therapy immediately and 6% to 40% require an additional surgical procedure within 5 years of surgery. Ablation of the endometrium is associated with fewer complications than hysterectomy and greater cost savings to the patient as well as the health care system.

First-generation endometrial ablation techniques include use of laser, roller-ball, or endometrial resection. These modalities are performed under hysteroscopic guidance and require careful fluid monitoring and advanced operator skill. Second-generation devices attempt to streamline the process of destroying the basalis layer of the endometrium. Although these modalities are faster and more user friendly, they are consequently more limited in their application to more complex cases involving fibroids or patients with previous uterine surgery.

A recent Cochrane review found a decreased operative time, increased use of local anesthesia, and increased rates of device malfunction with global devices in comparison to hysteroscopic ablative techniques. In addition, second-generation techniques were also associated with less fluid overload, uterine perforation, cervical lacerations, and hematometra, but more nausea, vomiting and uterine cramping.

Patient Selection

Patients considering endometrial ablation for menorrhagia must have completed childbearing, as pregnancy after destruction of the endometrial lining is contraindicated. Patients may have tried and failed medical therapy or be limited by contraindications to medical treatments. Women must be willing to accept some degree of menstrual bleeding as amenorrhea does not ensue for all patients.

Preoperative Evaluation and Preparation

Patients must be carefully evaluated to exclude an underlying premalignant or malignant cause of bleeding or underlying coagulopathy such as von Willebrand disease. Imaging should reveal an anatomically normal uterus with a cavity length of 6 to 14 cm depending on the device used. Assessment of the uterine cavity is needed ensure that bleeding is not related to intracavitary structural lesions such as submucosal fibroids or endometrial polyps. Saline infusion sonograph should be utilized to ensure the absence of intracavitary pathology. Additionally, TVUS should be considered after prior cesarean section to ensure that the lower uterine segment is >10 mm. Endometrial biopsy is recommended in women older than 40 years, or in those with risk factors for endometrial hyperplasia or malignancy. Patients should not have active genital or urinary tract infections at the time of the procedure and should have documentation of normal cervical cytologic appearance within the past year. Ablation is contraindicated in the postmenopausal woman. Patients will still require progesterone in combination with estrogen if therapy for menopausal symptoms is needed. Contraception is also necessary.

When hysteroscopic techniques are used, endometrial thinning improves visualization and can ensure full desiccation of the basalis layer with subsequent improved outcomes. All currently FDA-approved devices except Novasure required endometrial thinning in trial protocols usually by gonadotropin-releasing hormone (GnRH) agonist or mechanical curettage. The most inexpensive method for endometrial thinning is timing the procedure between cycle days 4 and 7 when the endometrium is less than 10 mm. Dilation and curettage (D&C) can serve to remove the superficial endometrium as well as to obtain a pathologic specimen. If microwave technology is utilized, then a D&C should not be performed prior to microwave endometrial ablation. Hormonal medical treatments, including GnRH agonists, danazol, progestogens, and oral contraceptive pills, may improve surgical results with variable efficacy. Administration of 200 to 400 μg of misoprostol orally or vaginally 8 to12 hours prior to the procedure can ease cervical dilation.

Surgical Techniques

Office Ablation Procedures

All modalities of global endometrial ablation are approved for use under general anesthesia as well as conscious sedation or local anesthesia. A comparison of available devices is shown in Table 12-3. New Current Procedural Terminology (CPT) codes now permit reimbursement for office ablation. Advantages of office procedure include saving time for physician and patient as well as more flexible scheduling. In most cases the procedure can be completed under local anesthesia, with use of preoperative NSAIDs, narcotics, antiemetics, and anxiolytics. Performance of a paracervical block can decrease pain in the office or operating room. Many different regimens for oral and injected pain medications are described in the literature with no evidence of superiority; therefore, each physician should choose and develop familiarity with the side effects and toxicities of a select few. Careful evaluation of the patient's co-morbid conditions, anxiety level, and comfort on routine pelvic examination and endometrial biopsy allows for selection of individuals who can successfully complete the ablation without general anesthesia.

Balloon Ablation

The ThermaChoice Uterine Balloon Therapy System (Gynecare, Somerville, NJ; Fig. 12-5) was the first global endometrial device and as such has the most robust clinical data regarding outcomes. The ThermaChoice III device consists of a 16 cm by 4.5 mm shaft with a silicone balloon catheter at its distal end enclosing an internal propeller to circulate fluid during the procedure. Initial FDA trials were conducted with the ThermaChoice I with a latex balloon that lacked the internal impeller. The newer devices have undergone significant modifications that have resulted in improved treatment of the uterine cornua and lower uterine segment with a noticeable clinical effect. A separate control unit monitors temperature, uterine pressure, and timing of the procedure. The balloon is inflated with up to 35 mL of 5% dextrose in water (D_5W) and the

Table 12-3 Comparison of Global Endometrial Ablation Devices

Device	Energy Type	Cervical Dilation	Cavity Size	Treatment Time	Pretreatment Used	Size of Intramural Fibroids Treated	Safety Features
ThermaChoice	Thermal balloon	4.5 cm	6–10 cm	8 min	Suction curettage	≤2 cm	Pressure and temperature shutoff
HerOption	Cryotherapy	4.5 cm	≤10 cm	15–20 min	GnRH agonist	≤2 cm	Ultrasound guidance
Novasure	Radiofrequency	8 cm	6–10 cm, 2.5 cm wide	1.5 min	None	≤2 cm	Cavity integrity check Measured tissue impedance
HydroTherm-Ablator	Heated fluid	8 cm	≤10.5 cm	10 min	GnRH agonist	≤3 cm	Hysteroscopic guidance Recirculated fluid monitoring
MEA	Microwave	8.5 cm	6–14 cm	2–5 min	GnRH agonist	≤3 cm	Intraoperative feedback, temperature Preoperative ultrasound and hysteroscopy

GnRH, gonadotropin-releasing hormone.

Figure 12-5 Balloon ablation: the ThermaChoice control unit and device.

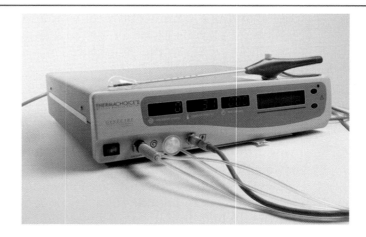

Figure 12-6 Her Option® Global Endornetrial Ablation unit.

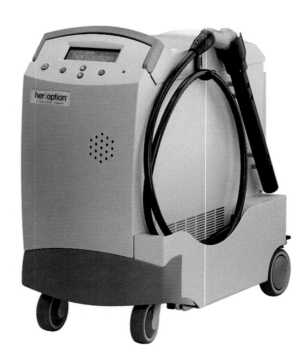

pressure is maintained between 160 to 180 mm Hg at a temperature of 87°C for 8 minutes followed by a cool-down phase. Subsequently the balloon is deflated and discarded.

ThermaChoice has also been used successfully in women with a fibroid uterus with a 10% rate of hysterectomy at 1 year. Data from case series yield an improved amenorrhea rate; and decreased premenstrual symptoms, dysmenorrhea, and need for pain medication during menses. The optimal uterine cavity for ThermaChoice is less than 10 cm and in trials the uterine cavity was pretreated by suction D&C. Minimal cervical dilation is required to allow passage of the 4.5mm device. It is important to slowly inflate the balloon to ensure accurate and appropriate pressures and adequate treatment of the entire uterine cavity.

Cryoablation

The Her Option® Global Endornetrial Ablation System (Cooper Surgical, Inc, Trumbull, CT) was approved in April 2001 (Figs. 12-6, 12-7). This device uses

Figure 12-7 Her Option® device.

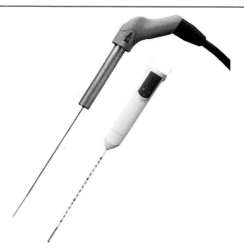

Figure 12-8 Her Option® in use under ultrasound. RT, Right; LT, left.

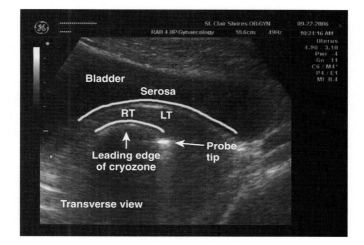

a cryoprobe that freezes the endometrium to −100 to −120 degrees Celsius, causing endometrial cell death. The cryoprobe measured 4.5 mm in diameter, requiring minimal cervical dilation and continuous transabdominal ultrasound monitoring is required (Fig. 12-8). The FDA protocol also required pretreatment with a single dose of 3.75 mg leuprolide acetate and consisted of a 4-minute freeze at one cornua, followed by a 6-minute freeze at the remaining cornua. In common usage, often a third freeze for 4 to 6 minutes in the lower uterine segment is performed, with a total treatment time of 15 to 20 minutes. Again, the optimal uterine cavity is less than 10 cm and minimal cervical dilation is required. This system provides a greater depth of tissue destruction to 9 to 12 mm.

Radiofrequency Ablation

The Novasure RF Ablation system (Cytec Corp, Marlborough, MA) consists of a gold-plated mesh electrode that conforms to the uterine cavity after deployment (Fig. 12-9). This system was FDA approved in 2001 and consists of the disposable device connected to a control unit, CO_2 tank, desiccant, foot switch, and power cord. Tissue impedance is continually measured and the procedure is stopped when 50 ohms is reached, which signifies that the endometrium has been vaporized and the device is contacting myometrium. Thus, a thicker endometrium will prolong the treatment time. The sheath measures

Figure 12-9 Novasure controller and device.

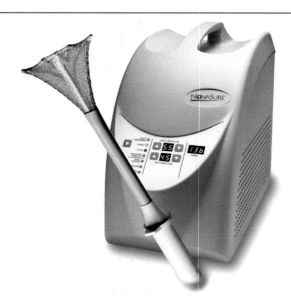

7.2 mm and use is advised for cavity size of 6 to 10 cm with a width of at least 2.5 cm.

In order to calculate the treatment time, the uterine sounding length and width of the uterine cavity is entered into the Novasure controller. The required power level is then calculated by the generator. By tapping the foot pedal, a cavity integrity check is performed to assess for uterine perforation. A second tap on the foot pedal initiates the treatment cycle, lasting from 40 to 120 seconds with 180 W of power at 500 kHz. During this time the suction device removes debris and moisture to achieve a treatment depth of 4.0 to 4.5 mm in the uterine body, with 2.2 to 2.9 mm at the uterine cornua. The device has the shortest treatment cycle and in FDA trials was used without endometrial pre-treatment on any cycle day. Additional trials have specifically evaluated the use of Novasure with polyps up to 2 cm and submucous fibroids with good results.

Hysteroscopic Thermal Ablation

The HydroThermAblator (HTA; Boston Scientific, Natick, MA) was approved in April 2001 (Figs. 12-10, 12-11). The device consists of a single-use 7.8-mm sheath with a 3-mm rigid hysteroscope that circulates heated saline in the uterine cavity under constant hysteroscopic visualization for 10 minutes. Fluid is maintained between 80° F and 90° F. The height of the fluid bag is adjusted to maintain the uterine pressure between 50 and 55 mm Hg, below the threshold for transtubal spillage. Overdilation of the cervix greater than 8 mm and the use of preoperative laminaria or misoprostol may increase the rate of transvaginal leakage. Use of a secondary or four-toothed tenaculum, a laparoscopic endoloop or even a cervical cerclage may be employed to avoid vaginal spillage and burns. The HTA sheath may also be fixed to the cervical grasping tenaculum using a cervical stabilizer device. Visualization of the cervix is necessary to identify a non–water-tight seal and adjust accordingly. The tip of the hysteroscope is kept just inside the cervical os.

Depth of endomyometrial necrosis ranges from 3 to 4 mm. The volume of fluid recirculated is monitored and the device shuts off if more than 10 mL is lost. A small amount of loss may be anticipated due to transcervical leakage or uterine relaxation; however, larger volumes are associated with uterine perforation. The FDA trial excluded women with any uterine anatomic anomaly and

Figure 12-10 HydroThermoAblafor (HTA) unit.

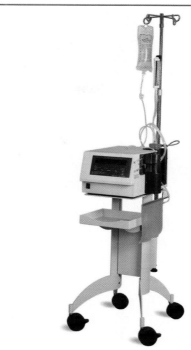

Figure 12-11 HydroThermoAblafor (HTA) device.

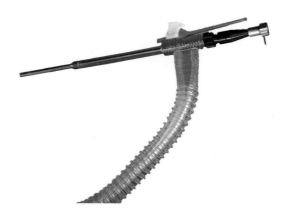

cavity length greater than 10.5 cm and required pretreatment with 7.5 mg of leuprolide acetate 3 weeks prior to the procedure. Retrospective trials have described the use of HTA in women with submucous fibroids 3 to 5 cm and müllerian anomalies, but further studies of efficacy are needed. HTA has also been associated with a temporary white discoloration of the cervix that resolves by 4 weeks.

Microwave Endometrial Ablation

The Microsulis MEA (FemWave, Microsulis Americas, Waltham, MA) was FDA approved in 2003 and uses microwave energy at a frequency of 9.2 GHz to destroy the endometrium (Fig. 12-12). The MEA has been used for patients with cavities up to 14 cm and in those with fibroids or polyps up to 3 cm that may distort the uterine cavity but still allow passage of the probe. Continuous temperature monitoring allows the surgeon to individualize treatment to each area of the cavity (Fig. 12-13). Microwave ablation treats to a depth of 5 to 6 mm and should be used only in areas where the myometrium is greater than 10 mm. In areas where the probe is not in direct contact with the

Figure 12-12 Microsulis unit and device.

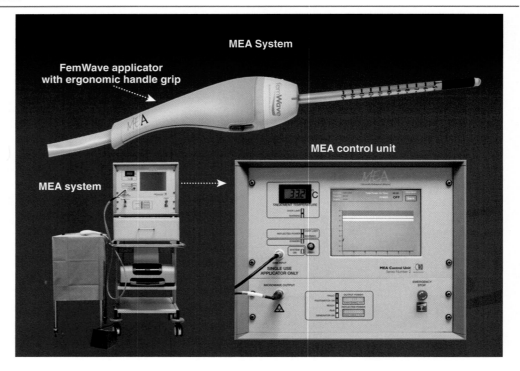

GUIDANCE THROUGHOUT TREATMENT

Consistencies across best techniques:

- Complete fundal treatment
- Treatment of each cornu
- Continuous sweeping of corpus adapting to irregularities
- Continued treatment in lower segment

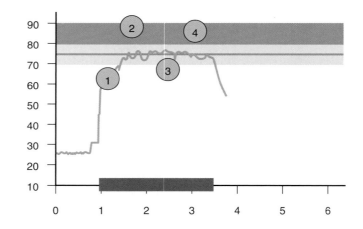

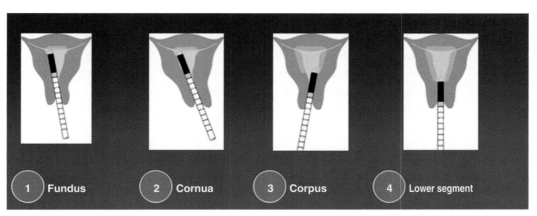

Figure 12-13 Microsulis treatment cycle.

endometrium the microwave energy still penetrates to a depth of 3 mm, allowing treatment of areas such as the tubal ostia. Overall treatment time is 2 to 5 minutes.

Hysteroscopy should be performed on the day of the procedure with careful attention to uterine landmarks. Dilation and curettage should not be performed. After cervical dilation is performed the 8.5-mm FemWave probe is inserted to the midfundus and swept across the fundus, while maintaining the temperature between 70° F and 80° F. Once the fundus is treated, both cornua are treated for an additional 5 seconds. Lastly the applicator is withdrawn using a sweeping motion to treat the remainder of the cavity while maintaining a constant temperature.

The conductive heating allows for a "spray paint" effect that allows treatment of distorted endometrium. The physician can ensure adequate treatment of each part of the uterine cavity using the data provided by the therapeutic band.

Selecting a Second-Generation Ablation Device

Current data have not demonstrated superior treatment efficacy or patient satisfaction with any single ablation system; therefore, choice of an ablation device should be dictated by provider comfort and experience. Other concerns such as cost, device size, need for cervical dilation, availability of technical and support staff, office or ambulatory setting, and length of procedure may also play a significant role.

Complications

Overall adverse events such as sepsis, blood loss, urinary retention, hemorrhage, blood transfusion, and vaginal vault and wound hematomas are less common with endometrial ablation than after hysterectomy, as are anesthesia complications. Complications during FDA trials were mostly minor and rare and included urinary tract infections, vaginal infections, fever, endometritis, thermal injury, abdominal pain, hematometra, and bacteremia. Adverse events occurring in general use are better represented by the Manufacturer and User Facility Device Experience (MAUDE) database maintained by the FDA. A review of the MAUDE events from 2003 to 2006 included more morbid effects such as bowel injury, CO_2 embolism, urinary tract injury, severe burns, laparotomy, hysterectomy, other major surgery, necrotizing fasciitis, cardiac arrest, and death. Minor complications reported in general usage include minor burns, pelvic infections, endocarditis, uterine perforation, postoperative bleeding, hematometra, pain, and failure of the device. The most common reported complication type varies among ablation devices. Major and minor burns were most common with HTA, bowel injury was reported most often with HerOption and MEA, possibly related to greater dependence on surgeon control. Adverse events resulting from physician error and out of protocol use were more common with MEA, and HerOption. ThermaChoice and Novasure had the highest number of complications relating to instrument or procedure errors.

Outcomes

Blood loss improves in 87% to 97% of women and amenorrhea results in 14% to 55%. Additional surgery for menstrual bleeding was required in 6% to 40% of women. Ablation is therefore initially less expensive than hysterectomy; however, the additional costs related to reoperation narrow this divide. Enhanced use of ablation in the office setting may further decrease costs.

Women in their late 40s have a lower reoperation rate than those in their early 40s. When reoperation is needed, it is most offen due to recurrent menstrual dysfunction, cyclic abdominal pain, or pelvic pain. Type of endometrial ablation, outpatient location, and presence of fibroids did not increase hysterectomy risk. Myomectomy at the time of ablation was associated with decreased risk for further surgery. Risk factors for hysterectomy also include grand multiparity, prior tubal ligation, adenomyosis, and history of dysmenorrhea.

New onset cyclic or chronic postablation pelvic pain can result from bleeding from intact islands of endometrium. Outflow of menstrual blood is prevented by the development of intrauterine adhesions, resulting in central or cornual hematometra. In women who have had a tubal ligation, retrograde menstruation causing distention of the proximal portion of the fallopian tube can also cause pain, termed postablation tubal sterilization syndrome (PATSS). PATSS may be difficult to diagnose as the hematosalpinx may not be visible throughout the cycle. Imaging with pelvic magnetic resonance (MR) during episodes of pain is most helpful. Conservative treatment for these complications is controversial and salpingectomy or hysterectomy may be required.

The potential for delayed or missed diagnosis of endometrial cancer is unknown, thus necessitating preoperative endometrial biopsy and hysteroscopy and avoidance of the procedure in high-risk individuals and those with complex endometrial hyperplasia with or without atypia. Additionally, evaluation of the endometrium after ablation is difficult or impossible due to poor visualization with TVUS and poor visualization hysteroscopically due to intrauterine firbrosis.

Despite preoperative counseling regarding the need for contraception following endometrial ablation, pregnancies have been reported. There have been maternal deaths reporter in women who conceived after endometrial ablation. The placenta can become markedly adherent, resulting in retained products of conception, infection, and hemorrhage. Postoperative changes can increase the difficulty of subsequent pregnancy termination. Perinatal complications include spontaneous abortion; preterm delivery; amniotic band syndrome; and placenta accreta, increta, and percreta, possibly requiring cesarean hysterectomy, among other complications. The patient's plan for lifelong postoperative contraception should therefore be carefully discussed prior to performing the ablation.

Conclusions

Although there is little difference in self-reported quality of life scores between patients with ablation compared to hysterectomy, patients in the latter group report greater satisfaction with their decision. This highlights the importance of careful patient selection and realistic preoperative counseling to ensure both optimal treatment success and patient experience. Women over 45 years of age have the least likelihood of failure or need for additional counseling. Thorough preoperative evaluation with an emphasis of excluding intracavitary lesions and hyperplasia is essential to improve outcomes, decrease failure, and decrease complications from endometrial ablation. For the right patient, endometrial ablation can provide an opportunity to treat menorrhagia with minimal disruption of routine activities while avoiding the morbidity associated with more invasive approaches.

Uterine Fibroid Embolization

Case Presentation

J.B. is a 43-year-old gravida 3, para 3 female, with three prior cesarean deliveries, who has been experiencing increasing menorrhagia and urinary frequency over the last 2 years. Her cycles are regular, every 28 to 30 days, without intermenstrual bleeding, but they are excessively heavy. Her quality of life has been affected. She occasionally misses work as a nurse, because of the need to change a pad and tampon every 45 to 60 minutes, and states that, "when the floor is busy, I can't get to the bathroom to change." In fact several times she has soiled through her white uniform, necessitating taking extra clothing to work. During the first several days, she also wears a Depends diaper, for the overflow bleeding that occurs. At night during her period, she awakens two or three times to change pads/tampon, and has "ruined" her mattress. She craves ice and feels fatigued. Her clothing is fitting tighter and despite regular exercise, her abdomen looks "pregnant" and she palpates a mass when lying flat. Finally, she notes urinary frequency and once had to be catheterized due to urinary retention. Her bimanual examination confirmed a 15- to 17–week-size pelvic mass. Ultrasound confirmed a 17.7 cm × 15.8 cm × 12.3 cm uterus. There were four leiomyomas with sizes ranging from 4 to 7 cm. Both ovaries were normal and there was no hydronephrosis. She is mildly anemic with hemoglobin level of 8.4 g/dL and hematocrit of 28.7%, and has a normal platelet count. Her TSH, recent Pap test, and HPV test are normal.

After appropriate counseling and review of options, the patient was interested in pursuing uterine fibroid embolization (UFE) as a treatment modality. Informed consent from her gynecologist and ACOG patient literature was given to the patient. She underwent pelvic magnetic resonance imaging (MRI) with gadolinium and had standard preoperative UFE laboratory tests drawn (CBC with platelets, blood urea nitrogen [BUN], creatinine, prothrombin time [PT], partial thromboplastin time [PTT]). MRI demonstrated multiple intramural fibroids ranging in size from 3 to 6 cm, no intracavitary component, and all fibroids enhanced. There were no adnexal masses, adenomyosis, or hydronephrosis. All laboratory tests were normal, except for evidence of anemia. Once these results were available, the patient was contacted and referred to interventional radiology for counseling, informed consent, and scheduling of the procedure. The patient was scheduled approximately 5 days after her period. She had an uneventful procedure and stayed in short-stay unit for 23 hours. Her 6-day recovery at home was without complications. She returned for postprocedure evaluation 1 month later and had final check-up at 6 months. At her final checkup, menorrhagia was resolved as well as bulk symptoms. Her anemia also resolved. Final uterine size with bimanual examination was 11- to 13-week size. Patient was very pleased with resolution of her symptoms.

Uterine fibroid embolization (UFE), also known as uterine artery embolization (UAE), is an emerging nonsurgical minimally invasive therapy that, with accruing clinical experience, is gaining widespread acceptance in North American and in Europe as a safe and effective treatment for reducing the symptoms of uterine leiomyomas. An estimated 300,000 UFEs have been performed worldwide since 1995, when this procedure was first utilized by Ravina and colleagues, and approximately 25,000 are performed annually in the United States.

UFE is performed by a trained interventional radiologist, ideally collaborating with a gynecologist who has determined that the patient is an appropriate candidate for the procedure. Particulate emboli to occlude the uterine arteries, thereby disrupting the blood supply to fibroids and leading to devascularization and infarction, has been reported to be effective in alleviating fibroid-related symptoms. The result is improvement in fibroid-associated symptoms, preservation of the uterus, avoidance of general anesthesia, and obviation of the potential complications and lengthy recovery associated with surgery. UFE is a safe, effective, and durable nonsurgical alternative to hysterectomy.

Indications and Patient Selection

The Task Force on Uterine Artery Embolization and the Standards Division of the Society of Interventional Radiology (SIR) and ACOG recommend that UFE

Table 12-4 Critical Questions for the Patient before Referral for Uterine Fibroid Embolization (UFE)

- Does the patient have fibroids? Could symptoms be related to adenomyosis or other factors?
- Are the symptoms related to the fibroids?
- Does the patient want children?
- Do the symptoms require treatment?
- Are there anatomic factors that predispose the patient to treatment failures or indicate the need for adjunctive evaluation to ensure treatment success?
- Are there gynecologic or nongynecologic medical conditions that predispose the patient to UFE or surgical risks?
- Are there other reasons why the patient does not want surgery?

be offered only to women with symptomatic uterine leiomyomas who are of reproductive age but who are not interested in childbearing. In this patient subpopulation, UFE is indicated for individuals with clinically documented fibroids and fibroid-related symptoms who wish to avoid surgery, particularly hysterectomy and who refuse blood transfusion for health or religious reasons; and who have failed medical or surgical therapy. Contraindication to general anesthesia may be another consideration.

Of the numerous treatment options available, patient selection for UFE is generally based on such factors as bulk symptoms, bleeding symptoms, dysmenorrhea, and desire for uterine preservation. A patient's ultimate choice among available fibroid therapies may depend upon the fibroid-related impact on her HRQOL, the length of convalescence that is acceptable to her, and the importance she assigns to tolerable invasiveness and symptom resolution. A list of critical questions to ask before referral for UFE is shown in Table 12-4.

Crucial to the success of UFE is the partnership and collaboration between gynecologists and radiologists in the global care of the patient. A cooperative relationship between the obstetrician/gynecologist and interventional radiologist is essential for effective diagnosis, treatment, management of complications, and follow-up of patients who are potential candidates for UFE, and the combined efforts of these specialists contribute to the establishment of optimal clinical guidelines for patient care. Collaboration begins with the screening and selection of patients, as both specialists must contribute their skills when choosing appropriate candidates. Although counterintuitive, gynecologists who embrace UFE referrals often increase the number of fibroid-related cases referred to their gynecology clinical practice. Not all patients with fibroids are candidates for UFE. Reasons may include patients who desire future pregnancy, who have unrealistic expectations, or who have MR findings that contraindicate the procedure (marked calcification, ovarian collateral blood flow, pedunculated fibroid on a stalk <3 cm, and abnormal appearing leiomyomas with ill-defined borders). A knowledgeable gynecologist can confidently determine which patients are suitable candidates. Those who do not meet the criteria are retained in the practice and other invasive fibroid therapies or hysterectomy are offered.

Procedure

Generally, UFE is performed by an experienced interventional radiologist (IR) in an interventional radiology suite. A dedicated nurse is an important component of the team. Ideally, the IR has admitting privileges to monitor the patient after the procedure. UFE requires approximately 60 to 90 minutes and is performed with conscious sedation and local anesthetic. Using fluoroscopic guidance, the interventional radiologist performs UFE from a single common femoral artery puncture site, usually on the right. The use of alternative arterial approaches may be considered in patients when the femoral artery is not accessible. The operator directs a catheter over the aortoiliac bifurcation into the contralateral (left) internal iliac artery and selective arteriography of this vessel is performed. This identifies the major nontarget branches and clarifies the configuration of the origin of the uterine artery. The uterine artery is easily identified angiographically by its characteristic tortuosity and medial course. In the case of uterine fibroids, it is usually markedly hypertrophied and its enlarged terminal branches splay over and penetrate the substance of the fibroid masses. A catheter is advanced deep into the uterine artery. When a secure position is confirmed, embolization may proceed.

Most practitioners currently use polyvinyl alcohol (PVA) beads or PVA microspheres, or a gelatin-coated tris-acryl polymer microsphere which are available in various size ranges. Particles of diameter 355 to 500 µm and 500 to 700 µm are commonly used. The smaller particles tend to cause more rapid tissue necrosis, and may be associated with greater postembolization discomfort. Recently tris-acryl plastic spheres (500–900 µm) (Emblospheres, BioSphere Medical, Rockland, MA) have become increasingly popular for UFE. Cited advantages include homogeneity of particle size, absence of interparticle clumping, and greater penetration into the vascular network feeding the fibroid.

The particles are injected under fluoroscopic observation, progressively occupying the fibroids' vascular bed. The catheter then is pulled back into the left internal iliac artery and postembolization angiography performed to confirm the resultant vascular occlusion. A catheter is then guided into the right uterine artery and an identical process of embolization is performed. Best results are obtained when both uterine arteries are catheterized. The catheter and vascular sheath are removed.

In 2% of cases, bilateral UFE is not possible. Causes of failure may include (1) anatomic variations or arterial spasm that is unresponsive to nitroglycerin or other vasodilators, (2) inability to catheterize one or both uterine arteries, (3) fibroids that may receive collateral blood flow from sources other than uterine artery (ovarian collaterals), and (4) embolic material that may clump and deliver insufficient embolic material to cause ischemia or the creation of false appearance of occlusion. It is considered a technical failure if bilateral procedure could not be performed. Current SIR guidelines aim for less than 2% technical failure rate. The overall radiation dose is equivalent to that of one or two computed tomography (CT) scans.

Postoperative Management

After procedure, patients typically experience uterine cramping that is managed by patient-controlled analgesia (PCA) pump. Most patients are admitted for 23 hours, although newer protocols are being evaluated for a 6- to 8-hour admission. It is important to provide optimal control of pain and monitor narcotic-related side effects in order to decrease length of stay and readmissions. In addition to a PCA pump, NSAIDs and antihistamines are also needed. Additionally, home-going medications should include antiemetics, stool softeners, laxatives, and narcotics.

Conditions for discharge include the ability to void spontaneously, control of pain medication with oral medications, and absence of nausea and vomiting. The most common indications for emergency room readmission are for this triad of symptoms. After 24 hours, most patients feel better and experience cramping for 3 to 5 days and are successfully managed by NSAIDs for 5 days and supplemental narcotic pain medication, as needed, for the first 1 to 3 days. Pain relief may be necessary for 6 to 14 days.

Constipation can result from narcotics and decreased ambulation. Patients may experience postoperative narcotic-induced constipation similar to postsurgical myomectomy or hysterectomy. Patients should be encouraged to remain well hydrated, minimize narcotic use, and use stool softeners.

Postprocedural follow-up protocol includes the following:

1. Avoidance of vaginal intercourse for 2 weeks, or until resolution of vaginal discharge.

2. Patients without any complications are seen within 1 month of the procedure by the gynecologist. Subsequent office visits are scheduled the first year at 6 and 12 months. One year after the procedure, annual visits are scheduled unless new symptoms occur. Most fibroid-related symptoms improve within 4 to 6 months after the procedure. Maximal fibroid shrinkage is obtained by months 4 to 6. In 10% of patients, additional fibroid shrinkage may occur up to 12 months after the procedure.

3. Patients with persistent symptoms of bleeding, pain, and fever should be evaluated immediately.

4. At each visit, bimanual examination should be obtained. Patients are asked about resolution of symptoms and their level of satisfaction with the procedure.

5. Repeat MRI of the pelvis if uterine fibroids continue to grow or if there is unusual pain that occurs.

6. When leukorrhea is persistent or serosanguineous discharge noted, office hysteroscopy is helpful in identifying discontinuity within the endometrium or necrotic prolapsing fibroids.

Complications

After UFE, most patients experience transient low-grade fever, and may also have night sweats and fatigue. This has been noted with embolization of other organs and is often referred to as postembolization syndrome (PES), which generally lasts for 3 to 5 days (or rarely, longer in some patients). The transient fever is generally not higher than 101.0° F and usually associated with mild leukocytosis.

Although PES does not signify an infection, clinicians may face difficulty distinguishing between PES and infection, although patients with PES generally do not feel acutely ill and do not have severe rigors, chills, or drenching sweats. Fortunately, infection immediately after UFE is quite rare. Most patients also will note some vaginal spotting that will last for a few weeks after the procedure. A return to work within 7 to 14 days is commonplace. Overall, the rate of complications associated with UFE is very low, and most complications are transient. Transcervical leiomyoma tissue passage is the most common complication requiring surgical intervention; it occurs in approximately 2.5% of patients. The most serious complication associated with UFE is endometritis/uterine infection, with a reported incidence of approximately 2%.

The rate of hysterectomy subsequent to UFE ranges between 0.25% and 1.6% and is generally attributable to infection, pain, and bleeding. Uterine necrosis, a rare complication (fewer than 10 reported cases to date) following this procedure, also necessitates hysterectomy and treatment with antibiotics to prevent bacteremia, sepsis, and death. Patients should be made aware of possible emergency hysterectomy should such severe complications arise.

A study of 400 consecutive patients undertaken by Spies and associates (2002) found that, based on ACOG definitions, perioperative complications occurred in only 5% of UFE procedures for symptomatic fibroids. Such complications included allergic reaction to contrast medium, accidental injury to the femoral nerve or uterine artery, groin hematomas, endometritis, pulmonary embolism, and arterial thrombosis. A current and much larger study involving more than 450 patients at the Cleveland Clinic published by Park and coworkers in 2008, found a more substantial rate of minor complications—61 complications in 53 patients, or 11% of the cohort—following UFE, although the associated morbidity rate was still very low. Office hysteroscopy was utilized liberally to evaluate post-UFE complaints such as leukorrhea and abnormal vaginal bleeding. Researchers reported that the factors most likely to increase the risk for developing complications included prior myomectomy and the use of embolic particles 355 μg to 500 μg in size, that is, smaller than the typical 500 μm to 900 μm.

Through 2007, there have been only four reported fatalities related to UFE. Pulmonary embolism was the cause of death in two cases; the other two deaths were a result of septicemia and disseminated intravascular coagulation.

Outcomes

Symptoms of menorrhagia improve in 83% to 92% of patients, pain improves in 77% to 79%, and bulk-related symptoms improve in 79% to 92%. Leiomyomas continue to shrink for up to 1 year following embolization, and the reported percentage of uterine or fibroid volume reduction varies according to the length of follow-up. Two multicenter studies with combined cohorts totaling more than 2200 patients recently reported long-term follow-up data for UFE-treated symptomatic leiomyomas. Both support the conclusion that UFE is effective and safe, with durable symptom control, few complications, and improved quality of life. Other sizeable prospective studies of UFE with 5 to 7 years postprocedure follow-up found continued symptom control in 72% to 73% of patients and a high rate of patient satisfaction (surprisingly, even in women who needed an additional intervention). These investigations also revealed that 87% to 91.4% of patients treated with UFE would recommend the procedure to others.

Walker and Pelage (2002) reported pregnancy outcomes among a group of 1200 women who underwent UFE, of which 56 became pregnant. There was a significant increase in cesarean section (72.7%) and increases in preterm delivery (18.2%), postpartum hemorrhage (18.2%), and miscarriage (30.4%) for the subgroup of women who became pregnant compared with the general obstetric population. The study authors concluded that women are able to conceive after UFE, and that the majority of such pregnancies result in full-term deliveries; however, they recommended conservative management of pregnancies occurring after UFE until more is known about delivery outcomes. They also advised close monitoring of placental status to facilitate transfer of care to an appropriate treatment center if abnormalities are detected.

Rare instances of premature menopause have been reported in 2% to 3% of patients under the age of 45 and in approximately 8% of women ages 45 and older following UFE. Decrease in ovarian reserve and nontarget ovarian embolization also has been reported. For all these reasons, pregnancy rates after UFE may be decreased and fertility compromised compared with women who have undergone myomectomy.

Conclusions

For women with symptomatic fibroids, UFE appears to be safe, effective, and durable alternative to classic surgery. In selected patients UFE carries high success and low complication rates that are sustained in the long term. Regarding quality of life and patient satisfaction, UFE equals or surpasses surgery. However, for women who are actively trying to conceive, the role of UFE remains unclear; at present myomectomy to enhance fertility may be a better choice.

UFE is an option that all physicians may wish to discuss with all patients presenting with uterine fibroids who are being offered hysterectomy or myomectomy. A collaborative and multidisciplinary practice between gynecologists and interventional radiologists represents state-of-the-art care for women with fibroids. With such an approach, our patients can be given a truly informed consent.

MR-Guided Focused Ultrasound

Case Presentation

A 46-year-old gravida 2, para 2 female presents complaining of gradually increasing abdominal pressure, back pain, and urinary frequency. She also reports feeling a hard mass in her lower abdomen. Her periods are regular and she notes that her bleeding is heavier and she has begun passing clots. She has already been evaluated and was told that she has three uterine fibroids on MRI ranging from 4 to 6 cm with the largest located in the anterior uterine wall. On bimanual examination the uterus is enlarged to 16-week size with a prominent anterior fibroid. Due to her desire to avoid surgery and prolonged recovery, she has previously declined treatment, but now requests more information on MR-guided focused ultrasound (US). She denies history of prior surgery. She and her husband of 14 years state that they have completed childbearing and that her husband has undergone vasectomy.

Focused ultrasound therapy has been used in many other specialties for the ablation of soft tissue lesions and, when coupled with MRI, offers a new modality for the treatment of uterine fibroids. Magnetic resonance imaging–guided focused ultrasound (MRgFUS) allows for precise localization of the target lesion as well as thermal monitoring during the procedure. The ExAblate 2000 (InSightec, Haifa, Israel) is the first such device approved by the FDA in October 2004 for the treatment of fibroids and is now offered in limited locations in the United States and internationally as an outpatient procedure. During the treatments, or sonications, a high-intensity US beam is focused on the fibroid of interest and delivers thermal energy to produce coagulative necrosis at temperatures greater than 55° C. The available data indicate a significant reduction in fibroid symptoms, with a prompt recovery and low rate of adverse effects.

Indications

As the use of MRgFUS for fibroid ablation is still in its infancy, current evidence describes its use only in a limited patient population. The treatment is designed to provide ablation of symptomatic fibroids with a lesion-based approach. Careful discussion of patient symptoms and fibroid mapping is needed to assess if the patient is an acceptable candidate and what myomas should be targeted. As there are only a few case reports describing pregnancy after MRgFUS, currently the treatment should be offered only to women with no intention of future pregnancy and adequate contraception should be offered. Patients are attracted to the procedure as it is truly minimally invasive and does not require any hospitalization. Most patients can return to routine activities the following day. The procedure involves minimal pain as the fibroid undergoes immediate coagulative necrosis rather than prolonged ischemia as in UFE; however, no comparative trials have been performed to otherwise compare these two modalities.

Patient Selection

Criteria for choosing a patient who is most likely to achieve maximal symptomatic relief from MRgFUS are still evolving as the techniques move from research to general practice. Initial FDA treatment guidelines required that the planned treatment involve only 33% of the fibroid and not exceed 100 cm^3 per fibroid or 150 cm^3 if more than one fibroid is treated. Untreated margins of 1.5 cm from the edge of the sonication to the serosa or myometrium and a margin of 0.5 cm from the treated area to the fibroid capsule if abutting the serosa are suggested. These treatment guidelines were subsequently modified to allow treatment of 33% of submucosal fibroids and 50% of all other fibroids. A serosal margin of 1.5 cm was still required, but restrictions on endometrial and capsular margins were lifted. Maximum treatment time of 2 hours was extended to 3 hours and repeat sonications within a 14-day period were allowed. A comparison of patients treated under the original and modified guidelines revealed a significantly greater improvement in symptoms and corresponding decrease in need for subsequent alternative treatment. Of note, fewer adverse events were noted in the modified treatment group. Other studies indicate that the ideal candidate has intramural fibroids that are greater than 3 cm and low signal on T_2-weighted MR images signifying areas of decreased perfusion and that enhance with gadolinium contrast material. Multiple sessions may be needed if fibroids are greater than 7 to 8 cm, if there are multiple fibroids, or if the fibroids have higher signal intensity. Greater benefits are seen when larger fibroids are targeted and an increased size of the treatment volume results both in better relief and decreased need for further treatment.

First, a thorough patient interview must be conducted to assess the type and degree of symptoms and to evaluate whether treatable fibroids account for the patients symptoms. An MR with gadolinium contrast medium is crucial to determine the number of fibroids and location. Additionally, the MR can also serve to evaluate for intervening structures such as scar tissue and metal implants or adjacent organs including bowel, ovary, bone, and pelvic nerves. Research protocols thus far have excluded patients with a uterus larger than 20-week size or with individual fibroids larger than 10 cm, with other pelvic disease, extensive lower abdominal scarring, or uncontrolled systemic disease. Of note, in one series only 6% of patients were excluded from treatment based on MR findings. Patients should also not have any other contraindication to MR such as a pacemaker and must not exceed MR table weight limits. As the fibroids remain in situ with no tissue for pathologic diagnosis, the procedure should only be performed on patients with no suspicion of leiomyosarcoma. There is evidence that MR represents a very useful diagnostic modality for this rare cause of uterine enlargement. Laboratory studies to evaluate for anemia and need for iron supplementation are performed and normal findings on cervical cytologic examination and endometrial biopsy are required as indicated.

Procedure

The patient is asked to fast overnight, to shave all hair from her lower abdomen, and to avoid the use of lotion or creams on her skin. Informed consent is obtained and a negative pregnancy test is required. Sequential compression devices are applied and a Foley catheter is placed to keep the bladder decompressed. Prophylactic antibiotics are given and conscious sedation is administered to decrease patient discomfort and motion artifact but still allow the patient to describe any adverse symptoms. The sonication treatments take place within the radiology suite utilizing a focused ultrasound system built into the MR table. The patient lies prone on the MR table with the abdomen flat on a gel pad to enable acoustic coupling (Fig. 12-14). Variously shaped gel pads are available to best position the patient to displace bowel loops and bring the fibroids more directly into the treatment beam (Fig. 12-15). Some modification of patient positioning with gel pads as well as distention of the bladder may be needed to optimize accessibility of the fibroids. A pretreatment MR image is obtained and the treatment volume of the fibroids of interest is outlined. The beam route is then planned to avoid any abdominal wall scars, bowel loops, or bony structures. Test pulses are administered to confirm the location and the ability to monitor temperature change. Treatment sonications are commenced with 20-second pulses alternating with 1 to 2 minutes of cool-down time. The beam paths are monitored during the treatment with modifications as needed and the patient is asked to report skin warmth, back pain, or uterine cramping. Post-treatment gadolinium images are obtained to identify the area of nonperfusion produced by the sonications. The anterior abdominal wall is assessed on these images as well as visually to identify any thermal injury. Occasionally a second session is scheduled to complete treatment if the fibroids are particularly large or numerous. The patient is then observed while recovering from the effects of the sedation and discharged home with a friend or family member. Most patients require only a nonsteroidal analgesic for pain control.

Complications

Immediate complications of the procedure are skins burns that have been reported in about 5% of patients; however, this was limited to areas of

Figure 12-14 Magnetic resonance–guided focused ultrasound. (Courtesy of The Cleveland Clinic Center for Medical Art & Photography, copyright 2009. All rights reserved.)

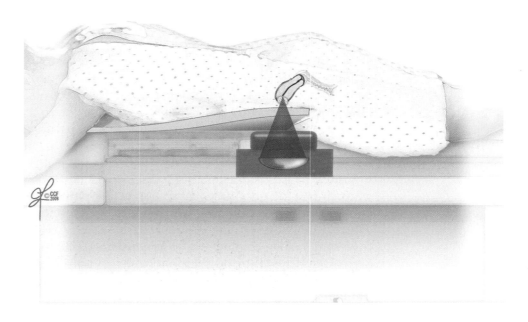

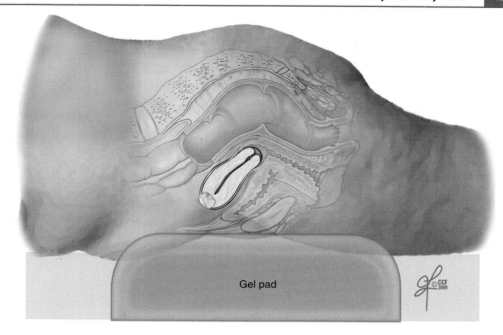

Gel pad

inadequate hair removal and can be minimized by shaving, cleaning the skin with alcohol, and limited treatment through abdominal scars. Inflammatory changes in the near field have been reported in 11% of patients. These cause minimal post-treatment discomfort and can be prevented by monitoring patient symptoms during treatment and thermal mapping during the procedure. Damage to adjacent organs is possible but rare. Bony and neural structures may lie in the far field of the treatment and a single case report of sciatic nerve palsy has led to modifications in the protocol to assess thermal effects beyond the target fibroid as well. The one reported patient's weakness and paresthesias had resolved by 12 months and no subsequent cases have been reported. Reports of postoperative fevers led to the routine administration of antibiotics. Isolated cases of venous thromboembolism have been reported and sequential compression devices now are recommended. Most patients need only minimal analgesia but some patients have required admission for postoperative pain or vomiting. Diarrhea and vaginal discharge have also been reported.

Outcomes

Published long-term outcomes are available from 24 months follow-up of 359 women (Stewart et al, 2007). Most of these subjects had participated in phase III trials, under limited FDA protocols. As these data represent the initial use of the technology, sequential patients may reflect changes in operator skills. Under a modified protocol allowing larger treatment, 90.5% reported significant improvement at 12 months. Due to the earlier limited protocols, 57% of these women had less than 20% of the targeted fibroid treated. The nonperfused volume (NPV) of the fibroid correlated well with necrosis observed in pathology specimens and is thus used as a representation of fibroid shrinkage. All patients reported significant improvement on symptom severity scales, with greater improvement seen in those who had more than 20% of the fibroid treated. The rate of re-treatment at 24 months with myomectomy, hysterectomy, uterine artery embolization, or any type of hormonal treatment was inversely related to the nonperfused volume. On Kaplan-Meier analysis, the probability of intervention-free survival was about 55% in those with low NPV compared to 75% in those with higher treated volumes. In women with a pretreatment hematocrit of less than 35%, significant increases in hematocrit were seen that also correlated with greater NPV. At 24 months, 9% of premenopausal women had transitioned to menopause and an additional 23% reported perimenopausal symptoms.

The MRgFUS procedure is not recommended for women who desire to attempt pregnancies, but solitary case reports have described uneventful term pregnancies after the procedure. Cost analysis based on preliminary data related to current costs and reintervention rates predicts that MRgFUS remains cost effective in 86% of simulations based on various assumptions. The available data show no signs of postembolization syndrome or other risks seen after UFE such as fever, leukocytosis, infection, leukorrhea, fibroid extrusion, and ovarian failure. The rate of additional complications if a hysterectomy is done after MRgFUS is unknown. The expansion of this procedure to women with larger fibroids and wider range of symptoms promises more data on outcomes in the near future. Outcome data are also likely to reflect protocol changes to increase post-treatment NPV and shorten sessions as well as increased understanding of which fibroids are most important to target. Identification of women at early onset of symptoms may allow treatment of fibroids while the lesions are small, allowing for more successful outcomes. The frontiers of this therapy include the expansion of criteria to include the treatment of women desiring future fertility and those with adenomyosis. First and foremost, there is great need for randomized controlled trials with direct comparison to other interventions for fibroid treatment and with longer duration of follow-up. Collaboration between gynecologists and radiologists is required to varying degrees depending on practice setting. Gynecologic involvement is currently somewhat limited by lack of CPT coding and reimbursement issues.

Discussion

Emerging technologies over the past 25 years have opened new avenues for the treatment of fibroids and menorrhagia. These efforts are driven by the desire to avoid both the morbidity and costs of definitive treatment by hysterectomy and to satisfy patient demand. Medical management often can be attempted as a first step in treatment. The availability of ambulatory surgical options with prompt recovery time minimizes patient experiences of pain and loss of productivity at home or work. While these new modalities can be offered as an alternative to hysterectomy, they do not represent interchangeable options. A thorough preoperative evaluation of the cause of excess bleeding is needed to tailor choice of therapy. Optimal outcomes are maximized by careful patient selection; with increased operator experience, long-term registry outcomes, and results of quality of life scores, these procedures may be offered to patients previously thought to be treated only by hysterectomy.

Selected Readings

Medical Management: Levonorgestrel-Releasing Intrauterine System

American College of Obstetricians and Gynecologists: Intrauterine Device. ACOG Practice Bulletin No. 59. Obstet Gynecol 2005;105:223–232.

Chrisman C, Ribeiro P, Dalton V: The Levonorgestrel-releasing Intrauterine System: An updated review of the contraceptive and noncontraceptive uses. Clin Obstet Gynecol 2007;50:886–897.

Kaunitz A: Progestin-releasing intrauterine systems and leiomyoma. Contraception 2007;75:S130–S133.

Lethaby AE, Cooke I, Rees M: Progesterone or progestogen-releasing intrauterine systems for heavy menstrual bleeding. Cochrane Database Syst Rev 2005;Issue 4:CD002126.

Mansour D: Modern management of abnormal uterine bleeding—the levonorgesterel intra-uterine system. Best Pract Res Clin Obstet Gynecol 2007;21:1007–1021.

Pakarinen P, Luukkainen T: Treatment of menorrhagia with an LNG-IUS. Contraception 2007;75:S118–S122.

Hysteroscopic Myomectomy

Bradley LD: Hysteroscopic resection of myomas and polyps (Chap 19). In Bradley LD, Falcone T (eds): Hysteroscopy: Office Evaluation and Management of the Uterine Cavity, 1st ed. Philadelphia, Elsevier, 2009.

Di Spiezio Sardo A, Mazzon I, Bramante S, et al: Hysteroscopic myomectomy: A comprehensive review of surgical techniques. Hum Reprod Update 2008;2:101–119.

Hart R, Molnar BG, Magos A: Long-term follow up of hysteroscopic myomectomy assessed by survival analysis. Br J Obstet Gynaecol 1999;106:700–705.

Jansen FW, Vredevoogd CB, van Ulzen K, et al: Complications of hysteroscopy: A prospective, multi-center study. Obstet Gynecol 2000;96:266–270.

Lasmar RB, Barrozo PR, Dias R, Oliveria MA: Submucous fibroids: A new presurgical classification to evaluate the viability of hysteroscopic surgical treatment—preliminary report. J Minim Invasive Gynecol 2005;12:308–311.

Murakami T, Tamura M, Ozaw Y, et al: Safe techniques in surgery for hysteroscopic myomectomy. J Obstet Gynaecol Res 2005;31:216–223.

Parker WH: Uterine myomas: Management. Fertil Steril 2007;88:255–271.

Phillips DR, Nathanson HG, Milim SJ, et al: The effect of dilute vasopressin solution on blood loss during operative hysteroscopy: A randomized controlled trial. Obstet Gynecol 1996;88:751–756.

Polena V, Mergui JL, Perrot N, et al: Long-term results of hysteroscopic myomectomy in 235 patients. Eur J Obstet Gynecol Reprod Biol 2007;130:232–237.

Vilos GA, Abu-Rafea B: New developments in ambulatory hysteroscopic surgery. Best Pract Res Clin Obstet Gynaecol 2005;19:727–742.

Wamsteker K, Emanuel MH, de Kruif JH: Transcervical hysteroscopic resection of submucous fibroids for abnormal uterine bleeding: results regarding the degree of intramural extension. Obstet Gynecol 1993;82:736–740.

Widrich T, Bradley L, Mitchinson AR, Collins R: Comparison of saline infusion sonography with office hysteroscopy for the evaluation of the endometrium. Am J Obstet Gynecol 1996;174:1327–1334.

Global Endometrial Ablation

ASRM Practice Committee: Indications and options for endometrial ablation. Fertil Steril 2008;90:S236–S240.

Deb S, Kulwant F, Atiomo: A survey of preferences and practices of endometrial ablation/resection for menorrhagia in the United Kingdom. Fertil Steril 2008;90:1812–1817.

Della Badia C, Nyirjesy P, Atogho A: Endometrial ablation devices: Review of a manufacturer and user facility device experience database. J Minim Invasive Gynecol 2007;14:436–441.

Dickersin K, Munro M, Clark M, et al: Hysterectomy compared with endometrial ablation for dysfunctional uterine bleeding. Obstet Gynecol 2007;110:1279–1289.

Dongen H, Van de Merwe AG, de Kroon CD, Jansen FW: The impact of alternative treatment for abnormal uterine bleeding on hysterectomy rates in a tertiary referral center. J Min Invas Gynecol 2009;16:47–51.

El-Nashar SA, Hopkins MR, Creedon DJ, et al: Prediction of treatment outcomes after global endometrial ablation. Obstet Gynecol 2009;113:97–106.

Fothergill RE: Endometrial ablation in the office setting. Obstet Gynecol Clin North Am 2008;35:317–330.

Gurtcheff SE, Sharp HT: Complications associated with global endometrial ablation: The utility of the MAUDE database. Obstet Gynecol 2003;102:1278–1282.

Lethaby A, Hickey M, Garry R, Penninx J: Endometrial resection/ablation techniques for heavy menstrual bleeding. Cochrane Database Syst Rev 2005;(4):CD001501.

Longinotti MK, Jacobson GF, Hung Yun-Yi, Learman LA: Probability of hysterectomy after endometrial ablation. Obstet Gynecol 2008;112:1214–1220.

McCausland AM, McCausland VM: Frequency of symptomatic cornual hematometra and postablation tubal sterilization syndrome after total rollerball endometrial ablation: A 10-year follow-up. Am J Obstet Gynecol 2001;186:1274–1283.

McGurgan P, O'Donovan P: Second generation endometrial ablation—an overview. Best Pract Res Clin Obstet Gynecol 2007;21:931–945.

Zarek S, Sharp HT: Global endometrial ablation devices. Clin Obstet Gynecol 2008;51:167–175.

Uterine Fibroid Embolization

Andrews RT, Spies JB, Sacks D, et al: Task Force on Uterine Artery Embolization and the Standards Division of the Society of Interventional Radiology. Patient care and uterine artery embolization for leiomyomata. J Vasc Interv Radiol 2004;15(Suppl 2, Pt 1):115–120.

Bradley LD: Uterine fibroid embolization: A viable alternative to hysterectomy. Am J Obstet Gynecol 2009;201:127–135.

Carls GS, Lee DW, Ozminkowski RJ, et al: What are the total costs of surgical treatment for uterine fibroids? J Womens Health (Larchmont) 2008;17:1119–1132.

Cura M, Cura A, Bugnone A: Role of magnetic resonance imaging in patient selection for uterine artery embolization. Acta Radiol 2006;47:1105–1114.

Dutton S, Hirst A, McPherson K, et al: A UK multicentre retrospective cohort study comparing hysterectomy and uterine artery embolisation for the treatment of symptomatic uterine fibroids (HOPEFUL study): Main results on medium-term safety and efficacy. Br J Obstet Gynaecol 2007;114:1340–1351.

Edwards RD, Moss JG, Lumsden MA, et al: Committee of the Randomized Trial of Embolization versus Surgical Treatment for Fibroids: Uterine-artery embolization versus surgery for symptomatic uterine fibroids. N Engl J Med 2007;356:360–370.

Gabriel-Cox K, Jacobson GF, Armstrong MA, et al: Predictors of hysterectomy after uterine artery embolization for leiomyoma. Am J Obstet Gynecol 2007;196:588.

Goodwin SC, Spies JB, Worthington-Kirsch R, et al: Fibroid Registry for Outcomes Data (FIBROID) Registry Steering Committee and Core Site Investigators: Uterine artery embolization for treatment of leiomyomata: Long-term outcomes from the FIBROID Registry. Obstet Gynecol 2008;111:22–33.

Hehenkamp WJ, Volkers NA, Birnie E, et al: Symptomatic uterine fibroids: Treatment with uterine artery embolization or hysterectomy—results from the randomized clinical Embolisation versus Hysterectomy (EMMY) Trial. Radiology 2008;246:823–832.

Homer H, Saridogan E. Uterine artery embolization for fibroids is associated with an increased risk of miscarriage. Fertil Steril 2009 Aug 8. [Epub ahead of print].

Isonishi S, Coleman RL, Hirama M, et al: Analysis of prognostic factors for patients with leiomyoma treated with uterine arterial embolization. Am J Obstet Gynecol 2008;198:270.

Lohle PN, Voogt MJ, De Vries J, et al: Long-term outcome of uterine artery embolization for symptomatic uterine leiomyomas. J Vasc Interv Radiol 2008;19:319–326.

Park AJ, Bohrer JC, Bradley LD, et al: Incidence and risk factors for surgical intervention after uterine artery embolization. Am J Obstet Gynecol 2008;199:671.

Ravina JH, Herbreteau D, Ciraru-Vigneron N, et al: Arterial embolisation to treat uterine myomata. Lancet 1995;346:671–672.

Scheurig C, Gauruder-Burmester A, Kluner C, et al: Uterine artery embolization for symptomatic fibroids: Short-term versus mid-term changes in disease-specific symptoms, quality of life and magnetic resonance imaging results. Hum Reprod 2006;21:3270–3277.

Spies JB, Cornell C, Worthington-Kirsch R, et al: Long-term outcome from uterine fibroid embolization with tris-acryl gelatin microspheres: Results of a multicenter study. J Vasc Interv Radiol 2007;18:203–207.

Spies JB, Spector A, Roth AR, et al: Complications after uterine artery embolization for leiomyomas. Obstet Gynecol 2002;100(Suppl 5, Pt 1):873–880.

Tropeano G, Amoroso S, Scambia G: Non-surgical management of uterine fibroids. Hum Reprod Update 2008;14:259–274.

Usadi RS, Marshburn PB: The impact of uterine artery embolization on fertility and pregnancy outcome. Curr Opin Obstet Gynecol 2007;19:279–283.

Walker WJ, McDowell SJ: Pregnancy after uterine artery embolization for leiomyomata: A series of 56 completed pregnancies. Am J Obstet Gynecol 2006;195:1266–1271.

Walker WJ, Pelage JP: Uterine artery embolisation for symptomatic fibroids: Clinical results in 400 women with imaging follow-up. Br J Obstet Gynaecol 2002;109:1262–1272.

Magnetic Resonance Guided Focused Ultrasound

Fennessy FM, Tempany CM, McDannold NJ, et al: Uterine leiomyomas: MR imaging-guided focused ultrasound surgery—results of different treatment protocols. Radiology 2007;243:885–893.

Gavrilova-Jordan LP, Rose CH, Traynor KD, et al: Successful term pregnancy following MR-guided focused ultrasound treatment of uterine leiomyoma. J Perinat 2007;27:59–61.

Hesley GK, Felmlee JP, Gebhart JB, et al: Noninvasive treatment of uterine fibroids: Early Mayo Clinic experience with magnetic resonance imaging-guided focused ultrasound. Mayo Clinic Proc 2006;81:936–942.

Hindley J, Gedroyc WM, Regan L, et al: MRI guidance of focused ultrasound therapy of uterine fibroids: Early results. AJR 2004;183:1713–1719.

Lenard ZM, McDannold NJ, Fennessy FM, et al: Uterine leiomyomas: MR imaging-guided focused ultrasound surgery—imaging predictors of success. Radiology 2008;249:187–194.

McDannold N, Tempany CM, Fennessy FM, et al: Uterine leiomyomas: MR imaging-based thermometry and thermal dosimetry during focused ultrasound thermal ablation. Radiology 2006;240: 263–272.

Rabinovici J, Inbar Y, Eylon SC, et al: Pregnancy and live birth after focused ultrasound surgery for symptomatic focal adenomyosis: A case report. Human Reprod 2006;21:1255–1259.

Rabinovici J, David M, Fukinishi H, et al: Pregnancy outcome after magnetic resonance–guided focused ultrasound surgery (MRgFUS) for conservative treatment of fibroids. Fertil Steril 2010;93:199–209.

Ren XL, Zhou XD, Zhang J, et al: Extracorporeal ablation of uterine fibroids with high-intensity focused ultrasound: Imaging and histopathologic evaluation. J Ultrasound Med 2007;26:201–212.

Samuel A, Fennessy FM, Tempany CM, Stewart EA: Avoiding treatment of leiomyosarcomas: the role of magnetic resonance in focused ultrasound surgery. Fertil Steril 2008;90:850.

Smart OC, Hindley JT, Regan L, Gedroyc WG: Gonadotrophin-releasing hormone and magnetic-resonance-guided ultrasound surgery for uterine leiomyomata. Obstet Gynecol 2006;108:49–54.

So MJ, Fennessy FM, Zou KH, et al: Does the phase of menstrual cycle affect MR-guided focused ultrasound surgery of uterine leiomyomas? Eur J Radiol 2006;59:203–207.

Stewart EA, Gedroyc WM, Tempany CM, et al: Focused ultrasound treatment of uterine fibroid tumors: Safety and feasibility of a noninvasive thermoablative technique. Am J Obstet Gynecol 2003;189:48–54.

Stewart EA, Gostout B, Rabinovici J, et al: Sustained relief of leiomyoma symptoms by using focused ultrasound surgery. Obstet Gynecol 2007;110:279–287.

Zowall H, Cairns JA, Brewer C, et al: Cost-effectiveness of magnetic resonance-guided focused ultrasound surgery for treatment of uterine fibroids. Br J Obstet Gynaecol 2008;115:653–662.

Teaching and Learning Gynecologic Surgery

13

Gouri B. Diwadkar M.D.
J. Eric Jelovsek M.D.

 Video Clips on DVD

13-1 Knot-Tying: A Guide to Tying Surgical Knots and Common Knot-Tying Mistakes

13-2 Feedback in Surgical Training

The results of learning to operate are observed in a surgeon's performance, but the process is much less obvious. The teaching model has historically been that a good surgeon is also a good teaching surgeon; although most of us do not always have a clear understanding of the best way to teach. The goal of this chapter is to help surgeon educators improve their teaching strategies. Understanding the factors that lead to effective learning should help us determine how we teach. Learning surgical skills primarily involves focused, repetitive practice and receiving appropriate feedback based upon valid and reliable assessment of performance. First, we will briefly review the educational theories that are applicable to teaching surgery. Then, each of the key components of effective teaching and learning, including practice, feedback, and assessment, will be explored in detail with the hope that surgeons may improve their teaching.

Educational Theory

A foundation in educational theory may help surgeons develop basic understanding of the principles and mechanisms behind how trainees learn to perform procedures in surgery. The theory of *behaviorism* is most closely associated with B.F. Skinner (1938) and involves the experimental analysis of behavior. Skinner contended that organisms exhibit certain behaviors in relation to their environment. He argued that we should look at what occurs before the behavior and the consequence of the behavior. Because the consequence reinforces or eliminates the behavior, Skinner proposed that learning is contingent upon reinforcement. If we apply behaviorist theory to the surgical setting, the only evidence we have that a trainee has learned to operate comes from the trainee's actual surgical performance. By observing this "behavior" in the operating room, skills can be improved or eliminated. For example, a trainee is more likely to operate if he/she knows all details of a patient's history

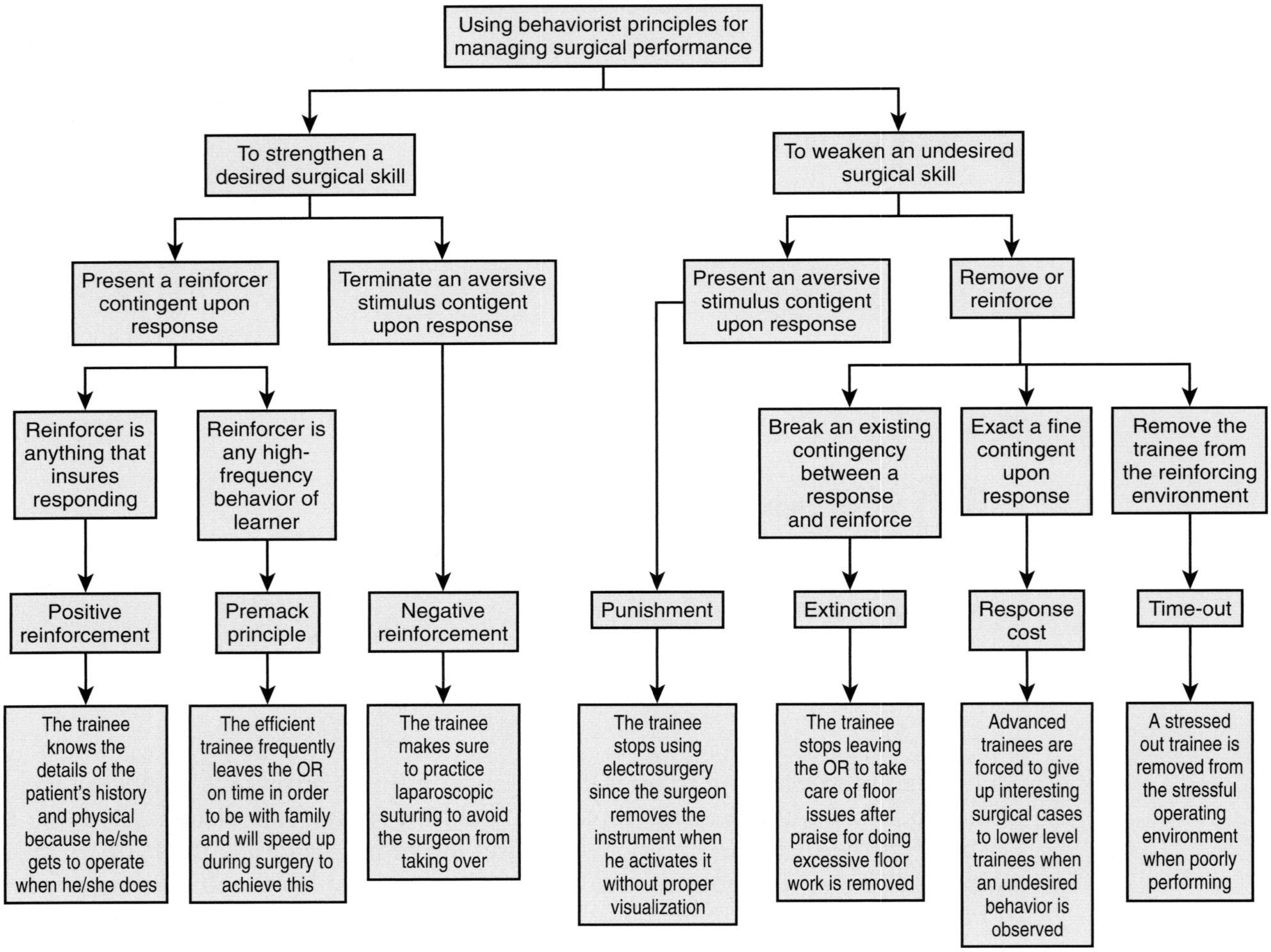

Figure 13-1 Behaviorist principles to managing surgical performance. The behaviorist principle to teaching surgery is based on strengthening or weakening a particular behavior by using reinforcers and aversive stimuli. Examples of each principle are illustrated.

and physical examination and has reviewed the relevant anatomy. Therefore, the specific behavior of thoroughly preparing for the case is positively reinforced with participation in the surgical case. Behaviorist principles and an example of their implementation in the surgical setting are illustrated in Figure 13-1.

To assume that we can only improve teaching by understanding what trainees do, rather than what they are thinking, is short sighted. Surgeon educators need to also understand what is going on in a trainee's mind during the performance of a surgical skill. Behaviorist principles fail to account for how the trainee processes the information that is to be learned. Therefore, it is helpful to understand some elements of cognitive information processing. According to the cognitive-information-processing view, learning is similar to the processor on a computer. Information is put in the mind from the environment, processed and stored in memory, and output is in the form of a learned behavior. Unlike behaviorism, there is an intervening variable that exists between the environment and the performance of the skill. That variable is the information processing system of the trainee. Atkinson and Shiffrin (1968) proposed a theory of memory which states that from the time information is received by the processing system, it undergoes a series of transformations until it can be permanently stored in memory. For example, while a trainee is performing a hysterectomy, an unclamped uterine vessel starts bleeding. Attention is drawn to this by the teaching surgeon, and the image of the bleeding vessel enters the trainee's sensory memory. The task of placing a clamp over the vessel is performed or rehearsed and becomes a part of the trainee's working memory. The desired response of improved bleeding (hemostasis) leads to this particular scenario becoming a part of the trainee's long-term memory.

Why is it important to understand how a trainee processes information? Because embedded into the information learned for new surgical procedures are critical cues that the experienced surgeon recognizes but a novice trainee has difficulty discriminating out of the large volume coming into the mind. For example, visual information decays after about 0.25 second and auditory information decays after about 4 seconds. It is currently unclear how long tactile information stays in sensory memory. Experienced surgeons already have stored the operations in memory and thus have learned to ignore most of this information as they relate it to normal parts of the procedure; therefore, they tend to focus on other aspects of the case such as variations and problems. As a result, experienced surgeons suffer from automaticity. An example of an overlearned skill that becomes automatic is knot-tying. Automaticity occurs when tasks are overlearned or incoming sources of information become habitual, to the extent that attention requirements are minimal. Experienced surgeons suffer from this because, when one's role is to teach techniques that have become automatic, it is difficult to recognize these techniques as important steps in the process of learning. For the experienced surgeon, when something out of the ordinary occurs during a procedure they shift out of a mode of automaticity and into a mode of selective attention. Selective attention is a surgeon's ability to select and process certain information while simultaneously ignoring other information. The teaching surgeon should draw attention to these critical cues that they have learned to recognize and help the trainee understand how to discriminate them from background information.

Obtaining Expertise

K. Anders Ericsson compiled at least two major advances in understanding how psychomotor skills are learned during acquisition and maintenance of expert skill performance. The first is the need for repetitive, focused practice. The second is the need for feedback. An expert's performance continues to improve as a function of increasing experience and deliberate, focused practice. Ericsson (2004) calculated that becoming an expert musician, master chess player, or expert athlete requires about 10,000 hours of deliberate and distributed practice. The importance of deliberate and repetitive practice can be applied to surgical trainees as well. The benefit from repetitive practice is not limited just to trainees early in the learning process. It is useful throughout a surgeon's career and may be particularly useful for the most senior surgeons. This is somewhat contrary to the long-standing belief that the most experienced surgeons deliver the highest quality care. A large systematic review by Choudhry and coworkers (2005) looking at the relationship between clinical experience and quality of health care suggests that surgeons who have been in practice longer may be at risk for providing lower-quality care if practice is not continued throughout one's career. Furthermore, aging appears to have a negative effect on the ability to learn new motor movement due to a decrease in mental encoding of motion. The motor cortex may not effectively reorganize and accommodate new information in surgeons older than 50 compared to younger individuals. Hand function and manual dexterity also deteriorate as a consequence of aging, as does the ability to control force with each finger. However, Voelcker-Rehage and Alberts (2005) demonstrated that older adults can reach performance levels comparable to younger adults but doing so requires extensive practice. This indicates that older physicians may need more quality improvement interventions and repetitive practice when maintaining and learning new surgical skills.

The second important principle is that even experts should be provided with immediate, direct, and relevant feedback on their performances. Together, time spent practicing a skill is most useful when trainees reflect on or receive feedback on their performance, and have numerous productive practice sessions distributed over time rather than the same number of hours compressed into one day's session. As a general rule, frequent practice sessions of any skill with intermittent rest periods appear to be better than mass training in a single session. Although this makes sense, this is not universally practiced in today's surgical training programs. The questions remaining are: What are the best methods of deliberate and repetitive practice? How does one provide appropriate feedback? What should be assessed, and what are the most useful methods of assessing that one has learned a surgical skill?

Deliberate Practice

Target Basic Automated and Correct Surgical Techniques

A usual starting point in skills teaching is to begin with surgical skills in which experienced surgeons have already achieved a level of automaticity. Suturing and knot-tying are examples of automated skills. That is, when tying a surgical knot, expert surgeons do not consciously think of the steps in order to accomplish the task. Once the surgeon reaches a phase of automaticity, it becomes increasingly difficult for surgeons not to overlook automated techniques when teaching. However, automated techniques are important for teachers to recognize because these techniques may be difficult to remedy once bad habits form. Therefore, it is essential that correct technique is demonstrated from the beginning of the learning process.

After choosing the skill to teach, one approach is to use error-training. This method begins by teaching correct technique. Once the trainee understands how a task is correctly performed, the next stage is to teach the trainee to recognize errors in technique and eliminate them during practice. Rogers and associates (2002) randomized 30 medical students to one of four training methods of tying two-handed surgical knots: (1) no instruction, (2) erroneous technique instruction, (3) correct technique instruction, or (4) combined correct and error technique instruction. The students were asked to perform a two-handed square knot, before and after viewing the instructional videotape. There was a significant improvement in assessment scores in the group receiving both the correct and error instructional techniques. This demonstrated that teaching trainees how *not* to perform a task, or common errors in performing the task, along with correct technique is more valuable that either method alone.

Common errors when learning basic knot-tying include the following:

1. *Failure to maintain tension:* It should be explained to the trainee that failure to maintain tension on the suture while tying increases the chance of slippage off the tissue and can be extremely dangerous when tying a vascular

structure. This error most likely occurs as the trainee gains speed in knot-tying, and it is helpful to have the trainee slowly perform the task while demonstrating correct technique.

2. *Air knots:* An air knot is caused by failure to push the suture past the knot. Failure to completely snug the knot down creates a space between consecutive knots. The space between knots compromises the security of the knot and may cause the knot to slip off the pedicle. Slowly performing the task may be helpful in evaluating this error.

3. *Holding the suture too close to the knot:* This compromises efficiency of movement by making it too difficult to pass the suture strand through the loop. This increases the time to place the knot and decreases efficiency of knot-tying. The suture should be held at least 5 cm away from the knot.

4. *Slip knot:* This knot is caused by incorrectly crossing the strands of a square knot or by failure to reverse the hands when placing horizontal tension after each throw. A slip knot is not a secure knot and can easily loosen.

See DVD Video 13-1, Knot-Tying: A Guide to Tying Surgical Knots and Common Knot-Tying Mistakes, for a correct demonstration of surgical knots and a demonstration of common errors.

Break Procedures Down into Manageable Steps

When preparing a lecture on a clinical problem one might outline the lecture beginning with epidemiology, pathophysiology, clinical presentation, treatments, and prevention. The topic of the lecture is broken down into concepts and by understanding the relationships between these concepts one can apply them to individual patients in the clinic. Similarly, in teaching procedural skills, it is helpful to break a procedure down into important tasks or manageable steps.

One important task during vaginal hysterectomy is clamping, cutting, and tying of a pedicle. See Table 13-1 for the manageable steps of a vaginal hysterectomy. Diwadkar and associates (2009) recorded 23 trainees during individual tasks of clamping, cutting, and suturing the left uterosacral ligament while performing a vaginal hysterectomy. Using motion analysis software to break down the procedure into discrete parts, differences in measurements such as time, angle, velocity, and hand trajectory of various steps emerged between novice and experienced surgical trainees. For example, at the start of suturing the uterosacral ligament pedicle, experienced trainees placed the Heaney clamp closer to a right angle to the vertical axis compared to novice trainees (Fig. 13-2). In this case, holding the Heaney clamp close to 90 degrees from

Table 13-1 Manageable Steps of a Vaginal Hysterectomy

Patient positioning
Bladder drainage
Incising the vaginal mucosa
Developing the plane between the anterior cervix and bladder
Entering the peritoneal cavity anteriorly
Entering the peritoneal cavity posteriorly
Clamping, transecting, and suturing the uterosacral ligaments
Clamping, transecting, and suturing the cardinal ligaments and uterine vessels
Clamping, transecting, and suturing the utero-ovarian ligaments
Suturing the vaginal cuff

Figure 13-2 **A** and **B,** Motion analysis: suturing the uterosacral ligament. At the start of suturing the uterosacral ligament, experienced surgeons placed the Heaney clamp closer to a right angle (96 degrees; **A**) to the vertical axis (represented by the bladder retractor) compared to novice surgeons (109 degrees; **B**). (Courtesy of The Cleveland Clinic Center for Medical Art & Photography, copyright 2009. All rights reserved.)

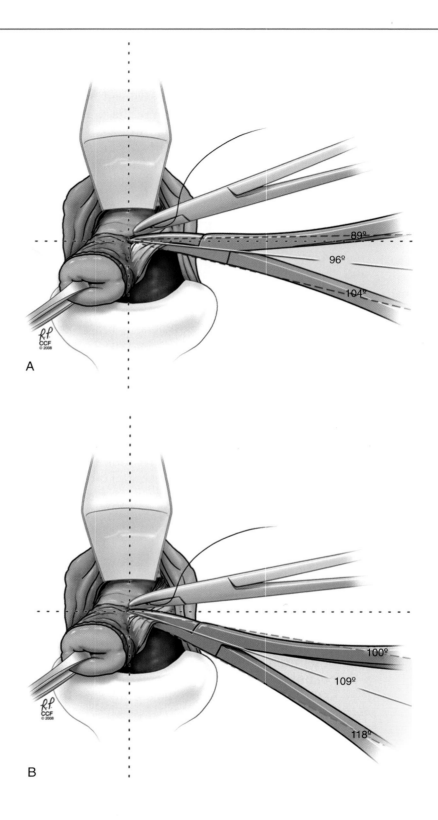

the vertical axis allowed for easier and faster suturing. It also allowed teaching surgeons to provide more deliberate focused teaching to the training surgeon. For example, this technique could then be communicated as, "Hold the Heaney clamp at a 90-degree angle to the bladder retractor, and it will be easier to see the needle as it passes through the tissue and will eliminate unnecessary passes of the needle."

Repetitive Practice

Simulation

Surgical simulation provides opportunity for repetitive practice of surgical skills outside the operating environment. Simulated surgical environments are gaining popularity due to several factors: poor teaching in high acuity and fiscal pressured operating rooms; work-hour restrictions on surgical trainees that result in decreased operating room exposure and less opportunity for repetitive practice; increased public awareness that surgeons demonstrate competency prior to operating on live patients; and public demand to minimize medical errors and iatrogenic injury to patients. The goals of surgical simulation are to create safe, controlled, reproducible environments that resemble real-life clinical situations and surgeries. Simulators clearly offer a compelling reason to reduce reliance on patients, cadavers, and animal models for surgical training, and some data suggest they may be just as good as other forms of surgical training. Moreover, surgical simulation in gynecology has been shown to be beneficial and superior to operating room experience alone. Studies have demonstrated that training in a skills laboratory may significantly shorten operating room time, increase patient safety, and reduce patient morbidity.

Low-fidelity simulators use less realistic materials and equipment, and are more useful for performing a simple task such as knot-tying or suturing. The American College of Obstetrics and Gynecology Surgical Curriculum includes examples of portable bench models that are easily constructed for teaching basic skills required for most common gynecologic procedures. For example, abdominal fascial closure can be simulated using a folded towel. Suture is used to reapproximate the towel edges with interrupted, continuous, and Smead-Jones stitches. Isolation and ligation of a vessel is simulated using a placenta and hemostats, scissors, and suture. This task evaluates the trainee's ability to isolate a vessel, clamp the vessel, divide the vessel, and tie both pedicles with square knots. The task can also be practiced with a tie on a passer. Ligation of a pedicle can be practiced with strips of bacon, Heaney clamps, and suture. This task evaluates the trainee's ability to place a Heaney clamp, place a Heaney stitch, and tie secure square knots.

Video box trainers are used for laparoscopic training, using real surgical instruments, endoscopes, and video screens. They provide an opportunity to practice basic skills required in any laparoscopic procedure, including eye-hand coordination, camera handling, grasping mechanisms, suturing, cutting, and clip applying. A study by Banks and coworkers (2007) randomized obstetrics and gynecology trainees to either laparoscopic simulation curriculum or a no-simulation group. Residents with simulation experience had higher scores than control subjects performing a tubal ligation on a live patient. Similar findings were reported by Coleman and Muller (2002) for the task of performing a salpingostomy for ectopic pregnancy. In gynecology, low-fidelity simulators exist for both vaginal and abdominal hysterectomy, cystoscopy, sacrocolpopexy, sacrospinous ligament fixation, colpocleisis, and obstetric sphincter laceration.

High-fidelity simulators use realistic materials, provide realistic cues to create a more realistic environment, and are used more often for surgical procedure training. High-fidelity simulators include animal models and virtual-reality simulators. Animal models, usually pigs, are useful for teaching complex laparoscopic techniques, but are limited by costs and availability. Similar to the video box trainers, virtual-reality simulators evaluate common laparoscopic skills, such as use of a 0-degree or 30-degree endoscope, eye–hand coordination, grasping, suturing, and clip-applying. Virtual-reality simulators create a more realistic scenario for laparoscopic techniques and procedures, record and save performance data, provide objective feedback, and allow the level of difficulty to be set. Disadvantages include costs and lack of haptic or tactile feedback.

Mental Imagery

Mental imagery can be a very effective means of encoding information, and there is some evidence that mental practice can improve surgical performance. Encoding refers to the process of relating incoming information to the concepts already in memory so that new material becomes more memorable. Mental imagery involves the cognitive rehearsal of a task with or without physical movement. The first theory behind mental practice postulates that muscle firing in the correct sequence strengthens muscle memory. The second theory is based on the development of mental blueprints that are rehearsed repetitively with mental practice, causing the behavior to become automatic. Widely used in sports, this technique has been shown to not only help a trainee acquire certain skills (cognitive imagery), but it can also help emotionally prepare a trainee to perform under stressful situations (motivational imagery). Mental practice in sports has been shown to be most effective when it is brief (no longer than 20 minutes) and when performed immediately before the task is to be performed. Prior to performing a hysterectomy, asking the surgical trainee to mentally rehearse each step of the procedure from abdominal incision to closure may be helpful. This may help trigger questions regarding portions of the procedure that are unclear so that they may be answered prior to starting the surgery.

There are also some data using mental imagery in surgical skills training. Bathalon, et al (2005) randomized 44 medical students to a 1-hour session on mental imagery, mental imagery with hand movement, or standard Advanced Trauma Life Support for the task of emergency cricothyrotomy. After 1 week, results on an Objective Structured Clinical Examination found that scores of the students who underwent mental imagery with physical movement were higher. Some surgeons incorporate mental imagery into the preoperative preparation of their trainees, reporting it to be a valuable addition to learning surgical procedures.

Feedback

In addition to repetitive practice, verbal feedback from an expert is a key factor in learning to correctly perform any skill. One study randomized novice medical students to a group that received computer-assisted instruction on knot-tying and a second group to receive a lecture using a slide presentation with individual live feedback while performing the task. Both groups were able to tie a square knot with no significant difference in total time, but the individual feedback group had better performance scores reflecting the quality of the technique and knots.

Feedback sessions should be an active dialogue between a trainee and a surgeon composed of skills or competencies relevant to the trainee's ultimate learning objectives. The following are general principles of providing formative feedback:

1. Useful feedback is timely, specific, and describes specific behaviors, knowledge, or attitudes that have been witnessed—not personal traits.

2. The surgeon's role is to help the trainee reflect on problems in a nonjudgmental way.

3. Whenever possible, the surgeon should ask questions rather than offer interpretations.

4. Feedback sessions should be mutually convenient.

5. Confidentiality of the trainee should be maintained.

It is also essential that feedback is provided early in the learning process to prevent learning of incorrect motor habits, which are difficult to remedy. Feedback can be given before, during, or after the skill is performed. It may occur at the end of the day in the operating room or at the end of a rotation.

Before practice it is critical to communicate what the objectives are and what level of performance is expected to achieve the objectives. (For examples of writing clear learning objectives, the reader is directed to Merrill, 1983, and Gagne et al, 1992.) The trainee then needs an overview of the skill and how it would be performed by an expert either by demonstration or examples. After practice, a trainee needs to be given feedback on selective items of the performance and the results of that performance. In general, this feedback should be constructive and immediate.

In our experience, starting the feedback process can make the surgeon and trainee feel somewhat uncomfortable, as it may feel out of the normal routine, and the trainee may feel as though you are scrutinizing his/her performance. Taylor (2008) suggests beginning the process by describing the difference between "quick" and "formal" feedback and how and when each occurs. Formal feedback is usually associated with assessment, and quick feedback is more associated with teaching. Although the aim of both is to improve performance, the observations that are made in formal feedback are more global and usually cover a period of time. Formal feedback often includes a comparison between early and current skills/knowledge. Quick feedback addresses observations "in the moment." Remind the trainee that they can initiate the feedback process by asking specific questions. Finally, discuss learning goals. For example, "While we are working together during this rotation, I will expect that you will ask a lot of questions. I will ask a lot of questions, too. From your answers, I'll get a sense of what you know and what you don't know yet. I am going to encourage you to periodically self-assess."

Giving immediate feedback can be difficult, especially in a busy, stressful operating environment. One model that can be used is the Ask-Tell-Ask Model, described by Taylor. This model is an effective template for providing feedback that focuses on learners' self assessment, giving you the opportunity to reinforce appropriate behavior (behaviorism) and correct faulty reasoning or technique. This model should be used before and after a surgical procedure. With this model of feedback, you ask trainees to assess their performance. If they have a concern about their performance, briefly address that concern. By focusing on the learners' concerns, you help them develop self-assessment skills while providing corrective feedback. The model is as follows:

ASK

- Ask for the trainee's self-assessment. Be specific, but leave room for comments about all tasks assigned. For example, "That was a difficult surgical case. How do you think the procedure went?"

TELL
- Acknowledge and address the trainee's concerns.
- State your observations.
  - Provide feedback on at least one task that the trainee performed well.
  - Address a maximum of one or two other areas for improvement.
- Provide focused teaching.

ASK
- Check the trainee's understanding.
- Discuss a plan for improvement.

See DVD Video 13-2, Feedback in Surgical Training, for a demonstration of the Ask-Tell-Ask feedback technique.

The most effective feedback is explicit, literal, and detailed. An example of poor feedback is, "Drive your needle through the uterosacral pedicle, not the uterine sidewall." A more effective statement is, "Hold the Heaney clamp at a 90-degree angle to the bladder retractor. This allows you to visualize your needle tip as you drive it through the tissue at the tip of the clamp, and prevents driving it through the uterine sidewall." Also, simply directing the trainee isn't necessarily the most effective way of teaching. When possible during surgery, it is often helpful to ask the trainee why a particular task or technique is essential, which may help the trainee understand the basis behind the technique and how the technique is performed. This process allows the trainee to relate the new information to existing knowledge, gain a deeper understanding of the skill, and may potentially improve retention and application of that skill to other associated scenarios.

Video playback has become another popular method of giving visual feedback. Video footage reduces subjectivity introduced with retrospective methods of feedback by allowing the instructor and learner to view the performance multiple times and evaluate the performance as if in real time. Video can also provide a means to break down the procedure into components or frames in order to examine every move the trainee makes, allowing the instructor to provide detailed feedback. Tsue and associates (2007) demonstrated how videotaped review of basic skills such as knot-tying can allow trainees to identify areas for improvement from their own performance allowing for practice on models or simulators prior to reattempting the task in the operating room.

Assessment

Assessment of the Trainee

Despite how much we improve our teaching abilities, it has been well established that assessment is a powerful driving force in what learners choose to learn. Assessment tools may be used for formal assessment or as a method of teaching by using the assessment to guide constructive formative feedback. For either approach, it is useful to be aware of commonly used assessment tools:

Case logs: Case logs reflect the quantity of cases and are easy to collect. This is the primary tool to document surgical competency. The primary limitation of case logs is they do not reflect the quality of the learning. Case logs lack content validity since they do not provide an accurate assessment of surgical skill for the individual performing the procedure. In addition, the numbers of cases to qualify as competent is not necessarily similar between two trainees given different rates of learning. Factors such as total time to perform the procedure and morbidity information do not provide any information on the difficulty of the case. Although it is recognized that this is a common form of assessment, case logs are not an ideal method for assessment.

Global rating scales and the objective structured assessment of technical skills (OSATS): The OSATS curriculum, first reported by Reznick in 1993, is based on the objective structured clinical examination (OSCE) and has been increasingly used in board certification examinations to determine clinical and technical competency. Initially developed for general surgery trainees, OSATS have reduced instructor subjectivity with the use of a procedure checklist and was determined by the Accreditation Council for Graduate Medical Education (ACGME) to be one of the better available methods of evaluating procedural skills. The scale requires trainees to rotate through stations in which they perform certain tasks in a set amount of time. Each trainee is evaluated by the same observer or multiple observers proficient in the task using objective criteria. The trainee's performance is scored with two methods. The first method uses a task-specific checklist of 10 to 30 surgical maneuvers that are essential elements of the procedure. The second is a score recorded with the use of a global rating scale that includes surgical behaviors such as respect for tissues, time and motion, and use of assistants (Appendix 13-1). The major weakness of the OSATS is that it requires time, equipment, and manpower. The global rating scale developed from the OSAT testing environment has been used to assess vaginal surgery.

Vaginal Surgical Skills Index (VSSI): A procedure-specific global rating scale, modified from the global rating scale of operative performance, has recently been shown to be valid and more reliable than the global rating scale described by Martin and coworkers (1997) for assessing vaginal surgical skills. This is a 13-item scale that measures technical skills used while performing vaginal surgery (Appendix 13-2). It should be noted that minimum cutoff scores for determining competence in performing vaginal hysterectomy have been determined for the VSSI (total score of 32) and global rating scale of operative performance (total score of 15). We estimated that after performing between 21 and 27 vaginal hysterectomies an average obstetrics and gynecology resident can reach these competency cutoff scores, although this will vary from individual to individual.

Dexterity analysis systems: These computerized systems have been developed to measure movement of sensors attached to the surgeon's hands while performing procedures. Currently, cost and lack of trained interpreters limit the use of such devices widespread.

Self-assessment: Recent studies focusing on surgical skills and self-assessment have demonstrated a correlation between self-assessment scores and other external measures. Mandel and associates (2005) found that self-assessment by residents on task-specific, overall, and global scores during open and laparoscopic surgery significantly correlated with faculty ratings on a six-station OSATS. Residents rated themselves lower than the faculty and had good insight into their deficiencies even when their skills were poor. Other studies have shown that self-assessment may be more effective after viewing a videotape of one's surgical performance. Ward and associates (2003) conducted a study that asked residents to rate their skill level after viewing of taping of themselves completing a laparoscopic procedure on a pig model. The residents were required to watch four tapings of expert surgeons performing the same task prior to completing the ratings. With the video footage, residents were able to analyze their skills without having to remember their performance at the time of the surgery. The resident ratings were found to correlate with the faculty ratings. Jowitt and associates (2007) found that computer-based video learning for knot-tying was effective in a self-directed learning environment among

ence and quality of health care. Ann Intern Med 2005;142(4):260–273.

Coleman RL, Muller CY: Effects of a laboratory-based skills curriculum on laparoscopic proficiency: A randomized trial. Am J Obstet Gynecol 2002;186(4):836–842.

Council on Resident Education in Obstetrics and Gynecology Surgical Curriculum. Available at: www. acog.org/departments/dept_web.cfm?recno=1. Accessed Nov. 2009.

Cuschieri A, Francis N, Crosby J, Hanna GB: What do master surgeons think of surgical competence and revalidation? Am J Surg 2001;182(2):110–116.

novice trainees. Novice trainees were asked to self-assess their knot-tying skills when learning to tie a one-handed square knot. They were randomized to cease practice or continue practice once they self-assessed themselves as proficient. Evaluations by experts revealed an improvement in post-test performance scores for both groups after viewing the computer-based video. Interestingly, there was no difference in scores between the group that ceased practice and the group that continued practicing after self-assessing proficiency. These find-

Datta V, Mackay S, Mandalia M, Darzi A: The use of electromagnetic motion tracking analysis to objectively measure open surgical skill in the laboratory-based model. J Am Coll Surg 2001;193(5): 479–485.

Diwadkar GB, Jelovsek JE: An assessment of the operating room educational environment: Measuring surgical trainess perceptions. J Surg Education 2010, in press.

Diwadkar GB, van den Bogert A, Barber MD, Jelovsek JE: Assessing vaginal surgical skills using video motion analysis. Obstet Gynecol 2009;114(2 Pt 1):244–251.

Driscoll MP: Psychology of Learning for Instruction. Boston, Pearson Education, 2005.

Ericsson KA: Deliberate practice and the acquisition and maintenance of expert performance in medicine and related domains. Acad Med 2004;79(Suppl 10):S70–S81.

Gagne RM, Briggs LJ, Wagner W: Principles of Instructional Design. Fort Worth, Harcourt Brace Jovanovich, 1992.

Grabe M: Attentional processes in education. In Phye GD, Andre T (eds): Cognitive Classroom Learning. Orlando, Academic Press, 1986.

Jelovsek JE, Walters MD, Korn A, et al: Establishing cutoff scores on assessments of surgical skills to determine surgical competence. Am J Obstet Gynecol 2001, in press.

Jowitt N, LeBlanc V, Xeroulis G, et al: Surgical skill acquisition with self-directed practice using computer-based video training. Am J Surg 2007;193:237–242.

Kanashiro J, McAleer S, Roff S: Assessing the educational environment in the operating room—a measure of resident perception at one Canadian institution. Surgery 2006;139(2):150–158.

Kaufman DM: Applying educational theory in practice. BMJ 2003;326:213–216.

Keller VF, Carroll JG: A new model for physician patient communication. Patient Educ Counseling 1994;23:131–140.

Knot-Tying Manual. Somerville, NJ, Ethicon, Inc., 2005.

Kopta JA: The development of motor skills in orthopaedic education. Clin Orthop Relat Res 1971;75:80–85.

Mandel LS, Goff BA, Lentz GM: Self-assessment of resident surgical skills: Is it feasible? Am J Obstet Gynecol 2005;193(5):1817–1822.

Martin JA, Regehr G, Reznick R, et al: Objective structured assessment of technical skill (OSATS) for surgical residents. Br J Surg 1997;84(2):273–278.

Merrill MD: Component display theory. In Reigeluth CM (ed): Instructional-Design Theories and Models. Hillsdale, NJ, Erlbaum, 1983.

Reznick RK: Teaching and testing technical skills. Am J Surg 1993;165(3):358–361.

Roff S: The Dundee ready educational environment measure (DREEM)—a generic instrument for measuring students' perceptions of undergraduate health professions curricula. Med Teach 2005;27(4):322–325.

Rogers RG: Mental practice and acquisition of motor skills: Examples from sports training and surgical education. Obstet Gynecol Clin North Am 2006;33(2):297–304.

Rogers DA, Regehr G, MacDonald J: A role for error training in surgical technical skill instruction and evaluation. Am J Surg 2002;183:242–245.

Skinner BF: The Behavior of Organisms: An Experimental Analysis. Englewood Cliffs, NJ, Prentice-Hall, 1938.

Smith SG, Torkington J, Brown TJ, et al: Motion analysis. Surg Endosc 2002;16(4):640–645.

Taylor C: ASK-TELL-ASK model for giving feedback. Personal communication, Cleveland Clinic, 2008.

Tsue TT, Dugan JW, Burkey B: Assessment of surgical competency. Otolaryngol Clin North Am 2007;40(6):1237–1259.

Van Sickle KR, Ritter EM, Baghai M, et al: Prospective, randomized, double-blind trial of curriculum-based training for intracorporeal suturing and knot tying. J Am Coll Surg 2008;207(4):560–568.

Voelcker-Rehage C, Alberts JL: Age-related changes in grasping force modulation. Exp Brain Res 2005;166(1):61–70.

Ward M, MacRae H, Schlachta C, et al: Resident self-assessment of operative performance. Am J Surg 2003;185(6):521–524.

Appendix 13-1 Global Rating Scale

Trainee's name:	Date of operation:

Procedure(s) the trainee performed:	Proportion of procedure that the trainee performed. *(Circle one)*
1. _____	≤50% *or* >50%
2. _____	≤50% *or* >50%
3. _____	≤50% *or* >50%

Global Rating Scale of Operative Performance

Please circle the number corresponding to the candidate's performance in each category, irrespective of training level. Performance is rated on a spectrum from 1 to 5, as shown.

Respect for Tissue

1	2	3	4	5
Frequently used unnecessary force on tissue or caused damage by inappropriate use of instruments		Careful handling of tissue but occasionally caused inadvertent damage		Consistently handled tissues appropriately with minimal damage

Time and Motion

1	2	3	4	5
Many unnecessary moves		Efficient time/motion but some unnecessary moves		Clear economy of movement and maximum efficiency

Instrument Handling

1	2	3	4	5
Repeatedly makes tentative or awkward moves with instruments		Competent use of instruments but occasionally appeared stiff or awkward by inappropriate use of instruments		Fluid moves with instruments and no awkwardness

Knowledge of Instruments

1	2	3	4	5
Frequently stopped operating and seemed unsure of the next move		Demonstrated some forward planning with reasonable progression of procedure		Obviously planned course of operation with effortless flow from one move to the next

Use of Assistants

1	2	3	4	5
Consistently placed assistants poorly or failed to use assistants		Appropriate use of assistants most of the time		Strategically used assistants to the best advantage at all times

Knowledge of Specific Procedure

1	2	3	4	5
Deficient knowledge Needed specific instruction at most steps of operation		Knew all important steps of operation		Demonstrated familiarity with all aspects of operation

Overall, is the trainee competent to safely perform this task unsupervised?   ❑ NO   ❑ YES

Comments:

Adapted from Martin JA, Regehr G, Reznick R, et al: Objective structured assessment of technical skill (OSATS) for surgical residents. Br J Surg 1997;84(2):273–278.

Appendix 13-2 Vaginal Surgical Skills Index (VSSI)

Trainee's name:				**Date of operation:**		

Procedure(s) the trainee performed:

1. _____

2. _____

3. _____

Proportion of procedure that the trainee performed: *(Circle one)*

≤50% *or* >50%

≤50% *or* >50%

≤50% *or* >50%

Please evaluate each trainee according to the criteria below and check the box that most corresponds to their performance.

Initial inspection *(Check one)*	☐ 0 Incomplete and unsystematic inspection of relevant pelvic and vaginal structures	☐ 1 Partially complete and unsystematic inspection of relevant pelvic and vaginal structures	☐ 2 Complete but unsystematic inspection of relevant pelvic and vaginal structures	☐ 3 Complete and somewhat systematic inspection of relevant pelvic and vaginal structures	☐ 4 Systematic and complete assessment of relevant pelvic and vaginal structures	☐ Not observed
Incision *(Check one)*	☐ 0 Does not perform appropriate incision(s) safely and does not use incision(s) effectively ensuring optimal exposure	☐ 1 Incompletely performs appropriate incision(s) safely and does not use incision(s) effectively ensuring optimal exposure	☐ 2 Performs appropriate incision(s) safely but does not use incision(s) effectively ensuring optimal exposure	☐ 3 Performs appropriate incision(s) safely and partially uses incision(s) effectively ensuring optimal exposure	☐ 4 Performs appropriate incision(s) safely and uses incision(s) effectively ensuring optimal exposure	☐ Not observed
Maintenance of visibility *(Check one)*	☐ 0 Almost never or never obtains appropriate exposure	☐ 1 A few times (less than half the time) obtains appropriate exposure	☐ 2 Sometimes (about half the time) obtains appropriate exposure	☐ 3 Most time (more than half the time) obtains appropriate exposure	☐ 4 Almost always or always obtains appropriate exposure	☐ Not observed
Use of assistants *(Check one)*	☐ 0 Almost never or never strategically used assistant(s) to the best advantage	☐ 1 A few times (less than half the time) strategically uses assistant(s) to the best advantage	☐ 2 Sometimes (about half the time) strategically uses assistant(s) to the best advantage	☐ 3 Most time (more than half the time) strategically uses assistant(s) to the best advantage	☐ 4 Almost always or always strategically uses assistant(s) to the best advantage at all times	☐ Not observed
Knowledge of instruments *(Check one)*	☐ 0 Almost never or never uses and is familiar with correct instruments	☐ 1 A few times (less than half the time) uses and is familiar with correct instruments	☐ 2 Sometimes (about half the time) uses and is familiar with correct instruments	☐ 3 Most time (more than half the time) uses and is familiar with correct instruments	☐ 4 Almost always or always uses and is familiar with correct instruments	☐ Not observed
Tissue and instrument handling *(Check one)*	☐ 0 Almost never or never appropriately handles tissue and instruments	☐ 1 A few times (less than half the time) appropriately handles tissue and instruments	☐ 2 Sometimes (about half the time) handles tissue and instruments appropriately	☐ 3 Most time (more than half the time) handles tissue and instruments appropriately	☐ 4 Almost always or always handles tissue and instruments appropriately	☐ Not observed
Electrosurgery *(Check one)*	☐ 0 Almost never or never uses electrosurgery safely and efficiently	☐ 1 A few times (less than half the time) uses electrosurgery safely and efficiently	☐ 2 Sometimes (about half the time) uses electrosurgery safely and efficiently	☐ 3 Most time (more than half the time) uses electrosurgery safely and efficiently	☐ 4 Almost always or always uses electrosurgery safely and efficiently	☐ Not observed
Knot-tying/ligation *(Check one)*	☐ 0 Almost never or never quickly and correctly performs suture ligation and knot-tying	☐ 1 A few times (less than half the time) quickly and correctly performs suture ligation and knot-tying	☐ 2 Sometimes (about half the time) quickly and correctly performs suture ligation and knot-tying	☐ 3 Most time (more than half the time) quickly and correctly performs suture ligation and knot-tying	☐ 4 Almost always or always quickly and correctly performs suture ligation and knot-tying	☐ Not observed

Appendix 13-2 Vaginal Surgical Skills Index (VSSI)—cont'd

Hemostasis *(Check one)*	☐ 0 Almost never or never exposes bleeders and uses correct technique to obtain hemostasis safely and effectively	☐ 1 A few times (less than half the time) exposes bleeders and uses correct technique to obtain hemostasis safely and effectively	☐ 2 Sometimes (about half the time) exposes bleeders and uses correct technique to obtain hemostasis safely and effectively	☐ 3 Most time (more than half the time) exposes bleeders and uses correct technique to obtain hemostasis safely and effectively	☐ 4 Almost always or always exposes bleeders and uses correct technique to obtain hemostasis safely and effectively	☐ Not observed
Procedure completion *(Check one)*	☐ 0 Almost never or never completely removes fluid and debris and thoroughly inspects for bleeding	☐ 1 A few times (less than half the time) completely removes fluid and debris and thoroughly inspects for bleeding	☐ 2 Sometimes (about half the time) completely removes fluid and debris and thoroughly inspects for bleeding	☐ 3 Most time (more than half the time) completely removes fluid and debris and thoroughly inspects for bleeding	☐ 4 Almost always or always completely removes fluid and debris and thoroughly inspects for bleeding	☐ Not observed
Time and motion *(Check one)*	☐ 0 Almost never or never efficiently performs movements with no awkward or unnecessary moves	☐ 1 A few times (less than half the time) efficiently performs movements with no awkward or unnecessary moves	☐ 2 Sometimes (about half the time) efficiently performs movements with no awkward or unnecessary moves	☐ 3 Most time (more than half the time) efficiently performs movements with no awkward or unnecessary moves	☐ 4 Almost always or always efficiently performs movements with no awkward or unnecessary moves	☐ Not observed
Flow of operation and forward planning *(Check one)*	☐ 0 Almost never or never demonstrates forward planning allowing for proper flow of the procedure	☐ 1 A few times (less than half the time) demonstrates forward planning allowing for proper flow of the procedure	☐ 2 Sometimes (about half the time) demonstrates forward planning allowing for proper flow of the procedure	☐ 3 Most time (more than half the time) demonstrates forward planning allowing for proper flow of the procedure	☐ 4 Almost always or always demonstrates forward planning allowing for proper flow of the procedure	☐ Not observed
Knowledge of specific procedure *(Check one)*	☐ 0 Almost never or never demonstrates familiarity with all aspects of the operation	☐ 1 A few times (less than half the time) demonstrated familiarity with all aspects of the operation	☐ 2 Sometimes (about half the time) demonstrates familiarity with all aspects of the operation	☐ 3 Most time (more than half the time) demonstrates familiarity with all aspects of the operation	☐ 4 Almost always or always demonstrates familiarity with all aspects of the operation	☐ Not observed

Overall, is the trainee competent to safely perform this task unsupervised?   ☐ NO   ☐ YES

Comments:

Index

A

Abdominal aorta, 45–48, 47f–49f
Abdominal bloating
  before and after hysterectomy, 90t
Abdominal hysterectomy
  anatomical considerations, 107–108, 107f, 116
  case studies, 104, 115, 117
  chronic pelvic pain case study, 115
  comparison chart with vaginal and laparoscopic, 85t
  complication rates, 84–85, 195–211, 196t
  difficult and special cases, 118–121
    cesarean hysterectomy, 121
    obesity, 120–121
    obliterated rectovaginal septum, 119–120
    scarring of vesicouterine septum, 120
    supracervical hysterectomy, 118–119, 119f
    unsuspected malignancy, 120
  evolution and history of, 2t–3t, 20–24, 25–29, 25f, 26f
  factors in choosing route, 85t, 103
  indications for, 103
  menorrhagia and fibroids case study, 117
  in patient with fibroids, 118
  statistics, 103
  statistics versus vaginal and laparoscopic, 77
  surgical procedures and steps
    anesthesia, 105
    difficult or special cases, 118–121
    incision types, 105–107
    pelvic anatomical exam, 105–107
    positioning, 105, 105f
    steps, variables and illustrations, 107–118, 108f–115f
  uterovaginal prolapse case study, 104
  versus vaginal approaches
    evolution and history of, 23–24, 25f
Abdominal supracervical hysterectomy
  as difficult abdominal hysterectomy, 118–119, 119f
  evolution of, 2t–3t, 27
  first surgeries on, 2t–3t
Abdominal wall
  contents of, 31–32, 33f
  surface illustration of, 32f
Abnormal uterine bleeding (AUB)
  case studies
    and endometrial hyperplasia, 180–181
    postoperative, 197–198
    and vaginal hysterectomy, 124
  endometrial ablation, 73
  as indication for hysterectomy, 70t, 73
Activities of daily living
  before and after hysterectomy, 90t, 92–93
  and health-related quality of life (HRQOL), 89, 90t, 92–93, 98–99
Adenomyosis
  as possible indication for hysterectomy, 70t
Adnexa
  anatomical description and illustration of, 41–42, 41f, 42f, 44f
  divided from uterus during oophorectomy, 166, 167f, 168f
  Sheth's adnexa clamp, 166, 168f

Adnexal disease
  determining hysterectomy route, 103, 123
Age
  as factor influencing hysterectomy rates, 66–67, 67f, 71t
  as hysterectomy complication/risk, 195, 199
  and preoperative assessment, 78, 80t
Algorithm
  for choosing hysterectomy route, 83f
Allis clamps, 138f
Alternative treatments
  to hysterectomy
    hysteroscopic myomectomy, 218–225, 218f, 219f, 220t, 221f
    levonorgestin-intrauterine system (LNG-IUS), 214–218, 215t
    microwave endometrial ablation, 232, 232f, 233
    MR-guided focused ultrasound (MRgFUS), 240–244, 242f, 243f
    overview of, 213–214
    uterine fibroid embolization (UFE), 213, 235–240, 236f
Ampulla, 41–42, 41f, 42f, 44f
Anatomy
  and abdominal hysterectomy, 107–108, 107f, 116
  in antiquity, 2t–3t, 3–5, 4f
  associated with uterine surgery, 31–59
    anterior abdominal wall, 31–32, 32f–33f, 34–35, 36f–37f, 38–39, 39f–40f
    cervix, 39–41, 41f, 42f
    lower urinary tract, 48, 50–53, 50f, 52f–54f
    nerves of pelvic cavity, 58–59
    pelvis spaces and avascular planes, 54–58, 55f–57f
    sigmoid colon and rectum, 53–54
    uterine corpus, 39–41, 41f, 42f
    uterine support structures, 42–43, 44f, 45
    vasculature, 45–48, 47f–49f
  evolution of, 1–29
  of pelvis to examine before hysterectomy, 107f
  timeline of milestones regarding, 2t–3t
Anesthesia
  for abdominal hysterectomy, 105
  complications with, 197t
  during early surgeries, 2t, 18
  examination under, 137–138
  history of, 2t–3t
  suboptimal throughout history, 1, 2t–3t
  for vaginal hysterectomy, 124–125
Anterior abdominal wall
  anatomical description and illustration of, 31–32, 32f–33f, 34–35, 36f–37f, 38–39, 39f–40f
Anterior cul-de-sacs
  anatomy of, 54–55, 55f
  entry causing difficult and challenging vaginal hysterectomy, 150–152
  entry during vaginal hysterectomy, 126–128, 127f–128f
Anterior superior iliac spines, 31, 32f

Antibiotics
  for infection control, 199–200, 200t
  prophylactic, 79–80
  vaginal hysterectomy, 124
Antiembolics
  vaginal hysterectomy, 124
Antimicrobial regimens, 200t
Antisepsis, 18
Anxiety
  improved with hysterectomy, 89, 90t, 98–99
Aorta
  supplying blood to pelvic structures, 45–46, 47f–49f
Arcus tendineus fascia pelvis (ATFP), 45
Aretaeus, 4
Arteries
  of pelvis, 45–46, 47f–49f
Asepsis
  suboptimal throughout history, 1, 2t–3t
Asherman syndrome, 217
Aspirin
  preoperative assessment of, 78
Atypical endometrial hyperplasia
  as possible indication for hysterectomy, 70t
Automaticity, 251, 252
Avascular planes
  and pelvis spaces
    anatomical description and illustration of, 54–58, 55f–57f

B

Back pain
  before and after hysterectomy, 90t, 92
Behaviorism, 249–250
Bellinger, John, 2t, 20–21
Benign conditions
  alternative treatments to hysterectomy, 213–244
  factors influencing route choices, 82t
  and hysterectomy complications, 195–211
  hysterectomy for, 77
  versus malignant and hysterectomy, 70t, 71f
Bilateral tube ligation, 170
Birth control
  as alternate treatment to hysterectomy, 91t, 92
  reducing risk of ovarian cancer, 170
Bivalving
  for enlarged uterus, 141, 142f
Bladder
  anatomical description and illustration of, 48, 50–53, 50f, 52f, 54f
  demarcation of, 150–152, 151f
  dissection off uterus
    during vaginal hysterectomy, 126–127, 128f
  function before and after hysterectomy, 97
  and incision precautions, 34, 38, 50–51, 125–126, 126f
  injuries (See bladder injuries)
  inside view of, 50f
Bladder cancer
  as indication for hysterectomy, 70t

Bladder injuries
    complications with hysterectomy, 196t,
        204, 205f, 206f
    cystotomy, 204, 205f, 206f
    with prior cesarean deliveries, 204, 205f
    sharp dissection required to prevent, 150,
        151f
Bladder integrity, 151–152
Bleeding
    before and after hysterectomy, 89, 90t,
        92–93
    case studies
        and endometrial hyperplasia, 180–181
        postoperative, 197–198
        and vaginal hysterectomy, 124
    excessive uterine, 70t, 73
    hysterectomy *versus* alternative treatment
        trials on, 91t, 92–93
Blood transfusion
    complication with or without
        oophorectomy, 168t
Bone mass
    and osteoporosis, 173
Bovie extender, 138f
Bowel function
    before and after hysterectomy, 97–98
Bowel injuries
    complications with hysterectomy, 196t,
        209–210
Breast cancer
    reduction with prophylactic
        oophorectomy, 171
Breastfeeding
    reducing risk of ovarian cancer, 170
Briesky-Navratil vaginal retractors, 138f
Broad ligament
    covering uterine corpus and upper cervix,
        40, 42f
    fibroid case study, 61–62
    grasping during surgery, 106–111, 108f
    illustration of, 43f
    during prophylactic oophorectomy
        surgery, 163–164, 164f, 167f
Burnham, Walter, 2t, 21

C

Cadavers, 6, 10
Camper's fascia, 31–32, 33f, 34f
Cancer
    breast
        reduction with prophylactic
            oophorectomy, 171
    as contraindication for intrauterine
        systems (IUS), 215
    endometrial, 171
    fallopian tubes, 171
    heredity nonpolyposis colorectal, 170
    ovarian
        as indication for hysterectomy, 70t
        prevention with prophylactic
            oophorectomy, 169–171
    peritoneal, 171
    preoperative assessment of, 78, 80t
    prevention *versus* surgical menopause
        decisions
        with prophylactic oophorectomy, 161
    statistics regarding hysterectomies and, 70t
    unsuspected malignancy
        causing difficult abdominal
            hysterectomy, 120
    vertical incisions, 106
"Candy-cane" stirrups, 124, 125f
Cardinal ligaments
    supporting uterus, 42–43, 44f, 45
Cardiovascular system
    and prophylactic oophorectomy, 172–173
Case logs, 258–259
Catheters
    ureteral, 207–208
    used in ancient times, 5–6

Cervical canal
    anatomical description and illustration of,
        39–40, 41f
Cervical cancer
    historical milestones in treatment of, 2t–3t
    as indication for hysterectomy, 70t
Cervical fibroids
    case study regarding, 59, 60f, 61
Cervical intraepithelial neoplasia (CIN)
    as possible indication for hysterectomy,
        70t
Cervicovaginal entry, 153, 154f
Cervix
    anatomical description and illustration of,
        39–41, 40, 41f, 42f, 44f
    bleeding after prior supracervical
        hysterectomy, 132
    blood supply to, 46–48, 47f–49f
    connective tissue supporting, 43, 44f, 45
    definition of, 40
    descent of, 137
    elongated causing difficult vaginal
        hysterectomy, 155–156
    evolution of the understanding of, 1–29
    historical milestones in understanding,
        2t–3t
    and laparoscopic supracervical
        hysterectomy, 179–180, 186–187
    preservation desires and fibroids, 186–187
    preservation with laparoscopic
        supracervical hysterectomy (LSH),
        180
    removal and quality of life, 98–99
    removal with abdominal hysterectomy,
        112–114, 114f
    risks and benefits of preserving, 99–100
    supracervical hysterectomy, 118–119, 119f
    trachelectomy, 133–134, 133f
    and uterus extirpation (*See* total
        laparoscopic hysterectomy [TLH])
Cesarean deliveries
    bladder injuries with prior, 204, 205f
Cesarean hysterectomies
    as difficult abdominal hysterectomy, 121
    evolution and history of, 2t–3t, 21–22
Chassaignac's Screw Ecraseur, 16f
Cherney, Leonid S., 3t, 23
Cherney incisions
    in abdominal hysterectomy surgery,
        105–107
    description and illustration of, 35, 38f
Chloroform
    history of, 2t–3t
Choppin, Samuel, 2t, 18–19
Chronic pelvic pain
    case study for abdominal hysterectomy,
        115
    as indication for hysterectomy, 70t, 72,
        74
Clamps
    early compression forceps, 2t, 19–20
    and retractors used in vaginal
        hysterectomy, 128f–131f, 129–134,
        133f
    used during abdominal hysterectomy,
        106–111, 108f, 109f–113f, 109f–114f
    used for difficult and challenging vaginal
        hysterectomy, 138, 138f
Clark, John Goodrich, 3t, 22
Colorectal cancer, 170
Colpotomy
    during total laparoscopic hysterectomy,
        185
Columbat's uterocepts, 15–16, 15f
Complications; *See* hysterectomy,
    complications
Compression forceps, 2t, 19–20
Concomitant salpingo-oophorectomy, 185
Connective tissue
    supporting uterus and vagina, 43, 44f, 45
    surrounding cervix, 40, 41f

Coring
    early method, 3t
    intrauterine, 141, 142f–143f, 144
Cornu, 41–42, 41f, 42f, 44f
Cost analysis
    of hysterectomies, 85
    of hysterectomies *versus* intrauterine
        systems, 217
Cryoablation unit
    HerOption, 227t, 228–229, 228f, 229f
Cryotherapy
    characteristics of, 227t, 228–229
Cul-de-sacs
    anterior and posterior, 54–55, 55f,
        126–127, 127f, 128f
    obliterated posterior endometriosis
        case study, 62, 62f
Cylindrical specula, 14f
Cystoscopy
    during abdominal hysterectomy, 113–114
    cost analysis of, 207
    intraoperative, 204, 205f, 206f, 207
    during vaginal hysterectomy, 151–152
Cystotomies
    and bladder injuries, 204, 205f, 206f
    preventing accidental, 126–127
    transvaginal repair of, 204

D

Da Vinci
    Leonardo, 6
De Graff, Regnier, 8–9, 9f
Decision-making
    algorithm for choosing hysterectomy
        route, 83f
    regarding prophylactic oophorectomy,
        85–86, 161–162, 174–176, 175f
Delpech, J.M., 3t, 20
Depression
    improved with hysterectomy, 89, 90t, 98–99
Dexterity analysis systems, 259
Diagnostic laparoscopy
    to diagnose endometriosis, 74
Distal segments of ureters
    anatomical description and illustration of,
        48, 50–53, 50f, 54f
Documentation
    of survival/recovery rates throughout
        history, 1, 2t–3t
Dorsal lithotomy position
    for vaginal hysterectomy, 124, 125f
Dysfunctional uterine bleeding (DUB)
    hysterectomy *versus* alternative treatment
        trials on, 91t
Dysmenorrhea
    causing difficulties in vaginal
        hysterectomy, 139
    as indication for hysterectomy, 70t, 72, 75
    and menorrhagia in nulliparous obese
        patient, 146

E

Electrocautery
    and laser hysteroscopic myomectomy, 223
Electrosurgical procedures
    for vaginal hysterectomy, 131–132
Elongated cervix
    causing difficult and challenging vaginal
        hysterectomy, 155–156
Endocervical canal, 40, 41f
Endometrial ablation
    as alternate treatment to hysterectomy,
        91t, 92–93, 213–214
    balloon ablation, 227–228, 227t, 228f
    complications, 233
    cryoablation, 228–229, 228f, 229f
    for excessive uterine bleeding, 73
    hysteroscopic thermal ablation, 230–231,
        231f

Endometrial ablation (Continued)
microwave endometrial ablation, 231, 232f, 233
office ablation procedures, 227, 227t
outcomes and conclusions, 233–234
overview of, 225–226
patient considerations, 226
preoperative evaluation and prep, 226–227
radiofrequency ablation, 229–230, 230f
surgical techniques and devices, 227–234, 227t
Endometrial cancer, 70t, 171
Endometrial cavity
anatomical description and illustration of, 39–42, 41f, 42f, 44f
Endometrial hyperplasia
statistics regarding hysterectomies and, 70t
Endometriosis
before and after hysterectomy, 93–95
and chronic pelvic pain, 115
determining hysterectomy route, 103, 123
diagnostic laparoscopy, 74
as indication for hysterectomy, 70t, 71f, 74–75
with obliterated posterior cul-de-sac, 62, 62f
statistics regarding hysterectomies and, 70t
Endometrium
anatomical description and illustration of, 40, 41f
Endopelvic fascia, 42, 44f
Enlarged uterus
bivalving or hemisection, 141, 142f
causing difficult and challenging vaginal hysterectomy, 139–141, 142f–143f, 144–147
intramyometrial coring, 141, 142f–143f, 144
lack of uterine descent, 147, 148f
myomectomy, 144, 146
preoperative procedures, 140–141
wedge morcellation, 144, 145f
Enseal Device, 191, 192f
Estrogen
and alternate treatments to hysterectomy, 91t, 92
following oophorectomy, 171–176
European Society of Gynecological Endoscopy (ESGE)
classifying myometrial penetration, 219–220
EVALuate trials, 96, 196t
Examination under anesthesia (EUA)
during vaginal hysterectomy, 137–138
Exposure
and suboptimal surgery throughout history, 1, 2t–3t

F

Fallopian tube cancer
as indication for hysterectomy, 70t, 171
Fallopian tube prolapse
complication with hysterectomy, 210–211
complication with or without oophorectomy, 168t
Fallopian tubes
anatomical description and illustration of, 40, 41–42, 41f, 42f, 44f
cancer, 70t, 171
concomitant salpingo-oophorectomy, 185
four areas of, 41–42, 44f
innervation of, 58–59, 60f
Fatigue
before and after hysterectomy, 90t, 92–93
Female reproductive system
historical timeline for understanding, 2t
Fertility issues
versus hysterectomy, 92
Fever
complication with hysterectomy, 196t, 198–199

Fibroids
case studies regarding
broad ligament, 61–62
cervical, 59, 60f, 61
and menorrhagia, 117
and cervix preservation desires, 186–187
classifying depth, location and penetration, 219–220, 221t
first successful removal of, 3t, 20–21
first surgeries on, 2t–3t
hysterectomy complications with, 195
hysteroscopic myomectomy, 218–225, 218f, 219f, 220t, 221f
as indication for hysterectomy, 70t, 71–72, 71f
levonorgestin-intrauterine system (LNG-IUS), 214–218, 215t
microwave endometrial ablation, 232, 232f, 233
MR-guided focused ultrasound (MRgFUS), 240–244, 242f, 243f
symptoms, 139
uterine fibroid embolization (UFE), 92t, 93, 235–240, 236f
Fimbria, 41–42, 41f, 42f, 44f
Flexible uterine sound, 138, 138f
Focused ultrasound therapy, 240–244
Follicles
anatomy of ovarian, 42, 43f, 44f
Forceps
used in ancient times, 5–6
Freund, William, 2t, 19–20
Fumigation apparatus, 8f
Fundus of the uterus
anatomy of, 39–40, 41f

G

Geographic variations
as factor influencing hysterectomy rates, 67–68, 67f
Gestational trophoblastic tumors
as indication for hysterectomy, 70t
Global rating scales
and objective structured assessment of technical skills (OSATS), 259, 263
Graafian follicles
historical timeline for understanding, 2t
Granulation tissue
complication with or without oophorectomy, 168t
Graves speculum, 13–14
Gynecologic surgery; See also individual types of surgery evolution and history of, 1–29, 2t–3t
abdominal hysterectomy beginnings, 2t–3t, 20–24, 25–29, 25f, 26f
abdominal versus vaginal approaches, 23–24, 25f
in antiquity, 2t–3t, 3–5, 4f
cesarean hysterectomies, 2t–3t, 21–22
eighteenth century, 2t–3t, 9–11, 11f, 12f
Heaney technique, 26–29, 27f–29f
laparoscopic hysterectomies, 28–29
Medieval period, 2t–3t, 6
nineteenth century, 2t–3t, 11–23, 13f–17f, 19f–20f
pelvic examinations, 12–14, 13f, 14f
Renaissance Period, 2t–3t, 6–7, 8f
Richardson technique, 24, 25f–26f
seventeenth century, 2t–3t, 7–9, 9t, 10f
timeline of milestones, 2t–3t
trachelectomy, 14–15, 15f–16f
twentieth century to present, 2t–3t, 23–29, 25f–29f
vaginal hysterectomy, 17–20, 17f, 19f–20f
teaching and learning
assessing learning environment, 260, 261t
assessing trainee, 258–260, 263–265

Graves speculum (Continued)
behaviorist theory, 249–251, 250f
deliberate practice, 252–253
educational theories, 249–251, 250f
error-training, 252–253
feedback, 256–258
fundamentals of teaching, 261t
manageable steps, 253–254, 253t, 254f
mental imagery, 256
obtaining surgical expertise, 251–253
psychomotor skill development, 251–253
repetitive practice, 255–258
simulations, 255–256
Gynecology
historical timeline, 2t

H

Harmonic scalpel technology, 191, 192f
Health assessments
preoperative, 77–78
Health-related quality of life (HRQOL), 89, 90t, 92–93, 98–99, 214
Heaney, Nobel Sproat, 3t, 26–27
Heaney clamps/retractors
illustration of, 168f
teaching the use of, 253–254, 254f
used during abdominal hysterectomy, 106–111, 108f, 109f–113f
used for difficult and challenging vaginal hysterectomy, 138, 138f
used in vaginal hysterectomy, 124, 126, 128f–131f, 129–134, 133f
Heaney technique
evolution and history of, 26–29, 27f–29f
Hemisection
for enlarged uterus, 141, 142f
Hemorrhages; See also abnormal uterine bleeding (AUB)
before and after hysterectomy, 89, 90t, 92–93
case studies
and endometrial hyperplasia, 180–181
postoperative, 197–198
and vaginal hysterectomy, 124
complication with hysterectomy, 196t, 197–198
complication with or without oophorectomy, 168t
excessive uterine, 70t, 73
hysterectomy versus alternative treatment trials on, 91t, 92–93
Hemostasis
and blood flow, 46–48
Heredity nonpolyposis colorectal cancer (HNPCC), 170, 171
HerOption cryoablation unit, 227t, 228–229, 228f, 229f
Hippocrates, 1, 4
History; See also uterine surgery, evolution of
of uterine surgery and gynecology, 1–29, 2t–3t
Hormone therapy
as alternate treatment to hysterectomy, 91t, 92
preoperative assessment of, 78
Hormones
activity in ovaries post menopause, 171–172
and osteoporosis, 173
Human oviduct, 2t
HydroTherm-Ablator, 227t, 230–231, 231f
Hypogastric nerves, 58–59, 60f
Hysterectomy
before and after symptoms/ results, 90t
alternative treatments to
for benign conditions, 213–214
endometrial ablation, 225–234
hysteroscopic myomectomy, 218–225, 218f, 219f, 220t, 221f

Hysterectomy *(Continued)*
  levonorgestin-intrauterine system
    (LNG-IUS), 214–218, 215t
  microwave endometrial ablation, 232,
    232f, 233
  MR-guided focused ultrasound
    (MRgFUS), 240–244, 242f, 243f
  overview of, 213–214
  uterine fibroid embolization (UFE),
    235–240, 236t
  anatomy associated with, 31–59
  benign *versus* malignant diseases and, 70t,
    71f, 77
  choosing route for
    algorithm for, 83f
    complication rates with different, 84–85
    disease complications, 83–84
    factors influencing, 82t
    gynecologic factors, 81–84, 82t, 83f
    operative laparoscopy, 84
    physician personal preferences, 82–83
    prophylactic oophorectomy during,
      85–86
    route comparison chart, 85t
    vaginal access factors, 81–84, 83f
  complications
    abdominal, vaginal and laparoscopic
      comparison chart, 196t
    antibiotics, 199–200, 200t
    bladder injuries, 196t, 204, 205f, 206f
    bowel injuries, 196t, 209–210
    case studies regarding, 197–198,
      201–202, 203f, 208–210
    eVALuate trials, 196t
    fallopian tube prolapse, 210–211
    fever, 196t, 198–199
    intraoperative conversion to laparotomy,
      196, 196t
    patient safety indicators, 197t
    perioperative hemorrhages, 196t,
      197–198
    perioperative infections, 199
    rates and statistics, 195–197, 196t
    recommended antimicrobial regimens,
      200t
    rectal injuries, 196t, 209–210
    risks *versus* benefits, 195–197
    surgical morbidity rates, 195–196
    surgical site infections, 199–200, 200t
    types of, 197t
    ureteral injuries, 196, 196t, 204,
      207–208, 207f
    urinary tract infections, 196t, 201–203,
      203f
    vaginal cuff evisceration, 209–210
  epidemiology of, 65–66, 66t
  evolution and history of
    abdominal hysterectomy beginnings,
      2t–3t, 20–24, 25–29, 25f, 26f
    abdominal *versus* vaginal approaches,
      23–24, 25f
    in antiquity, 2t–3t, 3–5, 4f
    cesarean hysterectomies, 2t–3t, 21–22
    eighteenth century, 2t–3t, 9–11, 11f, 12f
    Heaney technique, 26–29, 27f–29f
    laparoscopic hysterectomies, 28–29
    Medieval period, 2t–3t, 6
    nineteenth century, 2t–3t, 11–23,
      13f–17f, 19f–20f
    pelvic examinations, 12–14, 13f, 14f
    Renaissance Period, 2t–3t, 6–7, 8f
    Richardson technique, 24, 25f–26f
    seventeenth century, 2t–3t, 7–9, 9t, 10t
    timeline of milestones, 2t–3t
    trachelectomy, 14–15, 15f–16f
    twentieth century to present, 2t–3t,
      23–29, 25f–29f
    vaginal hysterectomy, 17–20, 17f,
      19f–20f
  factors influencing rates of
    age, 66–67, 67f

Hysterectomy *(Continued)*
    physicians, 69
    socioeconomic factors, 68–69
    world geographic variations, 67–68, 67f
  general preoperative considerations
    informed consent, 79
    preoperative health assessment, 77–78
    preoperative testing, 78–79, 79t
  indications for, 70–75, 70t, 77
    chronic pelvic pain, 70t, 72, 74
    dysmenorrhea, 70t, 72, 75
    endometriosis, 70t, 71f, 74–75
    excessive uterine bleeding, 70t, 73
    fibroids, 70t, 71–72, 71f
    pelvic organ prolapse (POP), 70t, 73–74
    uterine leiomyomas, 70t, 71–72, 71f
  laparoscopic hysterectomy
    comparison chart *versus* vaginal and
      abdominal, 85t
    defining types of, 179–180
    evolution and history of, 28–29
    laparoscopic supracervical or subtotal
      hysterectomy
      benefits of, 189–190
      case study, 186–187
      description of, 179–180
      rationale for surgery, 189–190
      surgical techniques, 187
    laparoscopic-assisted vaginal
      hysterectomy (LAVH)
      discussion of, 191
      surgical technique, 189
    rationale for different types, 189–190
    robotic-assisted total laparoscopic and
      supracervical hysterectomy
      overview of, 179–180
      port placement, 188f
      rationale for, 190
      surgical technique, 188–189
    single-port, 190–191
    staging of, 180t
    statistics and trends in, 179–180
    statistics *versus* abdominal and vaginal,
      77
    summary of, 192
    total laparoscopic hysterectomy (TLH)
      case study, 180
      description of, 179–180
      port placement, 182–184, 184f
      positioning, 181–182, 181f
      surgical technique, 181–186, 181f,
        183f, 184f
      uterine manipulators, 182, 183f,
        184f
    vessel-sealing technology, 191–182,
      192f
  outcomes of
    bladder function, 97
    bleeding, 89, 90t, 92–93
    bowel function, 97–98
    chart summarizing, 90t
    endometriosis, 93–95
    menstrual bleeding, 89, 90t, 92–93
    ovarian function, 96
    pelvic organ prolapse, 98
    pelvic pain, 90t, 93–95
    psychosocial function, 90t, 98–99
    quality of life, 90t, 98–99
    sexual function, 95–96
    in subtotal *versus* total hysterectomy,
      99–100
  perioperative considerations, 79–81, 79t
    mechanical bowel preparation, 81
    prophylactic antibiotics, 80
    ruling out pregnancy, 79, 79t
    venous thromboembolic risks, 80–81,
      80t
  positive *versus* negative outcomes of, 90t,
    92–100
  route comparison chart, 85t
  statistics and trends, 65–69, 75, 77, 84–85

Hysteroscopes, 219f
Hysteroscopic myomectomy
  basic procedural steps, 220–221, 221f
  case study, 218, 218f
  complications, 224–225
  distention media, 223–224
  fluid management, 224
  hysteroscopes, 219f
  indications and contraindications, 220t
  other techniques using, 222–223
  patient considerations/preferences, 220t
  preoperative evaluation, 219–220, 221t
  using electrocautery and laser, 223
Hysteroscopy
  indications and contraindications for
    operative, 220t

I

Iliac arteries, 31, 32f
Iliohypogastric nerve, 35, 39f, 40f
Ilioinguinal nerve, 35, 39f, 40f
Immunosuppression
  increasing hysterectomy risks, 199
Incisions
  for abdominal hysterectomy, 105–107
  used in gynecologic surgery, 35, 36f, 37f,
    38f
  vaginal hysterectomy, 125–126, 126f
Infections
  perioperative, 199
  surgical site, 199–201, 200t
  urinary tract, 196t, 201–203, 203f
Inferior hypogastric plexus, 58–59, 60f
Informed consent
  as preoperative consideration, 79
Inguinal ligaments, 31, 32f, 39f
Instruments
  early pelvic exam, 12–14, 13f, 14f
  hysteroscopes, 219f
  suboptimal throughout history, 1, 2t–3t
  used for difficult and challenging vaginal
    hysterectomy, 138, 138f
  used in ancient times, 5–6
  in vessel-sealing technology, 191–182,
    192f
Internal os, 40, 41f
Intra-abdominal cavity
  contents of, 31–32, 33f
Intramyometrial coring
  for enlarged uterus, 141, 142f–143f, 144
Intraoperative conversion to laparotomy
  causing complications with hysterectomy,
    196, 196t
Intrauterine systems (IUS)
  levonorgestin-intrauterine system
    (LNG-IUS)
    advantages and disadvantages of, 215t
    benefits of, 217–218
    indications for, 214
    insertion techniques, 215–216
    patient considerations, 214–215, 215t
    side effects, 217
Inverted triangular endometrial cavity,
  39–40, 41f
Isthmus, 41–42, 41f, 42f, 44f

K

Kidneys
  and ureteral obstruction, 201
Knot-tying, 252–253
Kocher clamps, 106, 108f
Koh colpotomizer system, 182, 183f, 184f

L

Lack of uterine descent
  causing difficult vaginal hysterectomy,
    147, 148f
Langenbeck, C.J.M., 2t, 17

Laparoscopic hysterectomy
  comparison chart *versus* vaginal and
      abdominal, 85t
  complications associated with, 195–211,
      196t
  defining types of, 179–180
  evolution and history of, 28–29
  laparoscopic supracervical or subtotal
      hysterectomy
    benefits of, 189–190
    case study, 186–187
    description of, 179–180
    rationale for surgery, 189–190
    surgical techniques, 187
  laparoscopic-assisted vaginal hysterectomy
      (LAVH)
    discussion of, 191
    surgical technique, 189
  rationale for different types, 189–190
  robotic-assisted total laparoscopic
      supracervical hysterectomy
    overview of, 179–180
    port placement, 188f
    rationale for, 190
    surgical technique, 188–189
  single-port, 190–191
  staging of, 180t
  statistics and trends in, 77, 179–180
  summary of, 192
  total laparoscopic hysterectomy (TLH)
    case study, 180
    description of, 179–180
    port placement, 182–184, 184f
    positioning, 181–182, 181f
    surgical technique, 181–186, 181f, 183f,
        184f
    uterine manipulators, 182, 183f, 184f
    vessel-sealing technology, 191–182, 192f
Laparoscopic supracervical hysterectomy
    or subtotal hysterectomy
  benefits of, 189–190
  case study, 186–187
  description of, 179–180
  rationale for surgery, 189–190
  surgical techniques, 187
Laparoscopic-assisted vaginal hysterectomy
    (LAVH)
  description and discussion of, 180, 191
  surgical technique, 189
Laparoscopy; *See also* laparoscopic
  conversion to
    causing difficult and challenging vaginal
        hysterectomy, 158–159
  and hysterectomy
    survival with or without ovarian
        preservation, 94f
  operative, 84
Laparotomy
  conversion to
    causing difficult and challenging vaginal
        hysterectomy, 158–159
Large fibroid uterus
  determining abdominal hysterectomy
      route, 103
Laser
  hysteroscopic myomectomy, 223
Left common iliac arteries, 31, 32f
Levonorgestrel-releasing intrauterine system
    (LNG-IUS)
  advantages and disadvantages of, 215t
  benefits of, 217–218
  indications for, 214
  insertion techniques, 215–216
  patient considerations, 214–215, 215t
  research on benefits of, 91t, 92, 94
  side effects, 217
Ligasure vessel-sealing technology, 192, 192f
Ligatures
  early example of prolapsed uterus, 17f
Lister
  history of, 2t–3t

Lower urinary tract
  anatomical description and illustration of,
      48, 50–53, 50f, 52f–54f
  structures of, 48, 50–53, 50f, 52f–54f
Lynch syndrome, 170, 171

M

Magnetic resonance imaging (MRI)
  guided focused ultrasound, 240–244, 242f,
      243f
Maine Women's Health Study
  on hysterectomy outcomes, 89–100
Malignant diseases
  versus benign and hysterectomy, 70t, 71f
  as contraindication for intrauterine
      systems (IUS), 215
Markov decision-analysis model
  regarding ovary removal, 172
Maryland Women's Health Study
  on hysterectomy complications, 195
  on hysterectomy outcomes, 89–100
Massive bivalve
  used in ancient times, 5–6
Maylard incisions
  in abdominal hysterectomy surgery, 105–106
  description and illustration of, 35, 36f
Mayo scissors, 126–127, 127f, 128f, 133, 138,
    138f
McCall culdoplasty, 132–134
Mechanical bowel preparation
  as perioperative consideration, 81
Medications
  as alternate treatment to hysterectomy,
      91t, 92
  preoperative assessment of, 78
Medulla
  anatomy of ovarian, 42, 43f, 44f
Menometrorrhagia
  causing difficulties in vaginal
      hysterectomy, 139
Menopause
  and osteoporosis, 173
  ovarian function following, 171–172
  and sexuality following oophorectomy, 173
Menorrhagia
  case study and vaginal hysterectomy, 124
  and dysmenorrhea in nulliparous obese
      patient, 146
  and fibroids case study, 117
  and hysterectomy, 73
  with previous pelvic surgeries, 148–149
Menstrual bleeding
  before and after hysterectomy, 89, 90t,
      92–93
  hysterectomy *versus* alternative treatment
      trials on, 91t, 92–93
Metrorrhagia
  and hysterectomy, 73
Metzenbaum scissors, 126–127, 127f, 128f
Microsulis MEA, 231, 232f, 233
Minimally invasive routes
  laparoscopic and robotic, 179–192
Monastatic medicine, 6
Morbidity rates
  with hysterectomy surgery, 195–196
Mortality rates
  with prophylactic oophorectomy, 174–176,
      175f
MR-guided focused ultrasound (MRgFUS)
  complications with, 242–243
  indications for, 213–214, 240–241
  outcomes, 243–244
  patient selection criteria, 241
  procedure, 242, 242f, 243f
Musculoskeletal system
  and prophylactic oophorectomy, 172–173
Myomectomy
  for enlarged uterus, 144, 146
  hysteroscopic (*See* hysteroscopic
      myomectomy)

Myometrium
  anatomy of, 39–40, 41f

N

Nationwide In-Patient Sample of Healthcare
    Cost and Utilization Project, 77
Nephrostomy, 203f
Nerves
  iliohypogastric and ilioinguinal, 35, 39f,
      40f
  of pelvic cavity, 58–59, 60f
Neurological system
  anatomy of, 58–59, 60f
  following prophylactic oophorectomy,
      173–174
Nonsteroidal anti-inflammatory drugs
    (NSAIDs)
  with birth control pills *versus*
      hysterectomy, 91t, 92
  preoperative assessment of, 78
Novasure, 227t, 229–230, 230f
Nulliparity, 146

O

Obesity
  causing challenges with abdominal
      hysterectomy, 120–121
  causing challenges with vaginal
      hysterectomy, 146
  increasing hysterectomy risks, 197–199
  and surgical site infection prevention,
      200t
  as venous thromboembolic risk, 80t
Objective structured assessment of technical
    skills (OSATS), 259, 263
Obliterated rectovaginal septum
  causing difficulties with abdominal
      hysterectomy, 119–120
Oophorectomy
  cancer prevention *versus* surgical
      menopause decisions, 161
  decisions regarding, 85–86, 161
  with endometriosis, 74–75
  and osteoporosis, 173
  outcomes and complications, 166, 167f,
      168tf, 169–174
    breast cancer reduction, 171
    cardiovascular risks, 172–173
    discussion, 174
    musculoskeletal outcomes, 172–173
    nononcological outcomes, 171
    ovarian cancer reduction, 169–171
    sexuality/neurological outcomes,
        173–174
  ovarian descent, 162–163, 163f
  preservation and survival rates, 94f
  prophylactic, 85–86
  risk assessment, 161
  risk-reducing *versus* prophylactic, 169
  surgical techniques
    abdominal approach, 163–164, 164f
    vaginal approach, 163–164, 164f
Operating Room Education Environment
    Measure (OREEM) Scores, 260, 261t
Operative gynecology
  historical timeline, 2t
Operative hysteroscopy
  indications and contraindications,
      220t
Oral contraceptives
  as alternate treatment to hysterectomy,
      91t, 92
  preoperative assessment of, 78
  reducing risk of ovarian cancer, 170
Osteoporosis, 173
Outer cortex
  anatomy of ovarian, 42, 43f, 44f
Ova
  anatomy of, 42, 43f, 44f

Ovarian cancer
  as indication for hysterectomy, 70t
  prevention with prophylactic
      oophorectomy, 169–171
Ovarian descent
  and prophylactic oophorectomy, 162–163,
      163f
Ovarian follicles
  historical timeline for understanding, 2t
Ovarian tumors
  surgical history, 2t
Ovarian vessels
  illustration of, 44f
Ovaries
  anatomical description and illustration of,
      41–42, 41f, 42f, 44f
  blood supply to, 46–48, 47f–49f
  concomitant salpingo-oophorectomy, 185
  contents of, 42, 43f, 44f
  function before and after hysterectomy, 96
  historical timeline for understanding, 2t
  innervation of, 58–59, 60f
  preservation and survival rates, 94f
  prophylactic oophorectomy
      and breast cancer reduction, 171
      cancer prevention *versus* surgical
          menopause decisions, 161
      cardiovascular risks, 172–173
      decisions regarding, 85–86, 161
      discussion, 174
      musculoskeletal outcomes, 172–173
      nononcological outcomes, 171
      outcomes and complications, 166, 167f,
          168tf, 169–174
      ovarian cancer reduction, 169–171
      sexuality/neurological outcomes,
          173–174

P

Paletta, G.B., 2t, 17
Papanicolaou (Pap) smear
  preoperative, 78
Paracervical blocks, 125
Paralytic ileus
  complication with or without
      oophorectomy, 168t
Pararectal spaces, 56f, 57–58, 57f
Paravesical spaces, 56–57, 56f, 57f
Parietal peritoneum, 31–32, 33f, 34f, 35, 36f,
      37f
Patient safety indicators, 197t
Pedicle and vessel-sealing technology, 191,
      192f
Pelvic abscess, 198–199
Pelvic adhesive disease
  determining hysterectomy route, 103, 123
Pelvic anatomy
  early understandings of, 3t, 22–23
Pelvic cavity
  nerves of, 58–59, 60f
Pelvic examinations
  evolution and history of, 12–14, 13f, 14f
Pelvic inflammatory diseases (PIDs)
  and IUS users, 217
  as possible indication for hysterectomy, 70t
Pelvic organ prolapse (POP)
  before and after hysterectomy, 98
  case study, 201–202
  as indication for hysterectomy, 70t, 73–74
Pelvic pain
  before and after hysterectomy, 90t, 92–93,
      93–95
  case study for abdominal hysterectomy, 115
  hysterectomy *versus* alternative treatment
      trials on, 91t, 93
  preoperative assessment of, 78
Pelvic surgeries
  history of, 1, 2t–3t
  multiple past
      causing difficult vaginal hysterectomy,
          148–149

Pelvic viscera, 42, 44f
Pelvis
  anatomy
      early understandings of, 3t, 22–23
      anatomy to examine before hysterectomy,
          107f
      blood supply to structures of, 45–46, 47f–49f
      illustration of, 43f
      spaces and avascular planes of, 54–58,
          55f–57f
      support structures, 42–43, 44f, 45
Pelvis spaces
  and avascular planes
      anatomical description and illustration
          of, 54–58, 55f–57f
Percutaneous nephrostomy, 203f
Perioperative considerations, 79–81, 79t
  hemorrhages as complication with
      hysterectomy, 196t, 197–198
  infections, 199
  mechanical bowel preparation, 81
  prophylactic antibiotics, 80
  ruling out pregnancy, 79, 79t
  venous thromboembolic risks, 80–81, 80t
Peritoneal cancer, 171
Peritoneal insufflation, 196
Peritoneum, 31–32, 33f, 34f, 35, 36f, 37f
Peritonitis
  complication with or without
      oophorectomy, 168t
Pfannenstiel incisions
  in abdominal hysterectomy surgery,
      105–106
  description and illustration of, 35, 36f
Physicians
  as factor influencing hysterectomy rates,
      69
  preferences for laparoscopic
      hysterectomies, 192
  route preferences of, 82–83
Plexuses
  of pelvic cavity, 58–59, 60f
Pneumonia, 198–199
Positioning
  for abdominal hysterectomy, 105, 105f
  for laparoscopic hysterectomy, 181–182,
      181f
  low dorsal lithotomy, 105f
  Trendelenburg, 2t, 154, 181–182, 181f
  for vaginal hysterectomy, 124, 125f
Postablation tubal sterilization syndrome
      (PATSS), 234
Posterior cul-de-sacs
  anatomy of, 54–55, 55f
  entry difficulties, 152–155, 154f
  sharp entry into, 126, 127f
Pregnancy
  as contraindication for intrauterine
      systems (IUS), 215
  reducing risk of ovarian cancer, 170
  ruling out as perioperative consideration,
      79, 79t
Preoperative considerations
  informed consent, 79
  preoperative health assessment, 77–78
  preoperative testing, 78–79, 79t
Presacral spaces, 56f, 57f, 58
Prescriptions
  preoperative assessment of, 78
Prevesical space, 56f, 57f, 58
  historical timeline for understanding, 2t
  paravaginal attachments, 45f
Prolapsed uterus
  early example of ligature, 17f
Prophylactic antibiotics
  as perioperative consideration, 79–80
Prophylactic oophorectomy
  cancer prevention *versus* surgical
      menopause decisions, 161
  case study, 161–162
  decisions regarding, 85–86, 161–162,
      174–176, 175f

Prophylactic oophorectomy *(Continued)*
  outcomes and complications, 166, 167f,
      168tf, 169–174
      breast cancer reduction, 171
      cardiovascular risks, 172–173
      discussion, 174
      musculoskeletal outcomes, 172–173
      nononcological outcomes, 171
      ovarian cancer reduction, 169–171
      sexuality/neurological outcomes,
          173–174
  ovarian descent, 162–163, 163f
  risk assessment, 161
  versus risk-reducing oophorectomy, 169
  surgical techniques
      abdominal approach, 163–164, 164f
      vaginal approach, 163–164, 164f
Psychosocial function
  before and after hysterectomy, 90t, 98–99
Pubic symphysis, 31, 32f, 38f, 39f
Pyelonephritis, 198–199
Pyrexia, 168t

Q

Quadrivalve
  used in ancient times, 5–6
Quality of life
  before and after hysterectomy, 90t, 98–99
  hysterectomy *versus* alternative treatment
      trials regarding, 91t, 92–93
  improved with hysterectomy, 89, 90t

R

Race
  and surgical morbidity, 195–196
Radical hysterectomy
  history of, 3t
Recovery rates
  throughout history, 1, 2t–3t
Rectal cancer
  as indication for hysterectomy, 70t
Rectal injuries
  complication with hysterectomy, 196t,
      209–210
  with posterior entries, 153–154
Rectovaginal space, 56f, 57f, 58
Rectum
  and sigmoid colon
      anatomical description and illustration
          of, 53–54
Rectus abdominis muscles, 31, 32f, 36f, 37f,
      38f
Rectus muscles, 31–32, 33f, 34f, 36f
Rectus sheath, 31–32, 33f, 34f, 36f
Renal function
  and ureteral obstruction, 201
Resuturing
  of old wounds, 168t
Retractors
  and clamping in vaginal hysterectomy,
      128f–131f, 129–134, 133f
  used for difficult and challenging vaginal
      hysterectomy, 138, 138f
Retroperitoneal extravasation, 203f, 207
Retropubic spaces, 45, 56f, 57f, 58
Richardson, Edward H., 3t, 24, 25t
Richardson technique
  evolution and history of, 24, 25f–26f
Right iliac arteries, 31, 32f
Robotic-assisted total laparoscopic
      supracervical hysterectomy
  FDA approval of, 179–180
  overview of, 179–180
  port placement, 188f
  rationale for, 190
  surgical technique, 188–189
Round ligament
  grasping during surgery, 106–111, 108f
  during prophylactic oophorectomy
      surgery, 163–164, 164f, 167f

Routes
  comparison chart, 85t
Routes of hysterectomy
  complications comparison chart, 196t
Rowlandson, Thomas, 10, 11f

S

Sacral plexus, 58–59, 60f
Scalpels
  in challenging vaginal hysterectomy, 138,
    138f
  used in ancient times, 5–6
Scarpa's fascia, 31–32, 33f, 34f, 36f
Scarring of vesicouterine septum
  causing difficulties with abdominal
    hysterectomy, 120
Self-assessment
  of surgical skills
Serosa
  anatomy of, 39–40, 41f
"Seven cell doctrine", 4
Sexual health
  before and after hysterectomy, 95–96
  following hysterectomy versus alternative
    treatment, 91t, 92–93
  following prophylactic oophorectomy,
    173–174
Sharp dissection
  situations requiring, 150, 151f
Sheth's adnexa clamp, 166, 168f
Shock
  complication with or without
    oophorectomy, 168t
Sigmoid colon
  and rectum
    anatomical description and illustration
      of, 53–54
Single-port laparoscopic hysterectomy, 190–191
Skin
  of abdominal wall, 31–32, 33f, 34f, 36f
Skinner, B.F.
  on behaviorism, 249–250
Sleep issues
  before and after hysterectomy, 90t, 92
Smooth muscle
  surrounding cervix, 40, 41f
Social function
  before and after hysterectomy, 90t, 92
Socioeconomic factors
  as factor influencing hysterectomy rates,
    68–69
Soranus of Ephesus, 2t, 4–5
Spaces
  and avascular planes of pelvis, 54–58,
    55f–57f
  pararectal, 56f, 57–58, 57f
  paravesical, 56–57, 56f, 57f
  presacral, 56f, 57f, 58
  prevesical, 56f, 57f, 58
  rectovaginal, 56f, 57f, 58
  retropubic, 56f, 57f, 58
  vesicovaginal, 56, 56f, 57f
Speculums, 138f
Staplers, 192
Steiner-Auvard speculum, 138f
Strachan, John B., 3t, 15
Subcutaneous fat
  of abdominal wall, 31–32, 33f, 34f, 36f
Subtotal hysterectomy
  or laparoscopic supracervical
    benefits of, 189–190
    case study, 186–187
    description of, 179–180
    rationale for surgery, 189–190
    surgical techniques, 187
  versus total hysterectomy, 99–100
Supracervical hysterectomy
  bleeding following, 132
  as difficult abdominal hysterectomy,
    118–119, 119f
  evolution of, 2t–3t, 27

Surgery; See also individual types
  evolution and history of, 1–29, 2t–3t
  morbidity rates, 195–196
  route comparison chart, 85t
  teaching and learning
    assessing learning environment, 260,
      261t
    assessing trainee, 258–260, 263–265
    behaviorist theory, 249–251, 250f
    deliberate practice, 252–253
    educational theories, 249–251, 250f
    error-training, 252–253
    feedback, 256–258
    fundamentals of teaching, 261t
    manageable steps, 253–254, 253t, 254f
    mental imagery, 256
    objective structured assessment of
      technical skills (OSATS), 259, 263
    obtaining surgical expertise, 251–253
    psychomotor skill development, 251–253
    repetitive practice, 255–258
    simulations, 255–256
Surgical blood salvage/autotransfusion
  system, 138
Surgical knot-tying, 252–253
Surgical morbidity rates, 195–196
Surgical site infections, 199–200, 200t
Surgical skills
  objective structured assessment of
    technical skills (OSATS), 259, 263
Survival rates
  of hysterectomy and laparoscopy
    with or without ovarian preservation,
      94f
  throughout history, 1, 2t–3t
Suture-litagation
  vaginal hysterectomy, 129, 130f–131f
Sutures
  suboptimal throughout history, 1, 2t–3t

T

Teaching and learning
  gynecologic surgery
    assessing learning environment, 260,
      261t
    assessing trainee, 258–260, 263–265
    behaviorist theory, 249–251, 250f
    deliberate practice, 252–253
    educational theories, 249–251, 250f
    error-training, 252–253
    feedback, 256–258
    fundamentals of teaching, 261t
    manageable steps, 253–254, 253t, 254f
    mental imagery, 256
    obtaining surgical expertise, 251–253
    psychomotor skill development, 251–253
    repetitive practice, 255–258
    simulations, 255–256
Tenacula, 138f
Testing
  preoperative, 78–79, 79t
Testosterone
  activity in ovaries post menopause,
    171–172
"The Anatomist", 11f
ThermaChoice, 227–228, 227t, 228f
Thermal balloon, 227–228, 227t, 228f
Thromboembolic disease
  as hysterectomy complication, 195
Timeline of milestones
  in uterine surgery, 2t–3t
Total hysterectomy
  versus subtotal hysterectomy, 99–100
Total laparoscopic hysterectomy (TLH)
  case study, 180
  description of, 179–180
  port placement, 182–184, 184f
  positioning, 181–182, 181f
  surgical technique, 181–186, 181f, 183f,
    184f
  uterine manipulators, 182, 183f, 184f

Total procidentia, 201–202
Trachelectomy
  case study, 132
  evolution and history of, 14–15, 15f–16f
  procedures, 133–134, 133f
Tracheloplasty technique
  history of, 3t
Trainees; See teaching and learning
Transcervical access, 153, 154f
Transcervical endometrial ablation, 217
Transverse incisions
  history of laparotomy, 3t
Trendelenburg position, 2t, 154, 181–182,
  181f
Trocar insertion, 196
Tubal tear
  complication with or without
    oophorectomy, 168t

U

Ultrasound
  preoperative assessment with, 78
Umbilicus, 31, 32f
Unsuspected malignancy
  causing difficult abdominal hysterectomy,
    120
Ureteral catheters, 207–208
Ureteral injuries
  case study, 201–202, 203f
  with hysterectomy, 196, 196t, 204,
    207–208, 207f
Ureteral kinking, 201
Ureterolysis
  with relaxing incision, 186f
Ureters
  anatomical description and illustration of,
    48, 50–53, 50f, 54f
  injury and duplications, 51–52
  pelvic course of, 51, 52f
Urethra
  anatomical description and illustration of,
    48, 50–53, 50f, 54f
Urinary incontinence
  before and after hysterectomy, 90t, 97
Urinary system
  structures of, 48, 50–53, 50f, 52f–54f
Urinary tract infections
  complication with hysterectomy, 196t,
    201–203, 203f
  complication with or without
    oophorectomy, 168t
Uterine adhesions
  causing difficult and challenging vaginal
    hysterectomy, 155
Uterine adnexa
  anatomical description and illustration of,
    41–42, 41f, 42f, 44f
Uterine cancer
  historical milestones in treatment of, 2t–3t
  as indication for hysterectomy, 70t
Uterine cavity
  anatomical description and illustration of,
    39–40, 41f
Uterine corpus
  anatomical description and illustration of,
    39–41, 41f, 42f
  removal with cervix preservation (See
    laparoscopic supracervical
    hysterectomy (LSH))
Uterine descent
  lack of, 147, 148f
Uterine displacement
  historical timeline for understanding, 2t
Uterine fibroid embolization (UFE)
  as alternative to hysterectomy, 92t, 93
  case study, 235
  complications with, 238–239
  indications for, 235–236
  outcomes and conclusions, 239–240
  patient questions and selection, 235–236,
    236t

Uterine fibroid embolization (UFE) *(Continued)*
  postoperative management, 237–238
  procedure, 236–237
Uterine fibroids; *See* uterine leiomyomas
Uterine leiomyomas
  case studies regarding
    broad ligament, 61–62
    cervical, 59, 60f, 61
  and cervix preservation desires, 186–187
  classifying depth, location, and penetration, 219–220, 221t
  first successful removal of, 20–21
  first surgeries on, 2t–3t
  hysterectomy complications with, 195
  hysteroscopic myomectomy, 218–225, 218f, 219f, 220t, 221f
  as indication for hysterectomy, 70t, 71–72, 71f
  levonorgestin-intrauterine system (LNG-IUS), 214–218, 215t
  and menorrhagia case study, 117
  microwave endometrial ablation, 232, 232f, 233
  MR-guided focused ultrasound (MRgFUS), 240–244, 242f, 243f
  statistics regarding hysterectomies and, 70t
  uterine fibroid embolization (UFE), 92t, 93, 235–240, 236t
Uterine manipulators
  Koh and RUMI, 183f
  types of, 182
  VCare, 184f
Uterine mobility
  assessment of, 136–137
Uterine prolapse
  historical milestones in treatment of, 2t–3t, 8f
  preoperative assessment of, 78–79
  statistics regarding hysterectomies and, 70t
Uterine support structures
  anatomical description and illustration of, 42–43, 44f, 45
Uterine surgery; *See also* hysterectomy
  evolution and history of
    abdominal hysterectomy beginnings, 2t–3t, 20–24, 25–29, 25f, 26f
    abdominal *versus* vaginal approaches, 23–24, 25f
    in antiquity, 2t–3t, 3–5, 4f
    cesarean hysterectomies, 2t–3t, 21–22
    eighteenth century, 2t–3t, 9–11, 11f, 12f
    Heaney technique, 26–29, 27f–29f
    laparoscopic hysterectomies, 28–29
    Medieval period, 2t–3t, 6
    nineteenth century, 2t–3t, 11–23, 13f–17f, 19f–20f
    pelvic examinations, 12–14, 13f, 14f
    Renaissance Period, 2t–3t, 6–7, 8f
    Richardson technique, 24, 25f–26f
    seventeenth century, 2t–3t, 7–9, 9t, 10t
    timeline of milestones, 2t–3t
    trachelectomy, 14–15, 15f–16f
    twentieth century to present, 2t–3t, 23–29, 25f–29f
    vaginal hysterectomy, 17–20, 17f, 19f–20f
Uterosacral/cardinal complex, 42–43, 44f, 45
Uterosacral ligament vaginal suspension, 132–134
Uterovaginal prolapse
  case studies, 63, 64f, 104
  causing difficult and challenging vaginal hysterectomy, 156–158, 157f
Uterovaginal support
  levels of, 44f
Uterus
  anatomy of
    anterior abdominal wall, 31–32, 32f–33f, 34–35, 36f–37f, 38–39, 39f–40f
    cervix, 39–41, 41f, 42f
    illustrations of, 41f, 42f, 44f

Uterus *(Continued)*
    lower urinary tract, 48, 50–53, 50f, 52f–54f
    nerves of pelvic cavity, 58–59
    pelvis spaces and avascular planes, 54–58, 55f–57f
    sigmoid colon and rectum, 53–54
    uterine corpus, 39–41, 41f, 42f
    uterine support structures, 42–43, 44f, 45
    vasculature, 45–48, 47f–49f
  blood supply to, 46–48, 47f–49f
  and cervix extirpation (*See* total laparoscopic hysterectomy [TLH])
  connective tissue supporting, 43, 44f, 45
  descent of, 137
  early definition of, 5
  early diagrams of surgery, 19f
  enlarged (*See* enlarged uterus)
  evolution of the understanding of, 1–29
  grasping during surgery, 106–111, 108f
  historical timeline for understanding, 2t
  removal and prophylactic oophorectomy surgery, 162–166, 164f, 165f
  removal of in abdominal hysterectomy, 112–114, 114f
  size and shape
    determining abdominal hysterectomy route, 103
    determining vaginal hysterectomy, 136
  supracervical hysterectomy
    as difficult abdominal hysterectomy, 118–119, 119f
    vaginal hysterectomy surgical procedures, 124–134, 126, 128f–131f, 133f

V

Vagina
  access factors in hysterectomy, 81–84, 83f
  anatomical illustrations of, 41f, 42f, 44f
  connective tissue supporting, 43, 44f, 45
  evolution of the understanding of, 1–29
  narrow size as contraindication to vaginal hysterectomy, 123
Vaginal access
  difficulties, 103
  factors in hysterectomy, 81–84, 83f
Vaginal approach
  to prophylactic oophorectomy, 163–164, 164f
Vaginal bleeding
  before and after hysterectomy, 90t
Vaginal cuff
  closure during abdominal hysterectomy, 113, 114f, 115f
  closure during total laparoscopic hysterectomy, 185
  dehiscence of, 210
  evisceration, 209–210
Vaginal cuff cellulitis, 198–199
Vaginal examinations
  early instruments for, 12–14, 13f, 14f
Vaginal hysterectomy
  anterior cul-de-sac entry, 126–128, 127f–128f
  case studies, 124, 132
  comparison chart with abdominal and laparoscopic, 85t
  complications associated with, 84–85, 195–211, 196t
  difficult and challenging situations
    case study, 139
    conversion to laparoscopy or laparotomy, 158–159
    difficult anterior cul-de-sac entry, 150–152
    difficult posterior cul-de-sac entry, 152–155, 154f
    elongated cervix, 155–156
    enlarged uterus surgery, 139–141, 142f–143f, 144–147

Vaginal hysterectomy *(Continued)*
    factors influencing, 136–137
    instruments used for, 138, 138f
    lack of uterine descent, 147, 148f
    multiple prior pelvic surgeries, 148–149
    obese patients, 146
    route selection and decisions, 135–138
    uterine adhesions, 155
    uterovaginal prolapse, 156–158, 157f
    vulvar slant, 136–137, 136f
  dorsal lithotomy position, 124, 125f
  electrosurgical procedures, 131–132
  evolution and history of, 17–20, 17f, 19f–20f
  perioperative antibiotics/antiembolics, 124
  positioning, 124, 125f
  as route of choice, 81–83, 82t
  statistics *versus* abdominal and laparoscopic, 77
  surgical procedures, 124–129, 130f, 131–134
    anesthesia, 124–125
    bladder dissection off uterus, 126–127, 128f
    clamping and retractors, 128f–131f, 129–134, 133f
    entry into cul-de-sacs, 126–127, 127f, 128f
    incisions, 125–126, 126f
    suture-litagation, 129, 130f–131f
  teaching with manageable steps, 253t
  trachelectomy procedures, 133–134, 133f
Vaginal shape
  determining abdominal hysterectomy route, 103
Vaginal speculum
  early example of, 10f
  used in ancient times, 5–6
Vaginal Surgical Skills Index (VSSI), 259, 264–265
Vaginal trachelectomy
  case study, 132
  evolution and history of, 14–15, 15f–16f
  procedures, 133–134, 133f
Vaginal wall
  connection to cervix, 40, 41f
Vasculature
  anatomical illustration of uterine, 45–48, 47f–49f
Vasoconstrictors
  before incisions, 124–125
Veins
  of pelvis, 45–46, 47f–49f
Venous thromboembolic
  risks, 80–81, 80t
Vertical midline incisions
  in abdominal hysterectomy surgery, 105–106
Vesalius, Andreas, 6–7
Vesicouterine septum
  scarring of, 120
Vesicovaginal spaces, 56, 56f, 57f
Vessel-sealing technology
  in laparoscopic surgery, 191–182, 192f
Vulvar slant, 136–137, 136f

W

Wedge morcellation
  for enlarged uterus, 144, 145f
Wertheim, Ernst, 3t, 23–24
World geographic variations
  as factor influencing hysterectomy rates, 67–68, 67f
Wound sepsis
  complication with or without oophorectomy, 168t
Wounds
  infections, 198–199, 199–201, 200t
  resuturing of old, 168t